THE COMPLETE BOOK OF
BONE HEALTH

THE COMPLETE BOOK OF

BONE HEALTH

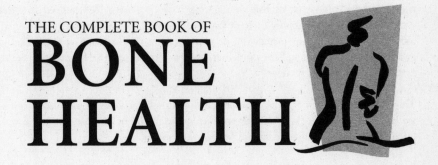

DIANE L. SCHNEIDER, MD

FOREWORD BY SALLY RIDE
ASTRONAUT AND CEO, SALLY RIDE SCIENCE

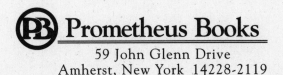

Prometheus Books

59 John Glenn Drive
Amherst, New York 14228-2119

Published 2011 by Prometheus Books

Photographs on page 55 courtesy of GE Healthcare (top and middle) and Hologic (bottom).

Illustrations by Tim Gunther, gunthergraphics.biz

Inquiries should be addressed to
Prometheus Books
59 John Glenn Drive
Amherst, New York 14228–2119
VOICE: 716–691–0133
FAX: 716–691–0137
WWW.PROMETHEUSBOOKS.COM

15 14 13 12 11   5 4 3 2

Library of Congress Cataloging-in-Publication Data

Schneider, Diane L., 1953–
    The complete book of bone health / by Diane L. Schneider.
        p. cm.
    Includes bibliographical references and index.
    ISBN 978–1–61614–435–7 (pbk.)
    ISBN 978–1–61614–435–7 (ebook)
    1. Bones. 2. Bones—Growth. 3. Osteoporosis—Prevention. 4. Osteoporosis—Treatment. I. Title.

QM101.S3476 2011
612.7'5—dc22

                                                                    2010054577

Printed in the United States of America

Dedication

To all the women and men worldwide who have participated in research studies to advance our knowledge about bone health.

To fellow bone researchers who ask the right questions and pursue the answers.

To the physicians whose contributions to my career made this book possible:

Mary G. Barry (Associate Professor [Clinical] of Medicine, University of Louisville), who started the journey with me in medical school;

H. Kenneth Walker (Professor of Medicine and Associate Vice Chair for Grady Hospital, Emory University), who shared his passion for teaching and compassion for patients;

Nelson Watts (Professor of Medicine, University of Cincinnati and Director of the University Bone Health and Osteoporosis Center), who introduced me to the area of osteoporosis during my training at Emory;

Joe W. Ramsdell (Professor of Medicine, Chief of General Internal Medicine, University of California, San Diego), who gave me the opportunity to become an epidemiologist as a junior faculty member; and

Elizabeth Barrett-Connor (Distinguished Professor of Family and Preventive Medicine, University of California, San Diego), who mentored me and shared not only research opportunities but life lessons.

CONTENTS

PART 4: THERAPIES FOR PREVENTION AND TREATMENT OF OSTEOPOROSIS

PART 5: THE BONE CONNECTION WITH COMMON PROBLEMS AND MEDICINES

Foreword

When I was an astronaut I got to experience the fun of being weightless—imagine being able to do twenty-four mid-air somersaults in a row, float across the room with a gentle push, or lift a refrigerator with one hand!

But weightlessness also carries some risks. For example, astronauts lose bone rapidly while they're in space. That's because their bones aren't stressed while they're weightless. This wasn't a problem for me on my 7–10 day space shuttle flights, but it is an issue for the astronauts who spend months on the International Space Station. Those astronauts don't have a problem while they're in space—after all, they don't need their bones while they're weightless—but it's something to be aware of when they return to Earth. As you might expect, bone density is closely monitored in astronauts who spend a long time in space. Fortunately, they gradually regain bone once they get their feet back on terra firma.

Astronauts aren't the only ones who lose bone. In fact, bone loss is one of the most pressing health issues for women today. But the issue that is so closely monitored in astronauts is often overlooked by the Earthbound public. It's easy to see why: bone loss is silent and invisible. It can sneak up on you without you knowing there's a problem—and that's what makes it insidious.

When I left NASA to join the faculty at University of California–San Diego, my UCSD colleague Dr. Diane Schneider became my primary care physician. She was a well-known bone researcher, and since I was a former astronaut we began talking about bone loss. That was many years ago, and she's still helping me understand and navigate the subject.

In this book, Dr. Schneider provides essential information for women and men of all ages. Preteens and teens build a foundation that must last a lifetime; older women must understand their options and take steps to avoid or minimize bone loss. Perhaps most important, she emphasizes the value of women educating themselves on the topic. In this case, knowledge really is power. There are many things that women and men can and should do, throughout their lives, to build and maintain strong, healthy bones.

It's important for the future of space travel for NASA to understand bone loss in weightlessness and to ensure that astronauts maintain healthy bones. It's just as important for women and men to understand this critical health issue and how to develop bone healthy habits.

—Sally Ride, PhD
Astronaut and CEO, Sally Ride Science
Professor of Physics, Emeritus, UCSD

11

Introduction:
To Your Bone-Healthy Life

Think about how much time and energy you spend trying to look good every day. Now estimate how much you focus on your bone health. Optimizing your bone health may not be a priority now, but regardless of your age, it needs to be a conscious part of your everyday routine. From day one, everything in your life impacts your skeleton.

Osteoporosis is *the* most common disease in women. You want to prevent the end result: fractures. One in two women over the age of fifty will break a bone. More women die due to broken hips and backs each year than from breast cancer.

Why don't you hear more about osteoporosis? No one says, "My osteoporosis is bothering me." It is considered an old woman's disease, but that is a total misnomer. Osteoporosis begins much earlier but it is silent and without symptoms. Men break bones, too. One in four men over the age of fifty will sustain a fracture and men are even more likely than women to die after having a hip fracture.

Fractures are not inevitable. You can make a difference. The goal of this book is to teach you *how*. You must start now, no matter what your age. It is never too late, even if you have already had one broken bone. On the other hand, it is never too early. Bone health is important for all ages from conception on. Prevention of fractures in later life is the goal. You *can* take charge and do something to change your course with simple measures.

> I always thought osteoporosis was just "an old woman's disease." By taking a seminar, I learned [that] for my age group it is real important to build bone mass. I need to build up my bone mass now so I can protect myself from fracture in the future.
>
> —Jennifer, age 21

Jennifer was an undergraduate student at the University of California, San Diego. She and her fellow classmates did a research project measuring bone density in collegiate women. They were astounded to find that many of the women had lower than normal bone density for their age, including Jennifer herself. She learned she had a chance to improve her bone mass, which peaks in one's late twenties or early thirties. Jennifer examined her lifestyle and made changes. By adding calcium, vitamin D, and regular exercise of running and weight training, she may ultimately reduce her risk for osteoporosis.

Your genes determine 60 to 80 percent of your bone health. You cannot pick your parents but you can adopt a bone-healthy lifestyle and make a difference in your life. You can lower your risk from genes and from the effects of aging and you can reduce your lifetime risk of fractures.

Unlike many women's health issues that have defined time frames, such as pregnancy or menopause, bone health is a lifelong endeavor for you and your family. Staying bone healthy is something you need to consider your whole life. Getting a healthy start is key to growing strong bones and establishing excellent lifelong habits.

Osteoporosis is a silent disease. For the majority of people there are no outward clues that it exists. The best analogy is the termite. Termites work slowly, breaking down the wood structure of your home. Little by little, small holes become larger and larger, creating weaker support structures. Usually, you cannot see their damage because it is hidden behind the walls. Everything looks normal—even the termite inspector does not see anything, until one day you strip off the dry wall during a remodel and you see the chewed-away wood. Worse, you have a structural failure and collapse: the bones of your house are breaking.

Osteoporosis is just like that. You cannot see it. You cannot feel it. Your doctors cannot tell it is there just by looking at you or asking you questions.

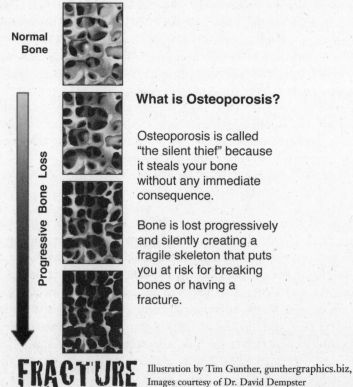

Normal Bone

Progressive Bone Loss

What is Osteoporosis?

Osteoporosis is called "the silent thief" because it steals your bone without any immediate consequence.

Bone is lost progressively and silently creating a fragile skeleton that puts you at risk for breaking bones or having a fracture.

FRACTURE

Illustration by Tim Gunther, gunthergraphics.biz, Images courtesy of Dr. David Dempster

Osteoporosis affects your bones not your joints. An eighty-four-year-old friend recently told me, "I have osteoporosis—my hips just wore out." No, what she has is degenerative arthritis, osteoarthritis, and the cartilage lining of her hip joint wore away. Her arthritis is a process totally unrelated to osteoporosis that required a total hip replacement to treat it.

How do you know if you have osteoporosis? It is a diagnosis usually reserved for women who are at least perimenopausal, which is late forties on average, and for men over the age of fifty. As a silent disease, a test must be done to detect osteoporosis before a fracture happens. Measurement of bone mass by dual energy x-ray absorptiometry (DXA) is the current standard test to determine if you have osteoporosis. If you have already had a fracture, even as a result of trauma, you most likely have osteoporosis.

Another common diagnosis is osteopenia. Osteopenia is not a disease; rather, it represents low bone mass. Thin bones do not necessarily mean weak bones. An assessment of risk factors for fracture along with bone-density testing will provide a more accurate picture of your fracture risk than bone-density testing alone. Management decisions should be based on a complete assessment of your fracture risk.

People always ask if I have osteoporosis because I am tall and thin, which are risk factors for the disease. No, I do not. My professional career has focused on bone health and osteoporosis. In the university setting, my research examined lifestyle and risk factors for bone loss and osteoporosis in both women and men. As an investigator, I participated in multicenter trials for new therapies for prevention and treatment of osteoporosis.

In addition, I have had health challenges that have required multiple back surgeries. Those experiences have helped me see life from the patient's perspective. They have taught me about how to seek out solutions when faced with a confusing and fragmented array of information and healthcare options, and then to take charge of my own health for the best quality of life.

This book puts everything about bone health into one resource. Utilizing the latest research, you will find solutions and practical help to aid in sorting out confusing and conflicting information. My goal is for you to feel as if you have a doctor in *your* house with up-to-date information based on scientific evidence to provide you with the answers you need for a bone-healthy life. As you read these chapters, pretend you are sitting down with me and having a friendly chat.

A few words on how to use the book: It is designed as a complete resource. Short individual sections condense vast amounts of information. Tens of thousands of research papers have been published on many of these topics; some scientists have spent their entire careers investigating one aspect of a single topic. The challenge is to summarize the latest research without oversimplification. Sometimes you may not find enough of what you are looking for, and in other places too much. Text boxes contain more technical information, and other boxed-text sections called "My Stories" are about my patients or individuals who have consulted with me about their challenges with bone health. Their experiences may be similar to yours.

While the book can be read from cover to cover, I have organized the information so that any section, or portion of the book, can be read separately to help you find the pertinent information and guidance you are seeking. Each section ends with a bottom-line summary of four to five points called "The Bare Bones." This final summary will aid you in scanning for a review of the section's content or for easy reference later. An appendix titled "Big Words: Medical Terms Broken Down" serves as a glossary of selected medical terms.

Medical terms can be confusing and may seem like a foreign language. Each time a medical term is introduced, I will define it in common words. You will become familiar with some bone-related words that will be helpful in understanding your bone health.

Throughout the book I use the term "doctor" as a representative term for all healthcare practitioners. Instead of using the awkward she/he in referring to a doctor, I use "he" only because male physicians still outnumber female physicians. However, the pronoun use is meant to be gender neutral.

No book is truly "complete." Medical knowledge is constantly changing with new research findings and knowledge. You can visit the website **4Bone Health.org** to stay abreast of the latest studies, tips, and news. You will find regular updates containing the latest bone-related headlines with expert commentary. The interactive tools are intended to help enhance a bone-healthy lifestyle. You can easily share the content with your family and friends. Check it out!

Finally, a reminder that this book is for informational purposes only. It is not intended to substitute for the professional medical advice or treatment recommendations provided by your doctor. You can use this book to help frame questions for your doctor, to ask your doctor's opinion about research findings or medications, and to help you understand your doctor's advice.

Sophocles, an ancient Greek playwright, said, "Look and you will find it— what is unsought will go undetected." Don't let that happen to you! Increase your awareness and make changes for a long life with good, healthy bones.

The Bare Bones
- Bone health is vital at all ages and stages of life.
- Osteoporosis is not inevitable, even with a family history.
- Whatever your age, simple measures can make a difference in your future fracture risk.
- A bone-healthy lifestyle is an important and imperative part of an overall healthy life.

PART ONE

BONE HEALTH BASICS

Building Perfect Bones: Timing Is Everything

Osteoporosis is truly a childhood disease. The problem with osteoporosis and fractures is that these do not occur until you are older. A misspent youth may place you at high risk for not only future fractures but for fractures as a preteen or teen. The window of opportunity to build the strongest bones begins during your mother's pregnancy and ends in your early adulthood.

You reach your skeletal maturity, called *peak bone mass*, by your late twenties to early thirties. Actually, the action occurs much earlier. For women, 90 to 95 percent of your peak bone mass is attained by age eighteen. This bears repeating: the majority of your bone mass is acquired by *age eighteen*. Men usually take a year or two longer to reach that level.

Think of your bones as your bank account or 401(k). You want to build up the balance as high as possible before you start making withdrawals. By age thirty you stop making deposits. Unlike a 401(k), the withdrawals start at a much earlier age. Penalties are accrued if you don't provide the supplies needed for bone maintenance.

The biggest drawback to reading this information now is that you are probably already older than thirty. But it is never too late to get on track with a bone-healthy lifestyle. Your bones require essential support every day. The basic tenets of bone health are true for your entire lifetime.

IT'S IN THE GENES

Building perfect bones begins with your mother and father: Your genes account for 60 to 80 percent of your potential adult bone mass. Lifestyle factors and sex hormones that kick in during puberty contribute the remaining 20 to 40 percent. While those percentages might sound discouraging, the good news is that you can make a difference of as much as 40 percent.

In addition, lifestyle factors may be underestimated when calculating the role of genetics. Environmental influences may affect the behavior of genes without altering DNA. Therefore, lifestyle choices play an important part in the way genes behave. This offers hope for people with a strong family history of osteoporosis. You should not hold a fatalistic attitude if you feel "doomed" by your family history.

Determinants of Peak Bone Mass

Multiple factors affect attaining peak bone mass, with genetic factors having the greatest influence. In order to reach your genetic potential, adequate levels of certain hormones along with healthy eating, adequate calcium and vitamin D, and exercise are essential.

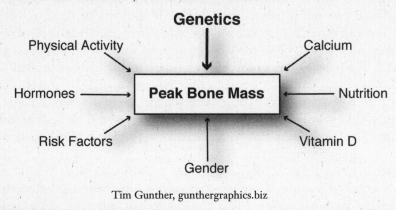

Tim Gunther, gunthergraphics.biz

IN THE BEGINNING: IS IT ALL OVER BEFORE IT BEGINS?

Growth of the skeleton is a complex process that begins in the womb and continues into early adulthood. Any problems during these years may result in reduced bone development leading to an increased risk of fracture later in life. Simply having poor vitamin D and calcium intake, or not maintaining a healthy weight during growth, can spell trouble in your golden years—or even earlier.

The first nine months, in your mother's womb, may shape the rest of your life, not just for your bone health but for your overall health. Calcium and vitamin D are required for development of the growing baby's bones. Addition of calcium starts midterm and increases in the third trimester, when the bones are growing rapidly. This corresponds to a daily calcium demand of about 250 to 300 milligrams (mg) during the third trimester. It is important that the mother's supply of nutrients is sufficient to match the baby's needs. The mother's absorption of calcium increases to meet the needs of the calcium transfer to her growing baby. Expectant mothers' calcium requirement is 1,000 mg a day. Higher levels of vitamin D supplementation may be required beyond the daily prenatal vitamins.

In one study, researchers found that low vitamin D levels in expectant mothers, measured in the third trimester of pregnancy, were associated with lower knee-to-heel lengths measured in their newborns at birth. In another study that followed about two hundred children from birth, lower bone mass at age nine was associated with their mothers' low levels of vitamin D in late pregnancy.

Low birth weight is associated with a higher risk of osteoporosis and other diseases, including heart disease. My patients were always surprised when I asked them for their birth weight. They thought it was a strange question. However, birth weight is correlated with the risk of fracture in later life. If you were a premature baby, you may have ended up with a smaller body size and smaller, less dense bones.

CHILDHOOD GROWTH

Immediately after birth, the rate of bone growth is high. Rapid growth occurs from birth to twelve months. Body mass generally triples and the growth in bone mass is similar. In the years between infancy and puberty, the most rapid growth in bone mass occurs from about ages one to four years. More rapid growth occurs in the bones of the arms and legs than in the trunk. Until puberty, bone mass is about the same in boys as in girls.

Genetic differences may have a role during this time period that explains much of the variability among different racial or ethnic groups. Some studies of Caucasian and African American children have found that bone mass is greater in African American children before puberty. Others observed that differences emerge in adolescence when African Americans gain more bone mass than Caucasians. Limited data from Asian and Hispanic youth show that their bone mass is similar to Caucasians or is intermediate between Caucasians and African Americans.

In the preteen years, the body begins revving up all of its systems for the rapid growth phase associated with puberty. At this stage, the skeleton of a preteen is more responsive to calcium, protein, and exercise than in later years. Young bones respond more to exercise than adult bones. Weight-bearing exercises are the most effective, particularly jumping and running.

PUBERTY: GROWTH SPURT

Growth hormones and sex hormones that kick in between childhood and puberty significantly alter bone mineral buildup. Peak bone growth lags behind peak height growth by approximately one year. Early prepuberty is the beginning of rapid bone growth. At puberty, with the secretion of sex hormones, growth of the trunk accelerates; the growth of the long bones of the arms and legs slows down until the growth plates fuse and linear growth stops.

Generally the growth spurt occurs between ages eleven and fourteen for girls and between thirteen and seventeen for boys. *Forty percent* of total adult bone mass is accumulated during these three to four years of rapid bone mass growth. The two years of peak skeletal growth occur approximately between the ages of eleven and a half and thirteen and a half for girls and between thirteen and fifteen for boys. However, changes follow maturity levels rather than exact chronological age. Bone mass approximately doubles between the onset of puberty and young adulthood, and it increases more in boys than in girls. The larger bone size in boys is probably a result of boys having a longer period of accelerated growth.

The increase in bone mass is primarily due to an increase in bone size with little or no change to the amount of bone tissue within the bones. This is what creates the increased risk of fracture during the puberty years.

These preteen and teenage years represent a critically important window of opportunity to build bones that are as strong and dense as possible. Illness in prepuberty or puberty may interrupt growth. The end result will be lower bone mass.

At the end of bone growth, individuals of the same age, same sex, and same height can have large differences in the amount of bone. Those differences can vary by up to a factor of two. For example, one girl may have 10 grams of bone mineral in one lumbar vertebra while another physically similar girl of the same age may have 20 grams. What accounts for this variation? Many factors influence bone mass accumulation, and these factors together account for the differences in peak bone mass among individuals.

Peak Bone Mass

- Peak bone mass is the maximum bone mass attained. At least 90 to 95 percent of peak bone mass is obtained by age eighteen in girls, and by age nineteen or twenty in boys. Genes play a major role. But the relative importance of the elements of nutrition, physical activity, vitamin D, and other risk factors is unclear.

- Genetics account for 60 to 80 percent of the variability in an individual's peak bone mass. Environmental and lifestyle factors, especially physical activity and, in teens, alcohol, smoking, and use of birth control pills, may interact with diet and nutrition to influence bone growth and development. The effects of lifestyle factors may depend on the stage of maturity. A less than ideal environment, including acute and chronic illnesses, may not allow a child to reach his or her optimal bone density.

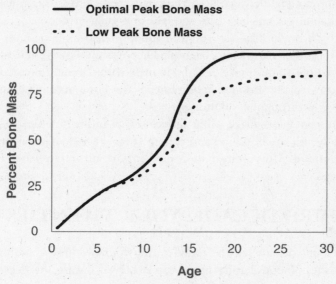

Tim Gunther, gunthergraphics.biz

UNHEALTHY LIFESTYLE

Even kids and teens who appear healthy might not reach their optimal peak bone mass. Blame their unhealthy lifestyles. As one parent expressed it, "Just when those hormones become supercharged we lose control over what our teenagers are going to do, eat, or say."

Most youths do not come close to meeting their daily recommended amounts of vitamin D or calcium. According to the latest figures, preteen and teen girls have the most serious deficiency, just at the time when more calcium is needed for growth. Only 15 percent of 9- to 13-year-old girls and 10 percent of 14- to 18-year-old girls met their daily requirements of calcium from diet alone. Meanwhile, 22 percent of 9- to 13-year-old boys and 42 percent of 14- to 18-year-old boys, met their daily recommended intake of calcium from foods. But still, the majority of boys consumed less than the recommended daily intake of 1,300 mg of calcium.

More time spent on the computer, playing video games, and watching television is usually at the expense of physical activity. Only about half of teenagers exercise on a regular basis. Inactivity is highest among girls, and Hispanic and African American teens.

Cigarette smoking continues to be adopted by teenagers. According to the Center for Disease Control (CDC), 20 percent of high school students smoke.

The rate is about equal between boys and girls. Teen smokers often have other poor health habits, such as bad diets and lack of regular exercise.

Unhealthy lifestyle may also result in suboptimal peak bone mass. Proper nutrition with sufficient calcium, vitamin D, physical activity, and hormonal support is essential to maximize peak bone mass within genetically determined bounds. These are the absolute requirements for bone accumulation during growth as well as throughout adult life.

Misspent youth can make a big difference to future fracture risk. Optimizing bone health in childhood and teenage years results in stronger, denser bones in adulthood. More immediate benefit may result in fewer fractures as a preteen or teen.

THE THIRD DECADE: YOUR TWENTIES

A little more bone density may be added during your twenties. Gains of 5 to 12 percent in bone mineral density have been observed during the decade. This time period is referred to as *consolidation*.

The potential for bone gain in the third decade should not be ignored. For example, a student-initiated class project at the University of California, San Diego, looked at young college women, ages eighteen to twenty-five. We were astonished to find lower than average bone density by DXA scan in many of the students. From the information on their questionnaires, it was apparent that their diets were practically devoid of calcium. They had stopped drinking milk and were subsisting on low calorie, nutrient-poor diets. We provided a year's supply of calcium supplements to all of the young women. Those who had been calcium deficient showed increases in their bone density after one year.

This finding, as well as other reports, suggests that young women of college age might be able to reduce the risk of fractures in their later years by being attuned to their bone health and by making simple changes earlier in life.

THE THIRTIES AND FORTIES:
WHAT GOES UP MUST COME DOWN

After reaching the maximum bone mass by age thirty, there is no nice plateau during middle age. Bone loss starts happening slowly with the process called *remodeling*, which is a little like climbing a mountain: You reach the summit, take some pictures to document your achievement, then slowly start to work your way down the other side.

Just as in growing your bone mass, the same supplies are essential to supporting bone remodeling, which is happening all the time. However, the bone remodeling process tends to result in a small net loss of bone.

If we go back to the 401(k) analogy, at retirement age you have no choice and you must make mandatory withdrawals. You try to be miserly by only making small withdrawals, and if you continue to provide all the essential supplies, it won't be too costly. But if you don't do your part in maintaining a healthy lifestyle, your savings may be raided: You might run out of money and end up bankrupt with a fracture.

Bone Mass over Lifetime

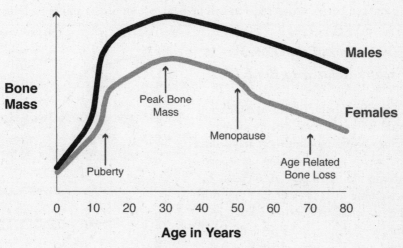

Tim Gunther, gunthergraphics.biz

MENOPAUSE

For women, the natural course of events means that the supply of estrogen ends as you transition into menopause. Bone loss will accelerate before you even stop having menstrual periods. Bone remodeling speeds up and the bone formation side of the remodeling process can no longer keep up with the breaking down of bone. You end up with a net loss that can be rapid in the first four to five years of menopause, followed by the slower loss of bone that is more associated with aging.

Women who are heavier and have more body fat tend to lose less bone mass. The fat produces a weak estrogen, called estrone, which provides some extra support for the bone. But there is a downside: Obese women are still at risk for suffering fractures of the upper arm, ankle, and lower leg.

AGE-RELATED BONE LOSS

Adult bone mass is a reflection of peak bone mass, age at menopause for women, and rate of bone loss. Those who acquire a greater bone mass balance during the first thirty years of life will be at lower risk for fractures later in life. Although osteoporosis is primarily a disease of older adults, building a strong, dense skeleton during the growing years may be the best way to prevent osteoporosis.

If bone mass can be maximized during growth and development, you will begin adulthood with optimal bone mass and will be less likely to develop osteoporosis in later years. The more bone mass you "bank" in childhood and adolescence, the better you will withstand the inevitable bone loss that comes with aging and the better protected you will be from osteoporosis and bone fractures.

Simulation of the Three Factors Related to Bone Loss

Optimizing bone health in childhood and teen years results in stronger, denser bones in adulthood and reduces the chances of developing osteoporosis later in life. A 10 percent increase of peak bone mass is estimated to reduce the risk of an osteoporotic fracture during adult life by 50 percent. Peak bone mass has more effect than your age at menopause or bone loss with aging.

Source: Hernandez CJ, et al. *Osteoporosis International.* 2003;14:843–847. Adapted from figure 2.

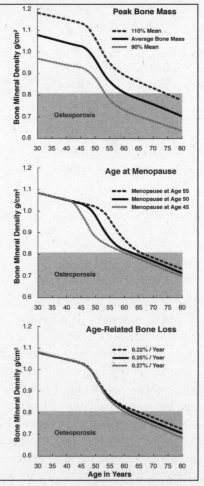

Now you should understand why *osteoporosis is truly a childhood disease that manifests in later life*. Increasing awareness and education about bone health in our children, grandchildren, and loved ones' lives is vital to prevention of fractures with aging. Improving modifiable factors of diet, physical activity, and calcium and vitamin D intake will result in maximizing bone growth. Achieving a high peak bone mass will lessen the impact of age-related bone loss and menopausal bone loss in women. A healthy lifestyle in childhood may have immediate beneficial effects by decreasing childhood fractures and by establishing healthy habits for one's lifetime.

The Bare Bones

- Low birth weight is associated with osteoporosis as an adult.
- Puberty starts the most important time for bone mass acquisition.
- Bone mass approximately doubles between the onset of puberty and young adulthood.
- Bone loss begins after achieving peak bone mass in the early thirties.
- In women, bone loss accelerates at menopause with loss of estrogen.
- Gradual and steady bone loss occurs with aging.

Fracture Facts: One Tough Break Leads to Another

If I collected a penny every time someone said that they had broken their wrist because they had fallen hard, I would have broken my piggy bank. Fracturing a bone when you fall is not normal. Your bones should not break when you fall.

Think of a piece of plastic when it is new. Although it is rigid, it still has some give to it. Over time, plastic tends to lose its bending ability so that it becomes more prone to crack. Bones are similar. With aging, bone becomes less bendable and more fragile. The force from a fall causes older bone to crack and fracture.

An arm or wrist fracture is a big red flag. It means that you are at risk for more fractures in the future—literally, a cascade of fractures. But fractures are not inevitable; by acting now you can prevent future fractures from happening. Recognition of risk is the first step. Unfortunately, the majority of people do not put two and two together.

A large international study of over sixty thousand women illustrates this point. In the Global Longitudinal Study of Osteoporosis in Women (GLOW Study), women from ten different countries in Europe, North America, and Australia were asked about awareness of osteoporosis. All were postmenopausal, with an average age of sixty-nine. Only one in five women thought her risk of osteoporosis was higher than other women of the same age.

The majority of women participating in the study who had been diagnosed with osteoporosis did not recognize that their condition could result in fractures. In fact, most of the women taking osteoporosis medicines did not think they were at high risk for fractures. Because they were being treated for the disease, they figured that they were in the safe zone and had the same level of risk for fractures as those who did not have osteoporosis. How wrong they were!

Osteoporosis is referred to as a silent disease. Fractures can break that silence. Interestingly, you may not even know you have had a fracture. Silent fractures occur in the spine. Most other fractures are caused by a fall. Fractures can have devastating consequences; they can lead to serious disability, and, yes, even death. The goal is to prevent fractures in the first place.

Based on the latest figures, more than two million adults break bones each year. Men account for 595,000 or 29 percent of the fractures. Although Caucasian men and women are predominantly affected, one in five men and one in eleven women are non-Caucasian.

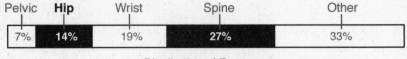

Pelvic	Hip	Wrist	Spine	Other
7%	14%	19%	27%	33%

Distribution of Fractures
Total Number = 2.05 Million (2005)

SOURCE: Burge R et al. *Journal of Bone and Mineral Research.* 2007;22:465-475.

Hip, spine, and wrist fractures are the classic fractures characteristic of osteoporosis. Fractures that include upper arm, rib, collarbone, kneecap, and lower leg are other sites of skeletal fragility. Of all fractures, the ones classified as "other" make up the largest proportion. Hip fractures that occur in the proximal femur, which is the bone between the hip and knee joints, account for one out of every seven fractures.

Wrist 3% Spine
Pelvic Other Hip

5%	6%	14%	72%

Cost of Fractures = $17 Billion (2005)

SOURCE: Burge R et al. *Journal of Bone and Mineral Research.* 2007;22:465-475.
Tim Gunther, gunthergraphics.biz

Fractures are costly. In 2005, the costs for new fractures in the United States were estimated at $17 billion. Hip fractures account for nearly three quarters of all fracture costs. Some projections show that hip fractures will be the top consumer of our healthcare dollars spent on the sixty-five and older age group. Already hip fractures account for about 20 percent of Medicare claims. The projected costs for more than 3 million fractures in 2025 are estimated at $25 billion.

A tsunami of fractures is expected with the graying of baby boomers. It is estimated that 40 to 50 percent of postmenopausal women and approximately 25 to 33 percent of men will eventually sustain a fracture. The numbers of fractures associated with low-energy falls are increasing with the expanding size of our aging population. Fractures of the hip and spine dramatically increase with age for both men and women. The rates of wrist fractures level off in women as they age.

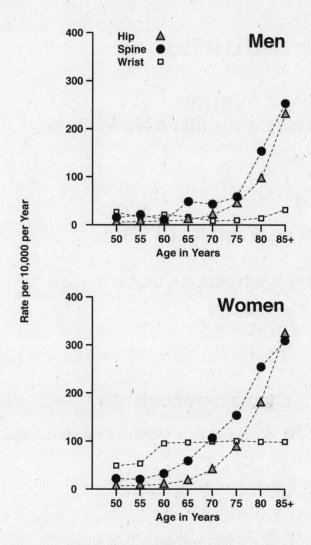

SOURCE: Burge R et al. *Journal of Bone and Mineral Research.* 2007;22:465-475.

Tim Gunther, gunthergraphics.biz

HIP FRACTURES

Hip fracture is the granddaddy of all fractures. The majority occur in individuals over age seventy-five. More than 40 percent occur in the eighty-five-and-over age group. If you are younger, hip fractures are usually not an immediate danger. The difficult part about prevention is thinking so many years ahead.

Hip Fractures

· **Every 2 minutes**
someone will suffer a hip fracture

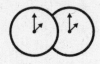

· **90%** are a result of a fall

· **1 in 4** hip fractures occur in men

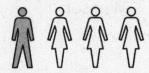

· Hip fractures may be deadly

1 in 3 men will die within a year after fracture

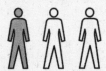

1 in 5 women will die within a year

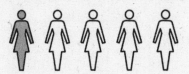

Tim Gunther, gunthergraphics.biz

Everyone seems to have a story about an older relative or friend who had a hip fracture:

"It was the beginning of the end."
"My grandmother never walked again."
"My grandfather never made it out of the hospital."
"My mother never recovered and died in a nursing home six months later."

Being in the hospital for whatever reason at an older age is fraught with danger. Major surgery, including repairing your broken hip, can result in disaster. Unfortunately, our organ systems in later years just do not have the reserve we have as younger adults. Older adults walk a balance beam without knowing it. Surgery knocks you off balance. Then it is a domino effect. One system goes, then another and another.

You want to avoid hip fractures in your golden years because you have a good chance of dying if you do have a fracture. Within one year of a hip fracture, 33 percent of men and 22 percent of women have died. Few medical diseases have such a high death rate. *Hip fractures are killers.*

Survivors after a year continue to have a higher death rate than their peers for ten or more years. Surviving does not equate to the same lifestyle as before the hip fracture. You are more likely not to return to your own home, but to instead end up in other residences that provide assistance.

YOUR STORIES...

Joan, age seventy-seven, got up early one morning to let out her dog. It was not quite light and she hadn't put on her glasses. She walked into her kitchen and hit a puddle of water from the dog's bowl, and her bare feet went out from under her. She landed hard on the tile floor with all of her weight on her right side.

Diagnosis: Hip fracture.

Fall-proofing your home will help decrease the likelihood of events like this.

SPINE FRACTURES (ALSO CALLED VERTEBRAL)

Not all fractures speak up. Only 20 to 30 percent of spine fractures are associated with a symptom, usually pain. These are called clinical spine fractures since they come to clinical attention. The ones that remain silent and are only identified through some type of x-ray imaging are called spine deformities or morphometric fractures.

No sex differences are observed in spine fractures. For both men and women, 27 percent of all fractures occur in the spine.

Spine fractures do not grab your attention like hip fractures. Few people end up in the hospital. Yet spine fractures may also have a tremendous impact on your life. You may have the image of a bent over older woman with a so-called dowager's hump or kyphosis. However, the majority of spine fractures may have only subtle clues, if any.

Height loss of two inches or more may indicate an underlying fracture. Back pain may be associated with a new fracture. In my experience, the patients who presented with back pain due to a fracture usually had a cause. They would report events such as: "I moved a heavy box of books"; "I lifted my grandson out of the crib"; and "I picked up a computer tower from under my desk."

The spine is made up of three regions: neck or cervical, trunk or thoracic, and low back or lumbar. Fractures do not occur evenly along the spine. The most common locations for spine fractures are below the shoulder blades (T7–8), the last two levels of the thoracic spine (T11–12), and the first two lumbar levels (L1–2). The curvature of the spine may contribute to fractures occurring in these locations. The transition from a rigid midback to a more mobile lower back may be another factor.

Once one spine fracture happens you are likely to have more. Your risk of a second spine fracture is highest in the year following your first. A spine fracture is also predictive of fractures occurring at other sites.

YOUR STORIES...

Anne, age sixty-nine, returned home exhausted and with back pain after spending several weeks at her daughter's house. The occasion of the visit was the birth of a granddaughter. It was a joyous time, but she was on the move all day and all night. Not only was she helping with the new baby, her biggest task was trying to keep up with her twenty-month-old grandson.

One time, she picked up her grandson after he had fallen and skinned his knee. Afterward, she felt intense lower back pain. She was almost incapacitated, but she managed the pain, until finally, six weeks later, she was forced to see her doctor. An x-ray revealed a fracture of her first lumbar vertebra. He prescribed physical therapy to help with pain relief, as well as to improve her body mechanics for lifting and other activities.

Having one spine fracture puts her at high risk for another fracture. Once her pain subsides and she can lie comfortably, a bone density scan will be scheduled. Examining all her risks and laboratory tests to look for common other causes of fracture is also planned before treatment is started.

WRIST FRACTURES

Fractures of the wrist follow an opposite age trend from hip fractures. Wrist fractures are more common in younger men and women (ages fifty to sixty-four) and then rates level off and decrease with aging.

The reason for the reverse age trend is reflexes. With an unexpected trip or fall, younger people are more likely to stick out their arm to break the fall. Although their wrist may break, the rest of the body is out of harm's way. Later, with aging, your arm does not get out fast enough, and whatever body part lands first gets the brunt of the forces and is at risk for breaking.

Women are almost two times more likely to break their wrists than men. The reason for the difference between the sexes is structure. Men have larger bone size than women. Larger bones are harder to snap than smaller bones.

Wrist fractures should have a big warning sign attached to them. If you have a wrist fracture, you have a two- to fourfold risk of fractures at other sites. Wrist fractures are your wake-up call. It's time to evaluate your risk and reduce your chances of another fracture.

Wrist fractures themselves may not be totally benign. In the Study of Osteoporotic Fractures, women over sixty-five who had wrist fractures showed significant functional decline. The activities of daily living that were compromised included meal preparation, heavy housekeeping, ability to climb ten stairs, shopping, and getting out of a car. The researchers equated the impact of wrist fracture in older women to those seen with other established risk factors for functional decline such as falls, diabetes, and arthritis.

SHOULDER FRACTURES

A shoulder fracture is of the upper arm or the bone called the humerus. The fracture of the shoulder is closely linked to hip fractures because the fall is similar. With a sideways fall, the shoulder hits first instead of the hip.

In fact, hip fractures are common within the year after shoulder fractures. A high risk of hip fracture follows a shoulder fracture. The risk decreases with time but remains higher than the risk for the general population of the same age.

If a shoulder fracture occurs, you need to be proactive and do everything you can to prevent a hip fracture.

OTHER FRACTURES

Fractures of the ribs, lower leg (tibia and fibula), collarbone, and kneecap are classified in the "other" category. Recent research has shown that these fractures are related to underlying osteoporosis, whereas in the past they were not considered to be a result of a fragile skeleton.

These other types of fracture account for the most common fractures in men, at 44 percent, and women, at 29 percent. They tend to be less severe, except that the pain with a rib fracture can be quite severe.

In the Osteoporotic Fractures in Men (MrOS) Study, rib fractures were the most common clinical fracture. Half of rib fractures were associated with a fall. In addition, men with rib fractures had classic risk factors for osteoporosis, including older age, low hip bone density, and history of fracture. A history of rib fracture predicted more than a twofold increase in risk of future fracture of the rib, hip, or wrist.

Interestingly, an ankle fracture in both men and women *does not* show the usual relation to age and bone mineral density as seen for other fragility fractures. However, the severity of many ankle fractures may be magnified by underlying skeletal fragility.

FRACTURES BEGET FRACTURES

The problem is that once you have one fracture the probability of another fracture is quite high. The increase in risk is not constant over time. The critical time is the first year after fracture, as the highest number of refractures occur in the first year after the initial injury. Up to one-third of men and women fracture again within one year. Risk decreases over subsequent years, but remains higher than the general population's risk for beyond ten years. Men are at higher risk than women of sustaining a subsequent fracture at any site after any type of first fracture, with the exception of an ankle fracture.

DEATH

Overall a higher rate of death following a fracture is observed in men than women. Since osteoporotic fractures are less common in men than women, they usually reflect a poorer underlying health. Other illnesses might be the cause directly or indirectly of the fracture event itself and also contribute to a poorer outcome after fracture.

Hip Fractures Are Not the Only Killers

Spine Fracture. The risk of death differs for spine fractures between ones that come to clinical attention with symptoms and those that are silent and are found on x-ray. In addition to all the problems with symptomatic spine fractures, those who feel pain associated with the fracture have death rates almost as high as the death rate for hip fractures. This is observed in both men and women.

For silent spine fractures, the association between fracture and risk of death is less clear because a minority come to clinical attention. In one ten-year follow-up of men and women with spine fractures diagnosed by x-ray, the risk of death was approximately twofold higher compared with those who showed no evidence of spine fractures.

Shoulder Fracture. The patterns for shoulder fractures are more difficult to interpret. A slight but significant excess in deaths is observed, which decreases with time; at five years after injury the risk was no longer greater than that of the general population.

A decreasing risk of death with time is a common feature of hip, spine, and shoulder fracture. In a sample of older Australian men and women, increased risk of death persisted for five years for all major fractures and for ten years after hip fractures. Subsequent fractures were associated with an additional five years of elevated risk.

Wrist Fracture. After a wrist fracture, studies show a similar risk of death to that of the general population. However, researchers found that people in their eighties who suffered a wrist fracture tended to be more physically active and robust. They were still spry enough to stick their hand out to break their fall instead of suffering a hip fracture. Wrist fractures in the eighty-and-older age group may be associated with an even lower mortality rate than that of their peers.

CHILDHOOD FRACTURES

Childhood fractures are rising. Why? Is it because of more risky behaviors? Or are children less bone healthy? I believe it is both.

One of my "adopted" French sons, Eddy, along with his brother, competes in motorcycle races called Supermoto. At age fourteen, Eddy had a major crash and broke both legs. That's an extreme example, I will admit, but not necessarily among those athletes who compete in today's action sports events.

Some evidence suggests that unhealthy lifestyle is a major cause. Less physical activity leads to the production of fat in the bone marrow instead of production of new bone-forming cells. The majority of preteens and teens do not meet the daily calcium and vitamin D recommendations. These factors may lead to making less bone, which results in lower peak bone mass.

What are the long-term consequences of a childhood fracture? There is conflicting evidence. Some evidence shows that you never catch up.

BIOMECHANICS OF FRACTURES

Numerically, more fractures occur in those with low bone mass than in those diagnosed with osteoporosis. In the Study of Osteoporotic Fractures, older women who had hip bone densities higher than the osteoporosis cut-off accounted *for more than half* of the observed hip fractures. Many factors play a role beyond what is measurable in bone density. Among them is bone strength, which includes density, structure, and material properties. In addition, nonbone factors such as muscle strength and the likelihood of falling also play large roles.

Microstructure

Young ⟶ Old

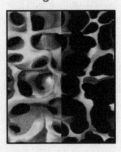

Geometry

Young ⟶ Old

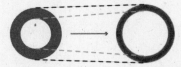

Loading Condition

Spine
Bending and lifting

Hip
Fall to side

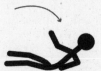

Tim Gunther, gunthergraphics.biz

A fracture occurs when the forces on the bone exceed its strength. The strength of the bone changes dramatically with aging. The microstructure of the bone becomes thinner and weaker. The geometry of the bone changes with thinning of the cortex and expansion of bone size. Forward bending movements increase the load on the spinal column and cause spine fractures. The impact of a fall to the side directly increases the force on the weaker bone and may result in a hip fracture.

The Bare Bones

- Although hip and spine fractures occur in older adults, fractures at any age increase the risk of future fracture.
- *Prevent the first fracture!* The risk of subsequent fractures is high, particularly in the first year after a broken bone.
- Hip, spine, and shoulder fractures increase your risk of death for five to ten years.
- Fractures occur when the force on the bone exceeds its strength.

Challenges and Choices:
What You Can and
Cannot Change

Our American *health*care system has been described as a *sick*care system. The problem is that our current system is all about crisis management and patching things up after the fact. Hundreds of billions of dollars are spent on pills, hospitalization, and disability for problems we can prevent. Sadly, we do not spend enough of our time and resources on prevention, which is our most difficult job. It is up to us to make healthy choices. An ounce of prevention is worth twenty pounds of cure!

In the prevention of fractures, your goal is to decrease your risk of silent bone loss. But you will have to wait many years to reap rewards. "Feeling better" is usually not a big motivator. For me, if I do not exercise every day, my back talks back. For osteoporosis, you do not have symptoms to alleviate. Rather, it is all about having a healthy lifestyle that is good for your overall health and reduces the chances of major chronic diseases.

You may not believe that the simple choices you make in your lifestyle can be as powerful as drugs, but they often are. Although certain risks are genetic, your lifestyle plays a big role in the expression of your genes. You do have some influence over some aspects of the factors that you think you cannot change.

The goal is to modify the risk factors over which you have control. The challenge is to sustain your motivation to make comprehensive changes so that healthy changes become part of your regular routine, and ultimately, your lifestyle.

Age. Age is the strongest of all risk factors. The older you are, the greater your risk of osteoporosis. Regardless of your bone density, the older you are, the more likely it is that you will suffer a fracture. If two women have the same bone density, but one is fifty-five and the other is twenty years older, the seventy-five year old has a greater risk of fracture. Bone microstructure becomes more fragile with age, putting the older woman at higher risk.

You cannot change the aging process, so the goal is to minimize age-related changes.

Sex. Women are definitely more likely than men to be at risk. More women than men sustain fractures because women start off with a smaller skeleton at peak bone mass. However, women do not have exclusive rights to osteoporosis. Men fracture, too. Osteoporosis is arguably the most understudied and underdiagnosed disease in men. One large research study, dubbed "MrOS," is following six thousand men, age sixty-five and older, trying to fill in the gaps.

Race and Ethnicity. Race and ethnicity make a big difference. Caucasians are at the highest risk. Asians, depending on heritage, have similar risk to Caucasians. African Americans have the lowest risk, but that does not make them immune. In general, Hispanics tend to be at intermediate risk. These are broad categorical statements that need to be individualized for your particular family heritage.

Previous Fracture. Once you have had one fracture, the chances of a later fracture are markedly increased. Usually, the previous fracture refers to one after the age of forty-five. However, recent research indicates that children who fracture may be at higher risk to fracture as adults. They may have lower bone mass and never catch up. Fractures in younger adults are also linked to fractures later in life.

Height and Weight. While undoubtedly you have some control over your weight, it is included here with height. A calculation using both height and weight produces body mass index (BMI). BMI is related to bone density. In general, those with lower BMI have a lower bone density and are more likely to be at risk for osteoporosis. The reverse is true as well. Those with higher BMI have a higher bone density and are less likely to be at risk for osteoporosis. BMI may be used as a rough measure in place of bone density, if bone density is not available.

Height and weight are individual risk factors as well. Although we think of small, petite women as being at risk, a height of five feet eight inches or taller is a risk factor. Height is related to the force of a fall—mass that falls from a greater height falls faster and with greater force. When the force is greater than the flexibility of bone, the bone breaks.

Weighing less than 127 pounds puts you at higher risk. You are less likely to have the cushioning on your hips, which helps to distribute the forces in a fall. Being a little bit heavier is better, but too much weight is a problem and may be related to lower bone quality and density, as well as higher risk of fractures of the upper arm, ankle, and lower leg.

Family History. The health history of your grandparents, parents, and sisters and brothers is extremely important. Sharing your maladies might get boring, but knowing the problems and diseases that run in your family is the key to understanding your risk.

In addition, you should be sharing this information with the generation or two younger than you. Although younger people tend to think of themselves as immortal, learning about their health heritage may make a difference in their current health habits.

For instance, if you share with your twenty-five-year-old daughter that her great-grandmother became bent over with age, that her grandmother had a hip fracture, and that you have osteoporosis, she may be more likely to eat more calcium-rich food, take a vitamin D pill, stop smoking, and start exercising.

Do not forget about the men! If your father broke his hip, that is an even stronger risk factor for you than your mother fracturing because men are less likely to fracture. The hip fracture your father had after slipping on ice was not because he fell hard but rather because he had fragile bones. Men are less likely to be diagnosed with osteoporosis.

Other Illnesses or Problems. Other diseases may be the cause of bone loss and osteoporosis. Common to rare disorders make up a long list of diseases that can cause or contribute to osteoporosis and fractures. The following list gives some of the common conditions.

Common Conditions Tied to Osteoporosis

1. Diabetes
2. Breast Cancer
3. Celiac Disease, also called gluten intolerance
4. Crohn's Disease
5. Depression
6. Early menopause before age 45
7. Epilepsy
8. Hyperthyroidism (overactive thyroid)
9. Rheumatoid Arthritis
10. Ulcerative Colitis

Although you may have a problem that contributes to bone loss, you can make a difference in your long-term bone health. For example, if you are diabetic, better control of your blood sugars will make a difference for your bone health. Even though you may have other diseases, taking care of yourself and keeping those problems well controlled will minimize their effects on bone, and overall, you will be in much better shape.

Medicines. Some medicines that are helpful in treatments of other diseases have harmful effects on bone. Steroids, such as prednisone, are the most common culprit. Recent observations found medicines commonly used may weaken bones.

> ### Common Medicines Tied to Osteoporosis
>
> 1. Arimidex® (breast cancer)
> 2. Actos® (diabetes)
> 3. Lexapro® (antidepressant)
> 4. Nexium® (heartburn and ulcers)
> 5. Paxil® (antidepressant)
> 6. Prednisone (multiple uses)
> 7. Prevacid® (heartburn and ulcers)
> 8. Prilosec® (heartburn and ulcers)
> 9. Prozac® (antidepressant)
> 10. Zoloft® (antidepressant)

Falls. Everyone falls. The risk of falls, and injuries from them, rises dramatically for those over age sixty-five. The majority of hip fractures are caused by falls. Falls may play a role in all other fractures, even those of the spine. Falls have multiple potential causes, and it takes a comprehensive approach to lower the risks. You need to "fall-proof" yourself and your home, which is where most falls occur.

Alcohol. As with everything else in life, we have supersized our alcoholic beverages. One "unit" of alcohol is the measure used in the new fracture risk assessment tool (see illustration on page 45). Three or more units a day gives you a black mark against your bones. The good news: One to two units of alcohol a day show a positive effect on bone and fracture risk. In fact, it is better for your bones if you drink moderately than if you do not drink at all.

Smoking. Of course, health reasons abound for not picking up cigarettes and cigars, and osteoporosis is only one of them. Smoking speeds up bone breakdown. In women, estrogen also tends to be lower when you smoke.

Sadly, our youth still view smoking as "cool." According to the latest survey from the Centers for Disease Control and Prevention (CDC), 20 percent of high school students smoke. They are doing this harmful activity before their bones have reached peak bone mass, so they may not reach their "optimal level."

Alcohol: "One Unit" Serving

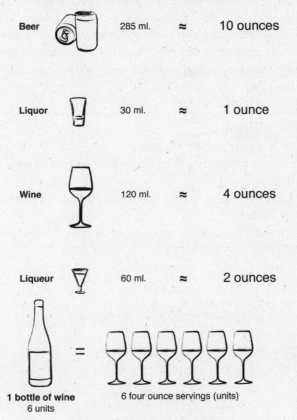

Beer	285 ml.	≈	10 ounces
Liquor	30 ml.	≈	1 ounce
Wine	120 ml.	≈	4 ounces
Liqueur	60 ml.	≈	2 ounces

1 bottle of wine
6 units

= 6 four ounce servings (units)

Tim Gunther, gunthergraphics.biz

Top Factors that Put You at Higher Risk of Fractures

1. Older age
2. Being a woman
3. Caucasian or Asian race
4. Weight less than 127 pounds
5. Previous fracture
6. Mother or father had a fracture
7. Steroids (oral prednisone)
8. Smoking
9. Alcohol (more than 2 drinks a day)
10. Rheumatoid Arthritis

Stacking up the risk factors may cause fractures earlier rather than later; add aging and falls to the other insults and it spells even more trouble in later years. The goal is to lessen the risk factors you can control. Lessen the impact of other diseases on bone health by controlling them. Decrease to the lowest possible dosing necessary medicines that also impact bones. Connect your family history and your bone health. Simple lifestyle changes will lessen your risk and promote a healthier lifestyle.

The Bare Bones
- Determine your risk for fractures.
- You can lower your risk even if you have a strong family history of osteoporosis.
- Not knowing you are in the "danger zone" for fractures is hazardous to your health.
- Take preventive measures to avoid bone fractures and serious injury.

The Bone Cycle: Cruise Control and Overdrive

The word *skeleton* brings to mind images of a Halloween decoration. However, this static picture of bones could not be further from reality. Through a process called remodeling, our bones are dynamic and ever changing. We may remodel our homes once or twice in our lifetime, but when it comes to our bones, the remodeling is constant and never ending.

Remodeling results from the interplay of three bone cell types: osteocytes, osteoclasts, and osteoblasts. More than 95 percent of the bone cells of an adult are osteocytes. Osteocytes are the cells buried in bone, and they maintain a dense network of connection with each other. They sense mechanical strain when the bone is bent or deformed, which happens all the time as muscles pull and tug on the bone. Higher mechanical strain is produced with exercise. Osteocytes are presumed to respond to this strain by sending signals that cause either new bone formation or existing bone removal.

Osteoclasts are the cells that break down bone. Osteoblasts are the cells that form new bone. These two types of cells work in concert to keep bone repaired and in good shape.

Bone resists breaking apart by relieving the stresses that develop from everyday life. These stresses cause tiny cracks called microcracks. Bone remodeling occurs in response to these microcracks in order to maintain the structural integrity of the skeleton and to serve its function as a storehouse of calcium.

Bone has a crack repair team that sets up bone remodeling units. Old bone is removed by the osteoclasts that dig around the cracks. They create actual pits or holes in the surface of the bone using acids to dissolve the old bone. The osteoblast cells migrate in and line the pits to form new bone. The bone is restored to its former level. Later, the new bone is hardened through a process called mineralization, so that the new bone becomes indistinguishable from the surrounding bone. It is similar to a painter filling in a hole in the wall with spackle and then painting over it.

Normal Bone Remodeling

new bone
matches amount
broken down

activation of
osteoclasts

bone formation
by osteoblasts

bone breakdown
by osteoclasts

transition

Tim Gunther, gunthergraphics.biz

Types of Bones

- There are two types of bone. Compact cortical bone makes up the outer shell of all bones and the shafts of the long bones of the arms and legs. It comprises about 80 percent of the skeleton. Spongy trabecular bone makes up the inner parts of the bones found in the spine (vertebrae), the pelvis, and the end parts of long bones.
- The spongy bone resembles a rigid sponge with a plate-like meshwork of beams. The plates within this kind of bone are called trabeculae; they act as cross braces to give support and prevent collapse of the structure.
- Remodeling occurs at different rates in the two types of bone. The spongy trabecular bone is metabolically faster than the dense cortical bone. This is a function of a greater number of cells in trabecular bone and a larger surface area where remodeling occurs. The spine therefore shows changes more quickly than the dense bone in the hip.

SPEED: CRUISE CONTROL

If the amount of new bone equals the amount being broken down, bone mass stays stable and does not change. A balance is maintained into your thirties and bones remain strong. Packets of old bone are replaced with packets of new bone in perfect synchrony.

Normal Bone Remodeling
- On average, your entire skeleton is renewed every ten years.
- Lifespan of an osteoclast is approximately three weeks.
- Lifespan of an osteoblast is approximately three months.
- One new remodeling site starts about every seven to ten seconds.
- Therefore, three to four million new bone-remodeling sites are initiated each year.
- One million sites operate at any given moment in your skeleton.

However, even at an early age, bone remodeling is not perfectly efficient. There is a small deficit in bone following each cycle. Given the number of bone remodeling cycles operating in the adult skeleton, this imbalance causes age-related bone loss that results in a bone deficit that probably increases with age.

SHIFT TO OVERDRIVE

Anything that increases whole-body bone remodeling will aggravate bone loss.

Menopause, with the accompanying loss of estrogen support, results in an increase of osteoclast activity. Bone breakdown happens much faster than the osteoblasts can form new bone. The rate of bone formation is unable to match the increased bone breakdown. This revving up of the cycle results in a net loss of bone tissue that can be significant. The plates of bone slowly become rod-like structures. The connections in the spongy trabecular bone become broken. Multiple areas of bone become structurally fragile and this eventually leads to increased fracture risk. The bones become thinner and weaker and are therefore prone to break more easily.

Many other factors, such as certain medicines and illnesses, may also accelerate bone breakdown so that the osteoblasts can't keep up.

Accelerated Bone Breakdown

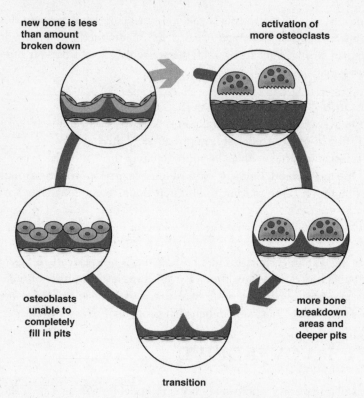

new bone is less
than amount
broken down

activation of
more osteoclasts

osteoblasts
unable to
completely
fill in pits

more bone
breakdown
areas and
deeper pits

transition

Tim Gunther, gunthergraphics.biz

Prescription medicines for osteoporosis are classified based on their action on bone cells. Most osteoporosis drugs target the activity of the osteoclast. Since the breaking down of bone is referred to as resorption, the medicines are called *antiresorptives*. Antiresorptives work by decreasing the action of osteoclasts, which decreases the rate of bone breakdown. Bone formation agents, on the other hand, work by activating the osteoblasts to increase the making of new bone. The response to therapy is based on rates of bone remodeling in different parts of the skeleton. For example, larger increases in bone density are seen at the metabolically more active spine than at the hip.

Microstructure in the Spine
Bone Loss with Aging

Bone Remodeling Cycle Imbalance
More bone breakdown than bone formation

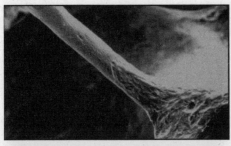

Single Trabecula

With bone loss, plate-like spongy bone becomes thinner and more rod-like in structure.

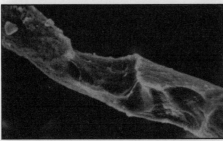

Remodeling Site

Deep bone remodeling cavity that almost penetrates the thin trabecula

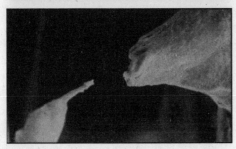

Disconnected Trabecula

Loss of connection

Images: Courtesy of Dr. Lis Mosekilde's family

Tim Gunther, gunthergraphics.biz

SYSTEM CONTROL: THE GOVERNATOR

Remodeling is regulated not only by hormones but also by local factors. A complex series of intricate steps activates the system. The hormones interact with local factors that regulate the repair. The two cell types, osteoclasts and osteoblasts, are functionally coupled. How they communicate with one another was discovered only in the mid-1990s.

Messenger System

Osteoblasts originate from bone marrow mesenchymal stem cells. Osteo-clasts are derived from blood-related stem cells. The development of osteoclasts is based on communication from osteoblasts. The osteoblast sends a messenger to deliver a signal to the osteoclast to grow up and get to work. This regulator of bone cycle has a long, complicated name: receptor-activating nuclear factor kappa B ligand, shortened to RANKL. This intermediary messenger binds to receptor sites on the surface of the immature precursors of osteoclasts called RANK.

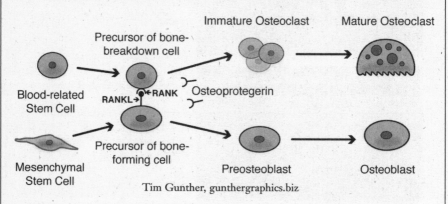

Tim Gunther, gunthergraphics.biz

Another factor called osteoprotegerin (OPG) is secreted by osteoblasts that bind RANKL and prevent it from stimulating the osteoclasts. Therefore, less osteoclast activity and less bone breakdown occurs with more OPG. It is as if the workers on the demolition team get a day off. These two factors produced by the osteoblasts regulate the creation of osteoclasts and their activity.

Identification of this messenger system lead to the development of a novel way to treat osteoporosis. Amgen's drug Prolia® has similar action to the body's own OPG. Prolia binds to RANKL to prevent the birth of new osteoclasts, to decrease the activity of osteoclasts, and to shorten the life span of osteoclasts. As a result, bone breakdown is dramatically decreased with a resulting increase in bone density and lower risk of fractures.

IS THE GUT REALLY IN CONTROL?

New research points to a Wizard of Oz manipulating bone growth from behind the scenes. The switches are controlled by an unlikely source—serotonin. Serotonin transmits signals between nerve cells in the brain but it cannot pass through a barrier to leave the brain.

Serotonin used in other parts of the body is produced mainly in the gut. Scientists at Columbia University found a gene called Lrp5 that regulates the production of serotonin in the gut. They found that bone cells take up serotonin like nerve cells. The serotonin signals bone to slow production of new bone. By turning off production of serotonin in the gut, the team could increase bone formation. In the lab, using mice that were undergoing menopause, the team was able to prevent the usual bone loss associated with menopause.

Stay tuned for more; it is a hot new area of research. Multiple research groups are investigating this approach for treatment of osteoporosis. Since only one medicine is available currently to increase bone formation, new therapies using this pathway to increase bone formation would broaden the choices for treatment of osteoporosis.

The Bare Bones
- Bone is constantly breaking down and building back up in a process called remodeling.
- The bone cells—osteoclasts and osteoblasts—work in concert to remodel the bone.
- When bone breakdown equals bone formation, bones remain strong.
- Bone loss occurs when bone breakdown exceeds formation.
- Women experience acceleration of bone loss at menopause with loss of estrogen.

PART TWO

ASSESSMENT OF BONE HEALTH

General Evaluation:
Visiting with Your Doctor

As an adult, you should be seeing your primary care doctor (that includes family practice, internal medicine, and obstetrics/gynecology doctors) at regular intervals, depending on your age and health. Everyone over the age of fifty should see his or her primary care physician once a year—no exceptions. Everyone under fifty who has a chronic ailment should also be seen at least once a year. Women of childbearing age should see a doctor who performs pelvic exams at least once a year. Everyone under fifty should undergo periodic health screenings at least every three years. Different disease screening and routine health evaluations are indicated at various age milestones. Health recommendations such as exercise or cessation of tobacco use that lower risks of heart disease, diabetes, and obesity, boost your bone health as well.

The performance of a regular history, physical examination, and laboratory will provide an overall assessment of your health. Your doctor may uncover clues that lead to further investigation. In general, bone health and general health measures go hand-in-hand. Evaluation focused on your bone health may include the following:

Height. When was the last time your height was measured? Chances are it has been a while. When asked, most people just give the height that is listed on their driver's license. In contrast, we usually keep track of our weight. However, you should keep track of your height, too.

Your parents may have put marks up along the doorframe when you were growing up. As we grow older, height needs to be followed in the same manner. However, the concern is that your height may be moving in the opposite direction—down. Measurement of your height using a fixed measuring device, like a wall-mounted device called a stadiometer, or by simply standing up against the wall should give an accurate value, but the attachment on the doctor's scale does not.

Compare your measured height with your driver's license height. For women, if you have lost two or more inches, and for men one or more inches, the concern is the possibility of silent, underlying, spine fractures. Height loss may be the subtle clue. To know, you must be measured once a year. Any loss from year to year should be further investigated.

Pills. You may be good about sharing information with your doctor about the prescription medicines you are taking, but what about everything else? What supplements and over-the-counter medicines are you also using? Let your doctor see what you are actually taking. Yes, I mean *see*. Don't just take a list. Bag them up and haul them in.

Some supplements or over-the-counter medicines may be promoting bone loss rather than helping. Go over all of your products with your doctor.

Leg Strength. The quadriceps is the large group of muscles on the front of your thigh. The strength of your quadriceps is an independent risk factor for fracture. These leg muscles are critical for walking, standing up, and sitting down. As we age, they tend to decrease in size and strength. A common way to test leg strength is to stand up from a chair without using your arms.

You can try this at home, too. Sit down in a chair that does not have arms. Put your back up against the back of the chair. Place your hands across your chest. Now, stand up. How did you do? If you had any problems, it is time to work on strengthening the quadriceps muscles.

Blood Test for Vitamin D. Low vitamin D is now a worldwide epidemic. Vitamin D may have many more health benefits than just those related to bone health. If you are not taking a vitamin D supplement, you most likely have low vitamin D blood levels. If you are taking a vitamin D supplement, that is good. However, so many factors influence your vitamin D status that the only way to know if you are taking enough is to have your blood level measured.

Unfortunately, because of the price gouging of laboratories, some regional Medicare carriers have restricted use of this blood test. Your doctor will know if this is a covered test or not. The cost has decreased in many places and ranges from a low of $30 to more than $150 depending on the contracts or the laboratory. If you would need to pay out-of-pocket for this test, find out ahead of time what the cost is so that you can make a careful decision about whether you can afford it. For the moment, in most places in the country, it is still covered.

Fracture Risk Assessment. Reviewing your risk factors for fracture will help determine if it is time for a bone density or DXA scan. To help quantify your risk, a tool called FRAX® is available online or as a smart phone application for your doctor. This assessment was developed by the World Health Organization (WHO) to estimate the ten-year probability of fracture. It was designed for men and women ages forty to ninety who have not received any osteoporosis medicines. The calculation uses clinical risk factors and bone density from a region of your hip (femoral neck). If a bone density scan has not been done, height and weight can be used as a substitute for bone density to estimate probability of fractures.

The US Preventive Services Task Force suggests using a tool like FRAX to help decide whether or not to screen with a bone density test in women under the age of sixty-five. It is recommended that all women sixty-five and older get a bone density test. Likewise, younger postmenopausal women at higher risk for fracture should also get a bone density scan.

MORE RISK FACTORS = HIGHER RISK OF FRACTURE

The risk of fracture increases as your risk factors accumulate. Here's an example using the FRAX tool to assess fracture risk using height and weight. Karen, at age sixty, is 5-foot-6 inches tall and weighs 140 pounds. Three risk factors are used for the example: parental hip fracture, rheumatoid arthritis, and previous fracture. Her ten-year probability of major fracture for different risk factors present is calculated using height and weight. The model calculates probability using body mass index (BMI) if bone density is not entered. The more risk factors she has, the greater the risk of major osteoporotic fractures.

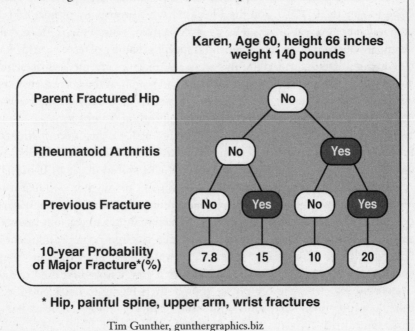

Karen, Age 60, height 66 inches weight 140 pounds

Parent Fractured Hip	No
Rheumatoid Arthritis	No / Yes
Previous Fracture	No / Yes / No / Yes
10-year Probability of Major Fracture*(%)	7.8 / 15 / 10 / 20

* Hip, painful spine, upper arm, wrist fractures

Tim Gunther, gunthergraphics.biz

In my opinion, these guidelines do not go far enough. Any perimenopausal or postmenopausal woman with risk factors and any man over the age of fifty with risk factors should have a bone density test. Why? Because research tells us that more than half of fractures occur in women and men who have low bone mass or osteopenia. On the other hand, if you are early postmenopausal and have no risk factors, a diagnosis of osteopenia may be associated with a low risk of fracture. The lower the bone density and the more risk factors present, the higher the probability of fractures. Early identification makes a difference in lowering the risk of future fracture. If you don't measure it, you may not be managing your bone health appropriately.

Your doctor does the FRAX calculation for you. Also, some of the new bone density machines have the software for FRAX and if one of these machines is used, it will be part of your bone density report. If you are Internet savvy, you can find the FRAX tool online by typing FRAX in the Google search box. The best use of FRAX is *after* you have had a bone density scan. Its use is indicated for those with low bone density who are not on medicines for osteoporosis or taking estrogen.

If a bone density DXA scan is ordered, an additional test on the same machine may be available to evaluate for spine fractures. This scan is called a vertebral fracture assessment (VFA). It is another tool that helps to assess fracture risk. If any silent spine fracture is identified, the risk of more fractures is high.

Fracture risk assessment may include a bone density scan (DXA), a scan of the spine for fractures (VFA), and the FRAX ten-year probability of fracture score. If your assessment reveals that you have low bone mass, a further look for contributing factors should be undertaken. There is no specified battery of tests; instead, your history and risk factors will guide this work-up. Doctors are medical detectives; we gather clues that lead us down various paths in search of the correct answers. The evaluation for low bone density and osteoporosis has to be individualized. Some tests may be done on most everyone; others will depend on your history.

One test I will mention that most experts agree is helpful in patients diagnosed with osteoporosis is a urine collection for twenty-four hours. Yes, an entire day. Every drop of urine is collected and stored in a jug. It needs to be refrigerated, so pick a convenient day when you can stay home. The urine may be measured for calcium, creatinine, and sodium. Sodium content will alert your doctor if your diet is too high in salt, which contributes to calcium loss. If your calcium is high, you may be taking too much calcium or your kidneys may be leaking calcium. Use of some diuretics or water pills called thiazides may help decrease the loss of calcium. If your calcium is low, a low vitamin D blood level or celiac disease may be the cause. Your body is trying to hang on to as much calcium as possible. The twenty-four-hour urine collection can be an inconvenience but it provides valuable information.

The Bare Bones

Evaluation of your bone health at your annual doctor's visit may include:

- Height measurement
- Review of prescription medicines, supplements, and over-the-counter medicines
- Quadriceps strength testing
- Vitamin D blood test
- Fracture risk assessment

Bone Density Scan: DXA 101

The field of bone health made a giant leap forward with the development of bone mass measurement devices. A standard x-ray can confirm the diagnosis of a fracture. However, an x-ray can only begin to detect low bone density after an estimated 30 percent loss of bone mass. Therefore, more sensitive devices have been developed.

The current best noninvasive test for bone mass measurement is dual-energy x-ray absorptiometry (DXA), commonly referred to as a bone density scan. It is a simple and painless test that uses low doses of radiation.

The amount of bone mass measured is called bone mineral density (BMD). Because minerals contribute to bone strength, bone mineral density serves as an important indicator for risk of a fracture. An estimated 60 to 80 percent of bone strength is related to bone mineral density. Lower bone mineral density predicts a higher risk of fractures; conversely, improvement in bone mineral density reduces the risk of fractures.

The best predictor for a specific fracture is to measure bone density at that skeletal site. Typically, bone density scans are done of the hip and the lower back (lumbar) region of the spine, which are sites of major osteoporotic fractures. The diagnosis of osteoporosis is based on results from the hip and spine, and in some circumstances, the forearm also may be used. Bone loss at the hip and spine may occur at different rates. Changes in bone density can be assessed with repeat scans, usually at intervals of two years or, if indicated, at shorter intervals.

WHAT DOES DXA MEAN?

The term DXA is short for dual-energy x-ray absorptiometry. The full name is descriptive of the technique. The dual-energy x-ray part of the name accounts for the use of two different energy levels of x-ray. Absorptiometry refers to the radiation passing through the various body tissues that have different patterns of absorption. The differences in the two beams of radiation that pass through your body's tissues allow the bone measurement to be subtracted from the surrounding tissues. The result is a calculated measure of bone mineral density quantified in grams per square centimeter (g/cm^2).

The DXA system that measures your hip and spine consists of a table, a radiation source usually beneath the table, a radiation detector above the table, and a computer. The DXA measures the lower area of the spine (lumbar spine, first to fourth levels) and hip (femur). The regions of the hip that are scanned and reported on vary a bit between scanners of different manufacturers.

The manufacturers of DXA machines most widely used in the United States are General Electric (GE) Healthcare and Hologic. A small number of Norland machines are also in use.

Many of these machines are also able to scan other parts of the body including the forearm and the whole body. The whole body scan also provides information on body composition, such as percent fat and lean muscle mass. Some scanners can provide a vertebral fracture assessment, which is a picture of the upper and lower spine that is used to discover silent spine fractures.

The amount of radiation exposure is extremely small and equivalent to about an hour-long flight on a jet airplane. The x-ray is a small beam that is focused on the table and does not scatter beyond it. Therefore, the technologist performing the test can stay in the room adjacent to the table. The test is safe and each site measured only takes a few minutes to complete.

Smaller portable units are used to scan the forearm, heel, shin (tibia), or finger. These may be useful in predicting fracture risk, but they are not used for diagnosis (except at the forearm).

HOW DO YOU KNOW IF YOU NEED A DXA?

Bone density scans are done in women near to menopause (perimenopause) or after menopause and in older men. In general, premenopausal women, with a few exceptions, do not need to be tested. However, a premenopausal woman may need a bone density scan if she is taking certain medicines such as steroids, has certain conditions such as celiac disease or an eating disorder, or is being evaluated for recurrent fractures.

If you are perimenopausal or postmenopausal, you should discuss with your doctor whether a DXA is an appropriate test for you. Men fifty and older should have the same discussion. The timing of your initial test depends on the presence of risk factors for osteoporosis and fractures. Recommendations for testing include:

1. *Screening.* If you do not have any known risk factors, a screening DXA is recommended at age sixty-five for women and at age seventy for men.

Similar to screening mammograms or colonoscopies, you get tested to check for the presence of a disease in the absence of symptoms. However, since most fractures occur in women with low bone mass, these screening recommendations may not go far enough in identifying women at higher risk for fracture. An earlier DXA following menopause may be helpful in establishing your baseline. Men have higher bone mass to start with and slower bone loss; therefore, the age for screening is set higher.

2. *At Risk.* If you do have risk factors for osteoporosis and fractures, a DXA test should be done earlier than age sixty-five for women and seventy for men. The goal is early identification and interventions to prevent fractures.

WHEN TO GET A DXA TEST

Screening
- Women age sixty-five and older
- Men age seventy and older

Risk Factors Present
- Women during the menopausal transition with risk factors for fracture
- Postmenopausal women under age sixty-five with risk factors for fracture
- Postmenopausal women discontinuing estrogen therapy
- Men under age seventy with risk factors for fracture
- Adults with a fracture after age fifty
- Adults with a disease or condition associated with low bone mass or bone loss
- Adults taking medicines associated with low bone mass or bone loss
- Anyone considering prescription medicines for treatment of osteoporosis
- Anyone being treated for osteoporosis to monitor treatment
- Anyone not receiving therapy in whom evidence of bone loss would lead to treatment

Sources: International Society for Clinical Densitometry and National Osteoporosis Foundation

HOW DO YOU SELECT WHERE YOU HAVE A DXA?

In most cases, you don't have a choice. Your doctor orders the test and you go to the location he uses. Your bone density results are determined by many factors that are in the hands of the center where your bone density is performed. Assurance of quality is important for accurate results.

Attempts at establishing a system for standardization of DXA centers have fallen flat after a pilot program. Unfortunately, no current standardization is in place for DXA tests as there is for other tests such as mammograms. This translates into wide variability in quality. However, technologists who run the DXA tests and physicians who interpret the DXA tests may have certification in bone densitometry. The International Society for Clinical Densitometry (ISCD) provides educational courses and a standardized testing process for clinicians and technologists. Those clinicians who successfully meet knowledge requirements are designated certified clinical technologists (CCD), and technologists are designated as certified bone density technologists (CBDT).

HOW DO YOU PREPARE FOR A DXA?

No special preparation is required. For comfort, you may want to wear pants without a zipper or metal closures. Often you will be asked to change into a patient gown. In the event that you have undergone a test in the radiology department that required oral contrast within two weeks prior to your testing date, you will need to reschedule your DXA. The contrast might not have fully cleared from your system, and this could influence the DXA.

HOW IS THE DXA DONE?

For a central DXA that includes imaging of your hip and spine, you will lie on a flat, padded surface.

Positioning for the hip depends on the DXA machine. Some machines have the capability of imaging both hips simultaneously. You will lie on your back for all machines. One foot or both feet are moved into a positioning device to hold your hip in place at the correct angle.

For the spine scan, you lie still on your back and your legs may be raised on a cushion to flatten your back against the table.

Examples of scans from Hologic and GE Healthcare DXA machines are shown on the following pages.

Bone Density - Hip

Name:	Sex: Female	Height: 60.0 in.
Patient:	Ethnicity: White	Weight: 114.0 lb.
DOB:		Age: 55

Referring Physician:

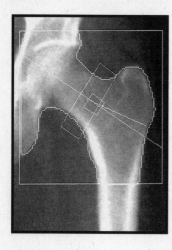

Scan Information:

Scan Date: ID:
Scan Type: f Left Hip
Analysis: Version 11.2
Operator:
Model: Delphi W (S/N 70517)
Comment:

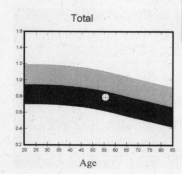

Total

Age

DXA Results Summary:

Region	Area (cm²)	BMC (g)	BMD (g/cm²)	T-Score	Z-Score
Neck	4.96	1.32	0.625	-2.0	-0.9
Troch	10.06	4.04	0.580	-1.2	-0.5
Inter	14.37	2.49	0.984	-0.7	-0.3
Total	**29.39**	**23.08**	**0.785**	**-1.3**	**-0.6**
Ward's	1.16	0.57	0.495	-2.0	-0.3

Total BMD CV 1.0%
WHO Classification: Osteopenia

Physicians Comment:

Reference curve and scores matched to White Female

Source: NHANES
Tim Gunther, gunthergraphics.biz

Hologic

Bone Density - Lumbar Spine

Name:	Sex: Female	Height: 60.0 in.
Patient:	Ethnicity: White	Weight: 114.0 lb.
DOB:		Age: 55

Referring Physician:

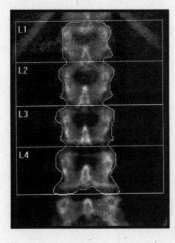

Scan Information:
Scan Date: ID:
Scan Type: f Lumbar Spine
Analysis: Version 11.2
Operator:
Model: Delphi W (S/N 70517)
Comment:

DXA Results Summary:

Region	Area (cm²)	BMC (g)	BMD (g/cm²)	T-Score	Z-Score
L1	10.78	7.84	0.727	-1.8	-0.8
L2	12.39	10.99	0.887	-1.3	-0.2
L3	12.51	11.51	0.920	-1.5	-0.4
L4	15.56	15.54	0.998	-1.1	0.1
Total	**51.25**	**45.88**	**0.895**	**-1.4**	**-0.3**

Total BMD CV 1.0%
WHO Classification: Osteopenia
Fracture Risk: Increased

Physicians Comment:

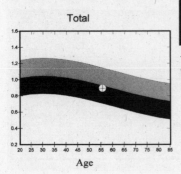

Total

Age

Reference curve and scores matched to White Female

Source: Hologic

Hologic

Tim Gunther, gunthergraphics.biz

Patient: Patient ID:
Birth Date: age 52   Referring Physician:
Height / Weight: Measured:
Sex / Ethnic: Female/White   Analyzed:

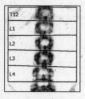

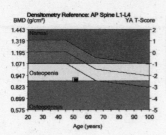

Densitometry Reference: AP Spine L1-L4

Region	BMD g/(cm²)	Young-Adult (%)	T-Score	Age-Matched (%)	Z-Score
L1	0.800	71	-2.8	73	-2.4
L2	0.874	72	-2.8	75	-2.4
L3	1.028	85	-1.5	88	-1.1
L4	0.857	72	-2.8	75	-2.5
L1-L4	0.893	75	-2.4	78	-2.1

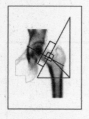

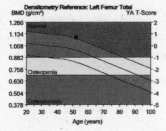

Densitometry Reference: Left Femur Total

Region	BMD g/(cm²)	Young-Adult (%)	T-Score	Age-Matched (%)	Z-Score
Neck	1.003	97	-0.2	107	0.5
Total	1.099	109	0.7	115	1.1

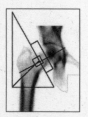

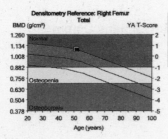

Densitometry Reference: Right Femur Total

Region	BMD g/(cm²)	Young-Adult (%)	T-Score	Age-Matched (%)	Z-Score
Neck	1.019	98	-0.1	109	0.6
Total	1.089	108	0.6	114	1.0

GE Healthcare

Tim Gunther, gunthergraphics.biz

Bone Density - Left forearm

Name:	Sex: Female	Height: 63.0 in.
Patient:	Ethnicity: White	Weight: 124.0 lb.
DOB:		Age: 79

Referring Physician:

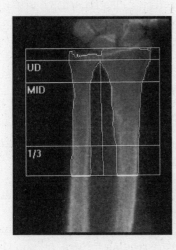

Scan Information:
Scan Date: ID:
Scan Type: a L. Forearm
Analysis: Version 11.2
       Left Forearm
Operator:
Model: Delphi W (S/N 70517)
Comment:

DXA Results Summary:

Results + Ulna	Area (cm²)	BMC (g)	BMD (g/cm²)	T- Score	Z- Score
UD	6.20	1.32	0.213	-3.9	-1.6
MID	11.30	4.04	0.357	-4.4	-1.1
1/3	5.30	2.49	0.471	-3.7	-0.6
Total	**22.80**	**7.85**	**0.344**	**-4.3**	**-1.2**

Total BMD CV 1.0%
WHO Classification: Osteoporosis
Fracture Risk: High

Total (Radius + Ulna)

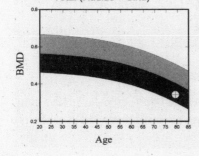

Physicians Comment:

Reference curve and scores matched to White Female

Source: Hologic

Hologic

Tim Gunther, gunthergraphics.biz

WHAT YOU NEED TO KNOW ABOUT YOUR DXA RESULTS

Test results may vary depending on the protocol from the DXA center. The majority of the time, only the report of the DXA is provided to you and your doctor. I encourage both you and your doctor to also get a copy of your complete bone density scan (what some people call "the pictures and the graphics") to review and keep for your records.

As an aside, keeping a copy of all your records, laboratory results, and reports is a good idea. Even with the move to electronic data records, your personal records will help you track your own information. You will have the comparison data readily available. It helps to stay informed and understand the measures of your health status.

If you were sitting down with me, I would systematically guide you through all the parts of the DXA scan printout and report. In this book, I am trying to do the virtual equivalent. And fortunately, we have the luxury of time. Don't expect your busy primary care doctor to do this. You will want to spend your time with him discussing what to do on the basis of the results. If you are not taking osteoporosis medicines, ask your doctor to calculate your FRAX score if it was not done as part of the DXA.

If you have a copy of the actual printout showing the images of your hip and spine, follow along with your papers out in front of you. On the other hand, if you have a summary report, you will find the descriptions helpful in giving you an idea of what the report is talking about. If you are reading for general knowledge, the accompanying pictures will illustrate each step. Examples are given from scans done on GE Healthcare and Hologic DXA machines.

STEP-BY-STEP

Step 1: Look at your identifying information.

Make sure all your demographic information is listed correctly. An inadvertent transposition of a birth date or selection of wrong race will throw off the results. This does happen!

- Your name
- Date of birth
- Age
- Race
- Height
- Weight

Step 2: Look at the image.

The image tells you right away which body site is being reported, hip or lumbar spine, or in some instances, forearm as well.

Hip

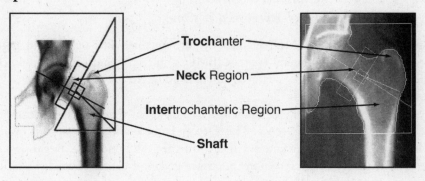

GE Healthcare   **Hologic**

Tim Gunther, gunthergraphics.biz

As shown on the images, the neck region (also known as the femoral neck) is the narrowest part of the hip. Other regions of interest that may be reported include the greater trochanter (troch) and intertrochanteric region (inter) or shaft. Depending on the manufacturer, the total hip is comprised of the neck, trochanter, and intertrochanteric, or shaft areas.

Lumbar Spine

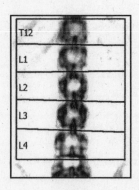
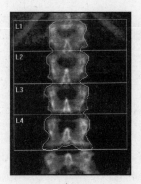

GE Healthcare   **Hologic**

Tim Gunther, gunthergraphics.biz

The first through the fourth lumbar vertebrae are scanned. The abbreviations L1, L2, L3, and L4 are used for each level. The total lumbar spine is referred to as L1–4. If fewer levels are used, the level not used is grayed out. A minimum of two lumbar levels are required for diagnosis.

Step 3: Look at the numbers—BMD and Standardized T-scores and Z-scores

Bone mineral density (BMD) quantifies your bone mass. It is a calculated measurement. The bone mineral content (BMC, a measurement of the amount of calcium) of each region is measured and divided by the area of that region. The resulting number is BMD.

Your BMD results are compared to two different reference populations to derive the T-score and Z-score. The T-score is the comparison of your results with young adults of the same sex at the time of peak bone mass. Regardless of ethnicity, you are compared to the reference group of young Caucasian women ages twenty to thirty. Men are compared to a reference group of young Caucasian adult males.

The Z-score is the comparison with individuals of the same age and ethnicity from a reference database. For example, if you are female, age fifty-five, and Asian, your BMD results for each region are compared to a reference group of fifty-five-year-old Asian women.

The conversion of BMD to standardized scores allows for a systematic assessment of results. The diagnosis of osteoporosis is based on T-scores for postmenopausal women and men age fifty and older. Z-scores are used for assessment of premenopausal women, men under the age of fifty, and children.

The summary data boxes give the numbers for each scanned region.

Region	BMD g/(cm²)	Young-Adult (%)	Young-Adult T-Score	Age-Matched (%)	Age-Matched Z-Score
Neck	1.003	97	-0.2	107	0.5
Total	1.099	109	0.7	115	1.1

GE Healthcare

Region	Area (cm²)	BMC (g)	BMD (g/cm²)	T-Score	Z-Score
Neck	4.96	1.32	0.625	-2.0	-0.9
Troch	10.06	4.04	0.580	-1.2	-0.5
Inter	14.37	2.49	0.984	-0.7	-0.3
Total	**29.39**	**23.08**	**0.785**	**-1.3**	**-0.6**
Ward's	1.16	0.57	0.495	-2.0	-0.3

Hologic

Tim Gunther, gunthergraphics.biz

As shown above, the regions of the hip displayed on the report vary between manufacturers, though all provide neck and total hip scores. For each region listed, look at the numbers one column at a time. On the GE report, the standardized scores follow the BMD column. The T-scores and Z-scores are expressed in two ways: by number and by percentage. The Hologic example provides area, BMC, BMD, T-score, and Z-score for each region of the hip.

Note the area of the hip called Ward's area or Ward's triangle. Many times, it is the lowest score. Ward's area does not have any clinical relevance and should not be used for diagnosis. This area is not included in the total hip. In short, you can ignore this measurement altogether.

Some machines have the capability of scanning both hips at the same time. Each side, left and right, is reported separately. In addition, the average or mean of both hips is given, as well as the difference between hips. The lowest scores are used for diagnosis.

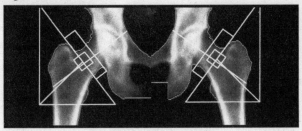

GE Healthcare

Tim Gunther, gunthergraphics.biz

Each level of the lumbar vertebrae is individually measured and scored. The average of L1–L4 or Total is given for all four vertebrae unless one or two levels are excluded.

Region	BMD g/(cm²)	Young-Adult (%)	Young-Adult T-Score	Age-Matched (%)	Age-Matched Z-Score
L1	0.800	71	-2.8	73	-2.4
L2	0.874	72	-2.8	75	-2.4
L3	1.028	85	-1.5	88	-1.1
L4	0.857	72	-2.8	75	-2.5
L1-L4	0.893	75	-2.4	78	-2.1

Region	Area (cm²)	BMC (g)	BMD (g/cm²)	T-Score	Z-Score
L1	10.78	7.84	0.727	-1.8	-0.8
L2	12.39	10.99	0.887	-1.3	-0.2
L3	12.51	11.51	0.920	-1.5	-0.4
L4	15.56	15.54	0.998	-1.1	0.1
Total	51.25	45.88	0.895	-1.4	-0.3

GE Healthcare   **Hologic**

Tim Gunther, gunthergraphics.biz

Step 4: Look at the graph.

Look at the top of the box to see which site is being displayed. These two examples are total hip. On the graph, BMD of the total hip is plotted by age. The reference curves are age-matched; therefore, the dots plotted represent the Z-score. The middle line represents the reference average equivalent to a Z-score of zero. On the GE graph, the upper line represents 1.0 standard deviation above average or a Z-score of 1.0. The lower line represents a Z-score of -1.0. For the GE example shown below, the total hip BMD result of 1.099 is plotted at age fifty-two and marked with a small box. This corresponds to a total hip Z-score of 1.1 and a T-score of 0.7.

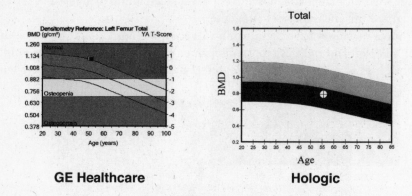

GE Healthcare   **Hologic**

On the Hologic graph, the reference curves are for 2.0 standard deviations above and below average. This printout shows the area between the average line and 2.0 filled in with a light shade and the area between the average line and -2.0 filled in with a darker shade. The symbol used is a plus sign within a circle. For the Hologic example, the total hip BMD of 0.785 is plotted at age fifty-five. This represents a Z-score of -0.6 shown below the average line in the dark shaded area.

Step 5: Look at the DXA report for diagnosis.

The physician who reads the DXA will make a summary report and give a diagnosis. The diagnosis is based on set of criteria that are used universally. The lowest of three sites—femoral neck, total hip, or lumbar spine—is used to make the diagnosis. It is common to have different results at the different sites of measurement. For example, in early menopause, it is common to see the spine lower than the hip. When estrogen levels drop, the spine loses bone faster than the hip.

Sites of Measurement for Diagnosis of Osteoporosis

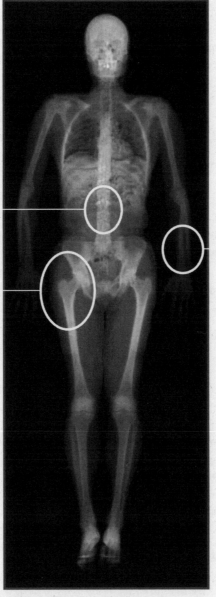

Image courtesy of GE Healthcare

Tim Gunther, gunthergraphics.biz

DIAGNOSIS OF OSTEOPOROSIS

In 1994, the World Health Organization (WHO) established the criteria for diagnosis of osteoporosis based on known fracture levels for white postmenopausal women. The T-score results are used to define the different categories.

Diagnosis	T-score
Normal	-1.0 and higher
Osteopenia or low bone mass	Between -1.0 and -2.5
Osteoporosis	-2.5 and lower
Severe Osteoporosis	-2.5 and lower with fracture

These criteria can only be applied to measurements of the lumbar spine, total hip, or the narrowest region of the hip called the femoral neck. The diagnosis is based on the lowest T-score among these sites. The forearm region called the distal one-third radius may also be used for diagnosis.

If a DXA scan of the hip and spine had the following T-scores,

Femoral Neck   -2.2
Total Hip   -1.8
L1–L4   -2.6

then the diagnosis would be osteoporosis based on the results of the lumbar spine.

In women prior to menopause or men under age fifty, Z-scores are used for diagnosis. A Z-score of -2.0 or lower is defined as "below the expected range for age." A Z-score above -2.0 is "within the expected range for age."

A low Z-Score (level lower than -2.0), at any age, may indicate that some other process or disease may be contributing to low bone density. An evaluation to look for the causes of low bone density may be indicated.

Step 6: Calculate FRAX for fracture risk if you have low bone density.

Some of the newer DXA machines have the software to calculate the FRAX after you have provided information for the risk factors. Otherwise, the FRAX may be calculated online (Google FRAX to find it). It also can be accessed via a dedicated smart phone application. An assessment of risk factors, along with your bone density, will provide a more complete picture of your fracture risk. Talk with your doctor to see if this is an appropriate evaluation for you.

Note: This tool is to be used in individuals with low bone mass who have not received any prescription osteoporosis medicines or estrogen therapy. The reason for this restriction is that the relationship between bone density and fracture risk changes with treatment. A small increase in bone density makes a much larger improvement in fracture risk. The FRAX tool is based on untreated women and men. *This is important.* Do not use it inappropriately; if you do, you will not get the correct information. There is currently no assessment tool for individuals who are already receiving treatment.

How does adding FRAX change your evaluation? Use of T-scores alone does not identify all the individuals at high risk for fracture, since not everyone at the same T-score is alike. Other factors must be taken into account. FRAX is a more comprehensive tool for identifying the individuals who will benefit most from treatment because it quantifies your fracture risk using the combination of risk factors and bone density.

For instance, age is a strong risk factor for fracture. If you are fifty years old and have a T-score of -2.0, your risk of fracture is much lower than the risk faced by an older woman with the same score. This relates to the microstructure or quality of bone. With age, there is more accumulated microstructure loss. Therefore, the quality of bone is poorer, making the bones weaker and more likely to fracture than in a younger person with the same score. The higher risk individual may benefit from prescription therapy even though she doesn't have the diagnosis of osteoporosis. On the other hand, someone at low risk of fractures does not need to go beyond the general measures.

The best way to illustrate this point is with an example.

My college girlfriend Kitty contacted me after having her first DXA scan. Without using FRAX to account for her risk factors, her physician had recommended she start prescription osteoporosis medication based on the results of the DXA scan. She wanted to know if this was the right thing to do. I told her, "Send me your information. After reviewing your bone density results, I will be happy to give you my opinion."

I asked her for a copy of the actual DXA scan. However, she was only able to get a copy of the radiology report, which she forwarded to me. Her findings were as follows:

The lumbar spine (L2–L4) BMD is 0.924 g/cm² with a T score of -1.10 and Z score of -0.76. The hip (femoral neck) BMD is 0.838 g/cm² with a T score of -1.27 and a Z score of 0.04 and the Ward's Triangle BMD score is 0.6398 g/cm² with a T score of -1.69 and a Z score of 0.07.

Based on the World Health Organization (WHO) criteria, her diagnosis is osteopenia, or low bone mass, as it is preferably called. To answer the question of whether Kitty needed to take medication, several other factors had to be taken into consideration. The overall goal is to prevent fractures.

Does Kitty have any risk factors that would contribute to a high risk of fracture? Looking into her personal and family health histories, she has never had a fracture, both of her parents are healthy and active into their late eighties, and her parents have neither experienced fractures nor been diagnosed with osteoporosis. In addition, Kitty has never taken steroids or smoked. She is healthy and has no chronic diseases such as rheumatoid arthritis. She does not take any medications that may be harmful to the bone. She is a social drinker (one or two glasses of wine per week) and she exercises regularly, mixing a gym routine with weights and walking. Her health history shows that she does not have any significant risk factors associated with osteoporosis.

I entered Kitty's information into the FRAX calculation tool for US (Caucasian), which included her weight (130 pounds converted to kilograms by the program), her height (66 inches converted to centimeters), her age (55), her gender (female), and answered "no" for the clinical risk factors of:

Previous fracture
Hip fracture in her mother or father
Current smoking
Steroid use
Rheumatoid arthritis
Secondary osteoporosis (this risk factor is not used in the calculation if
    BMD is entered)
Alcohol three or more units a day (one unit equals 10 ounces of beer, a
    one-ounce shot of liquor, or a four-ounce glass of wine)

Her femoral neck BMD was the last piece of information I entered. Then, I hit the "calculate" button. Note: If you forget to input any of the necessary information, an error message will be displayed.

A bright red box appeared, which showed the ten-year probability of fracture for the categories of major osteoporotic fracture and hip fracture. Four types of fracture comprise the major osteoporotic fracture category: forearm, shoulder, hip, and clinical spine fractures (these are the ones that are associated with symptoms, most commonly pain).

Kitty's ten-year probability of fracture with a femoral neck BMD T-score of -1.27 and no clinical risk factors for major osteoporotic fracture is 5.6 percent; and for hip fracture alone, her ten-year probability is 0.4 percent. Using the FRAX tool, Kitty's calculated ten-year risk of major osteoporotic or hip fractures is quite low.

Although the FRAX tool uses only one skeletal site of measurement, the femoral neck, the lumbar spine measurement should not be ignored. It needs to be taken into account as well. If the BMD at the lumbar spine is lower than at the hip, actual fracture risk may be higher than estimated by the FRAX score. For Kitty, the lumbar spine T-score of -1.10 was similar to the results of her femoral neck T-score.

The National Osteoporosis Foundation's treatment guidelines, which were released in 2008, incorporate the FRAX tool. For a postmenopausal woman with low bone mass (T-score of -1 to -2.5), FDA-approved therapies are recommended if the ten-year fracture probability for hip is 3 percent or greater or the ten-year fracture probability for major osteoporotic fractures is 20 percent or greater.

Based on these treatment recommendations, her lumbar spine BMD, and no other contributing risks, Kitty does not need to take any bone-specific drug at this time. She should continue with her bone-healthy regimen that includes adequate calcium, vitamin D, and exercise. A repeat DXA would be recommended in two to three years.

Armed with the information about risk, Kitty talked with her doctor, who agreed with the new assessment and plan.

Step 7: Make decisions.

Now that you have your T-score and ten-year probability of fracture, what should you do with the information?

Let's look at another example.

Leslie, age fifty-five, is five years postmenopausal and has just had her DXA. She, too, wonders: "Should I be taking a medicine for my bones?"

Because she is adopted, she does not know her family history. She is healthy, has no chronic problems, and takes no prescription medications. She takes a daily calcium supplement that includes vitamin D and a multivitamin for a total of 1,000 mg of supplemental calcium and 1,000 International Units (IUs) of vitamin D. She exercises regularly.

The results of her DXA are:

Region	BMD	T-Score
Left femoral neck	1.003	-0.2
Left hip total	1.009	0.7
Right femoral neck	1.019	-0.1
Right hip total	1.089	0.6
Lumbar spine L1–L4	0.857	-2.8

Leslie has quite different results at the spine and hip. Her spine bone density is much lower than her bone density at the hip. This is called skeletal discordance, which is a common occurrence, particularly in early menopause. Her spine BMD is lower than -2.5. Therefore, her diagnosis is osteoporosis. In addition, she had a lateral vertebral fracture assessment (VFA) that showed no evidence of any fractures.

Since the FRAX model only uses the femoral neck BMD to calculate the ten-year fracture probability, Lisa's fracture probability will be underestimated if the lumbar spine is not taken into account. Since Lisa's diagnosis is osteoporosis, it is not necessary to calculate her FRAX score.

This is one scenario where the fracture risk assessment tool is limited. In early postmenopausal women, because of rapid bone loss at the spine, the spine BMD commonly is lower than the BMD of the hip regions. Just as with any tool, the FRAX model has limitations, so you must consider your entire medical picture.

Lisa's vitamin D levels were reported to her as normal and other evaluations for bone loss did not yield any other factors. Her gynecologist recommended FDA-approved medicine options for her to consider.

TREATMENT GUIDELINES

The National Osteoporosis Foundation's guidelines for treatment using FDA-approved medicines for postmenopausal women and men fifty and over include:

1. History of a hip or spine fracture;
2. Osteoporosis by T-score at the hip or spine; or
3. Low bone mass (T-score of -1.0 to -2.5)
        AND
   ten-year fracture probability (FRAX score)
   for hip fracture of 3 percent or greater OR
   for major osteoporotic fractures of 20 percent or greater

WHAT OTHER DXA EVALUATION MAY BE ORDERED FOR ASSESSMENT OF YOUR BONE HEALTH?

The newer DXA machines are able to scan the upper and lower areas of the spine in order to detect spinal fractures. This test is referred to as a vertebral fracture assessment (VFA). Since the majority of spine fractures are silent, identification of a fracture through this imaging would change your risk profile. The VFA information combined with results of your DXA, plus the evaluation of risk factors, will provide a comprehensive picture of your overall risk.

If you have the test done on a Hologic machine, their scan is called instant vertebral assessment (IVA). The GE Healthcare machine refers to their test as dual-energy vertebral assessment (DVA).

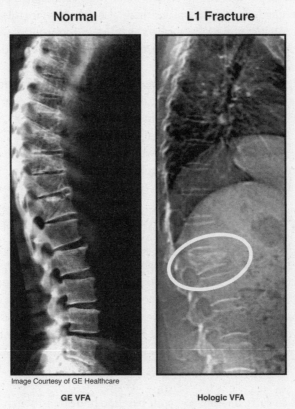

Normal **L1 Fracture**

Image Courtesy of GE Healthcare

GE VFA **Hologic VFA**

Tim Gunther, gunthergraphics.biz

In the example with fracture of the first lumbar vertebra, this level would also be seen on the regular DXA spine scan. If the fracture were located in the thoracic spine, then vertebral fracture assessment would identify the spine fracture that the lumbar DXA would have missed.

POSSIBLE LIMITATIONS OF THE LUMBAR SPINE DXA

The lumbar spine DXA may give results for bone mineral density that appear to be good numbers but actually are not. Particularly with aging, degenerative changes may occur that distort the vertebral bodies. A good example of this would be arthritis, which shows up as higher bone density, giving a misleading reading. Calcifications in other places may also falsely increase density results. For example, calcification in the aorta, which lies just in front of the spine, would do this. A fracture of one of the lumbar vertebrae, if not excluded, would also show up as a denser bone when, in fact, it is not.

If underlying problems are identified, one or two of the four levels of lumbar vertebrae that are scanned can be omitted from the analysis, but a minimum of two levels are necessary for a valid evaluation. In some situations, the spine bone density results may not be useful because the changes take place in three or all four of the vertebral bodies (L1-L4), which necessitates reliance on the hip site only. In addition, the nondominant forearm can be scanned as an alternative site to the lumbar spine.

WHAT DXA SCANS DON'T TELL YOU

Bone density results from a DXA are two-dimensional and do not adjust for bone size. However, bone size matters. If you have a small frame, your bone density tends to be lower than the bone density of someone taller with a larger frame.

Bone mineral density is a static measure. For your first bone density, it is not known how you arrived at your present level. Did you start out with much better bone and then lose bone to get to your present point, or have you had low bone density for quite a while? You may have started with less than optimal peak bone mass.

If you are in early menopause, your baseline bone density may look great but your bone turnover may be high, putting you at risk for fast bone loss. The baseline scan tells your past history, but it does not give any information about the current rate of loss. The rate of bone loss is an independent risk factor for fracture.

Bone quality or microstructure is not evaluated. Two individuals with the same bone density may not have the same fracture risk. If one is age fifty-five and the other is seventy-five, the older person has a much greater risk. This is where fracture assessment is helpful, since bone density DXA scans provide no direct measurement of bone quality.

Nevertheless, DXA is the best test for assessing bone density. Newer technologies with increased capabilities are under development that will go beyond quantifying bone density and will examine the quality of the microstructure. These newer technologies will expand and improve the capabilities of bone mass assessment.

<u>The Bare Bones</u>

- The bone density scan called DXA is the best current test for assessing bone mineral density.
- Bone mineral density predicts fracture risk.
- Diagnosis of osteoporosis is based on measurement of the spine, hip, or forearm.
- The FRAX tool incorporates results of the hip (femoral neck region) bone density with your personal risk factors to calculate your ten-year fracture probability.
- Results of DXA plus fracture risk assessment assist in making better intervention decisions than would be made using DXA alone.

Other Measurements: The Alphabet Soup of Imaging

Bone mineral density assessed by DXA scan is the current gold standard of bone mass measurement; however, DXA does not directly measure bone structure and strength. In fact, the majority of people who sustain a fracture do not have a diagnosis of osteoporosis by DXA. There is considerable overlap in bone density between individuals with and without fractures. Bone density measurements do not identify the changes in bone microstructure that influence true fracture risk. In addition, small improvement in bone density with bone-specific treatment does not explain the large decreases that occur in fracture risk.

I do not want to overemphasize the negatives of DXA, since it is a good measurement tool. However, I am using the limitations of measuring bone density by DXA to point out the factors for development of other imaging tools. Research has focused on determining factors beyond bone density that affect bone strength and fracture risk.

The ideal bone quality measure has so far eluded researchers. Until recently, bone biopsy was the only way to look at bone microstructure. The biopsy procedure involves the removal of a small sample of bone from your pelvis. New methods of bone imaging are being investigated that provide a look at bone's intricate structure without relying on biopsy. The perfect imaging would differentiate type of bone (dense cortical bone versus spongy trabecular bone), provide three-dimensional geometry, and measure properties of bone that could predict how much loading force will likely cause fractures.

QUS: Quantitative Ultrasound

If you are of childbearing age, the mention of ultrasound probably makes you think of the first pictures of your child. If you are older, ultrasound might mean getting a glimpse of your gallbladder or liver. Quantitative ultrasound (QUS) estimates bone mineral density.

No radiation is used. Instead, a pulse of high frequency sound waves is directed across the bone. The speed of sound is used to estimate bone mineral density. In normal, well-connected bone, sound travels through the bone at high speed. Osteoporotic bone with larger spaces and gaps shows a slower speed of transmission across the bone.

Small portable units are designed to make measurements at the heel, shin, or fingers. The heel ultrasound is the only validated device in the United States. The sound waves it generates are unable to penetrate the spine or the hip to make accurate measurements. However, the heel (calcaneus) is similar to the spine in composition, as both are primarily composed of spongy trabecular bone.

Ultrasound machines are attractive because they are small, portable, relatively inexpensive, and do not use radiation. They are used at health fairs, in doctors' offices, and in pharmacies. Ultrasound may be used for screening at-risk individuals, but it *cannot be used to diagnose osteoporosis or to monitor response to therapy*; however, ultrasound is predictive of fractures in women and men. If DXA imaging is available, it is a more precise way to quantify your bone density.

There was considerable interest in the new ultrasound devices when they were introduced in the 1990s. It was hoped that ultrasound would measure actual bone quality, which is something different from bone density alone. I was part of the ultrasound research boom and had the opportunity to test out the finger ultrasound device manufactured by an Italian company and approved in Europe but not in the United States. Now, many years later, the interest has waned, and the ultrasound has taken a backseat role in the United States.

The exciting diagnostic advances in CAT scan (CT) and magnetic resonance imaging (MRI) are now in the driver's seat of new imaging for bone structure.

QCT: Quantitative Computed Tomography

Total body CTs have become a popular test in some parts of the country. In San Diego, three centers offering whole body CTs are doing a booming business. Usually a bone density is thrown into the package deal. I am referring here to cash-pay, elective whole body tests that are heavily advertised.

The CT bone density consists of the measurement of the first or second lumbar vertebra. In most clinical settings, the test is done using single-energy mode, which does not distinguish between increased bone marrow fat and decreased bone. In addition, results are based on the diagnostic criteria for DXA scans. From my experience, the majority of people are told they have osteoporosis, when in fact they don't. This is the result of a misapplication of the DXA T-scores. The standardized T-score by QCT is about one standard deviation lower than the T-score from a DXA scan. Therefore, the same criteria for diagnosis *cannot* be applied to the QCT.

Many times the results of the CT scan then lead to the ordering of a DXA scan. So much for the wise use of your healthcare dollars! If you have a whole body CT, with the bone density provided along with your heart calcium scores, just be aware that the interpretation of the results may be incorrect.

On the other hand, QCT densitometry of the spine, properly evaluated, can be used to predict fracture and monitor therapy, although the amount of radiation is significantly higher than the exposure with DXA. CT devices tend to be used more in Europe than in the United States. The CT scans of the forearm (called pQCT) are common in Europe.

Research Tools: High Resolution MRI and QCT

The advances in computer technology are also reflected in imaging. Just like we have high definition (HD) television, the CT and MRI scanners have progressed to high resolution. If you have had the opportunity to watch a movie using Blu-ray technology, which offers an unprecedented HD experience, seeing the vibrant, new images of bone is similar. The detail is amazing! It is like having a noninvasive bone biopsy.

High resolution imaging by QCT or MRI provides a better visualization of structure. Measurements of the microstructure can be taken in much the same way as those of a bone biopsy. So far, the devices are developed for use at the wrist and sites on the leg, but not the sites of major fracture, the hip, and the spine.

FEA: Finite Element Analysis

Engineers using QCT images have modeled bone structure as a collection of finite elements. The models compute strength and can estimate other structural performances just like they would do for bridge construction. Use of FEA may prove to be able to assess fracture risk and predict if you can survive a fall without a fracture. The examination of biomechanical risk of fracture for clinical use should be available in the near future.

Newer imaging techniques that go beyond the DXA scan and can provide doctors with novel information on bone structure are exciting. These technologies hold great promise for predicting fracture, assessing response to treatment, and giving an accurate picture of bone quality. With data from clinical trials becoming available in the coming years, these advanced technologies are anticipated to become common clinical tools for assessment and monitoring of bone health. For now, though, the DXA scan is the best measurement device available for assessment of bone health.

The Bare Bones

- Heel ultrasound is a portable device useful for screening risk of fracture, but it cannot be used for the diagnosis of osteoporosis.
- QCT of the spine has the same ability as DXA to predict fracture risk, but T-score criteria used in DXA cannot be applied to diagnose osteoporosis on QCTs.
- Research using high-resolution MRI and QCT of the wrist and sites in the leg provide information about bone microstructure.
- A modeling technique using results of bone density can predict mechanical failure of the bone that would result in fracture.
- An array of new ways to look at bone are under development.

Bone Turnover Markers: Dynamic Assessment

Osteoporosis is diagnosed based on an assessment of bone density. However, the results only provide a past history rather than a snapshot of what is happening today. It is much like a house remodeling project. You can't judge what activity is going to happen on the job site today by looking at the building. You can only measure progress in the work completed so far.

The bone cells—osteoclasts and osteoblasts—are constantly remodeling bone. The speed of their activity is called bone turnover. To see how fast or slow they are working, markers of bone turnover can be measured in the urine or blood. There are bone turnover markers that measure osteoclast function (bone breakdown) and different markers that measure osteoblasts function (bone formation).

Bone turnover markers do not establish a diagnosis; rather, they reflect the activity of bone remodeling. High marker levels predict bone loss and fracture risk. A high level of a turnover marker indicates a risk of fracture similar to that of a bone density score in the osteoporosis range (T-score lower than -2.5). Therapies that slow down bone breakdown make these marker levels decrease. Medicines that stimulate bone formation do the opposite.

Low bone density in the hip and high levels of markers of bone breakdown together are more predictive of fracture than either measure alone. Bone markers used in combination with bone density may be helpful to provide an overall picture of your bone health status. For example, at the menopausal transition and into early menopause, bone loss is accelerated with the loss of estrogen. Markers may be useful in the prediction of bone loss at menopause and may help in making a decision about whether to take preventive medicines or not.

However, these markers have not been used widely. They are more likely to be checked if you see a specialist. Most of the time, the reason you are seeing a specialist is for an in-depth investigation of your bone status. High levels of these markers indicate that additional assessment is needed to find any underlying causes of the high bone turnover.

Some doctors are promoting the use of bone turnover markers for assessing the risk of side effects from certain medicines used to treat osteoporosis. However, there is no convincing data showing a link between levels of bone turnover and occurrence of side effects. For instance, in the case of jaw problems related to the use of some bone medicines, individuals who develop the problem may not have extremely low bone turnover or so-called oversuppression.

Markers may be helpful in monitoring therapy. In contrast to waiting two years to get a follow-up bone density scan or, if indicated, one year, the differences in markers are almost immediate. For most medicines, the markers show the maximal level of effect from the prescribed treatment within three months of beginning treatment. For someone who may be at risk for fast bone loss, such as with high-dose steroid therapy, markers may help in evaluating the effect of osteoporosis medicines in counteracting the bone loss much sooner than a follow-up bone density scan. The failure of bone marker values to respond appropriately means that further evaluation is needed to find out if the medicine is not working and, if it is not working, why.

After long-term treatment with bisphosphonate medicines like Fosamax®, sometimes treatment is temporarily stopped. Bone turnover continues to be decreased for some years after stopping the medicine with a slow increase of markers. Therefore, the markers may help decide when to restart therapy. Once the bone turnover markers increase toward a pretreatment level, therapy should be restarted, if indicated.

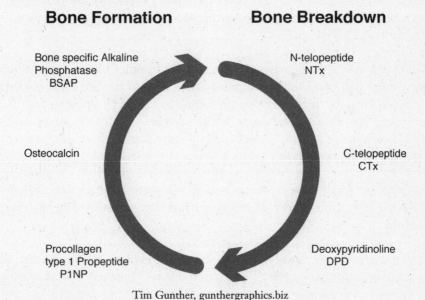

Tim Gunther, gunthergraphics.biz

MARKERS OF BONE BREAKDOWN

Bone tissue resembles reinforced concrete. The osteoclasts drill a hole into the hard concrete tissue, which is a hard bone matrix that is made up of inflexible calcium and phosphate minerals. It is reinforced by flexible fibers of collagen, a protein substance that plays a role similar to steel rebar. Fragments of collagen are released during bone breakdown.

The markers of bone breakdown measure parts of these collagen fragments in the urine or blood. The tests that your doctor might order include N-telopeptide (NTx), C-telopeptide (CTx), or deoxypyridinoline (DPD). You may be asked to collect a urine specimen in the morning the second time you urinate while still fasting. This urine sample gives a snapshot of the bone turnover during the time of highest activity. The analysis can also be done on a full day's collection of urine (twenty-four-hour urine) or a blood sample.

MARKERS OF BONE FORMATION

Bone is formed by the osteoblasts. The bone formation markers are the direct or indirect products of this type of bone cell. Some of these products are enzymes or other proteins that are secreted by osteoblasts. Others are byproducts of new collagen being deposited. All bone formation markers are measured from a blood sample. The ones most commonly measured are bone-specific alkaline phosphatase (BSAP), osteocalcin, and procollagen type 1 propeptides, referred to as P1NP.

Alkaline phosphatase is an enzyme that originates in other tissues in addition to bone. About half of total alkaline phosphatase is from the bone and the other half is produced by the liver. Measurement of alkaline phosphatase is part of your liver function tests on routine laboratory chemistries. A separate analysis called bone-specific alkaline phosphatase differentiates the bone-origin enzyme from the liver-origin enzyme.

Osteocalcin is a small protein synthesized by osteoblasts. Osteocalcin correlates with bone formation. However, the exact function of osteocalcin in bone is unknown.

P1NP is a measure of newly formed collagen in the bone. P1NP is a sensitive marker of bone formation rate. This test is the bone formation marker of choice when evaluating response to treatment.

Bone remodeling activity does not occur at the same rate throughout the day or from day to day. The workers need some down time. Levels of bone turnover markers are highest in the early morning and lowest in the afternoon and evening. Levels of urinary markers can vary 20 to 30 percent from the highest to the lowest values of the day. The challenge to checking these markers is the inherent biologic variability of activity of the osteoclasts and osteoblasts. The markers of bone formation appear to vary less from day to day than they do during any one day.

The Bare Bones

- Markers of bone turnover indicate the activity of bone remodeling.
- Higher levels are associated with faster bone loss.
- Markers are independent predictors of fracture risk and are useful in combination with bone density for assessment of fracture risk.
- Bone markers may be helpful in monitoring response to treatment sooner (within three months) than bone density (usually two years).

Monitoring with Follow-Up DXAs: NOT One and Done

When should you get another DXA scan after your first one? There are no cut and dried recommendations because the decision needs to be individualized. A lot depends on your expected rate of change.

In general, if you started an osteoporosis medicine, a follow-up bone density is recommended after two years of therapy. The improvement with treatment is expected to increase bone density, particularly at the lumbar spine site where the greatest changes are observed. These changes will exceed the small variability of the DXA machine.

Because most osteoporosis medications are so effective, there is some debate about whether a follow-up bone density is even needed after starting medication. However, I believe that it is important to know whether you are responding with favorable bone density changes or stable bone density instead of bone density loss.

If no treatment is indicated after your first DXA scan, the follow-up is dependent on the results of your first DXA and the expected change. For example, if you are early menopausal, the rate of change may be rapid, from two to five percent a year, on average. If your baseline DXA is in the normal range, you will not be losing bone at a rate significant enough to make a difference in your fracture risk. The follow-up period could be three or four years.

On the other hand, if you start out with a lower measured baseline DXA, you have less to lose. The same rate of bone loss from a smaller total amount of bone could make a difference and place you in a higher risk category. The follow-up period should be shorter and a follow-up scan would be appropriate in two years.

Also, all other risks need to be factored in. Are you taking a medicine that accelerates bone loss like aromatase inhibitors or steroids? If so, your physician may want to obtain bone density tests at one-year intervals to monitor the effects of an FDA-approved osteoporosis drug or to closely follow your bone density if you are not on medicine for your bones.

Your insurance coverage may have a say in the answer as well. Medicare coverage is set for two years. Most commercial insurers are in line with Medicare coverage. For a shorter interval, your doctor may need to file an appeal to get approval for the test.

Bottom line, there is no set answer. The follow-up interval depends on many factors. Talk with your doctor about the appropriate time to have your next DXA scan.

SAME PLACE, SAME MACHINE

Repeating your DXA scan is like using a scale to weigh yourself. You always try to use the same scale at the same time of day to monitor change. To know if there is a change in bone density, you need to use the same device. However, other factors may come into play:

- Your insurance coverage or health plan changes.
- You move to a different community.
- The DXA center is no longer in business.
- The DXA machine may be upgraded to a new machine or replaced with a different manufacturer's machine.
- Your doctor sends you to a different DXA center within the same system.

These barriers are not insurmountable. In the case of upgrade to new equipment from the same manufacturer, most centers do a special evaluation in order to have the new machine calibrated with the old one. Whenever possible, try to go to the same place for a repeat DXA, even if a new clinic location is more convenient.

If the same exact machine is not used, you *cannot make a direct comparison* and certainly cannot calculate the rate of change. Each manufacturer has proprietary acquisition of data and software. Even the region of interest may vary. For instance, measurement of the neck region of the hip is derived differently by each manufacturer. There are also differences in the placement of the femoral neck box, detection of the bone, and method of dual-energy production.

Nevertheless, if on the same day you had a hip scan on two different manufacturers' machines, each one would yield similar results. However, you cannot compare change in bone density over time with different machines.

DO NOT COMPARE T-SCORES

The most common error in interpreting results is comparing T-scores to monitor change. The correct approach is to monitor the absolute change in bone mineral density expressed as g/cm^2. The physician who reads your DXA should look at the absolute change in BMD. The change is usually calculated for the lumbar spine and the total hip. If both hips are scanned (dual femur), sometimes the "mean" (or average) of both hips is used. Measurement of the small area of the neck region of the hip (femoral neck) is not as precise, so calculation of change usually is not based on the neck region.

Is this a significant change? The interpretation is based on the variability of the individual machine. Did your change exceed the variability of the machine, which is called the least significant change or LSC? The report should indicate if your measured change is "statistically significant" based on exceeding the LSC. If your bone density change is statistically significant, it means that a biologic change happened that is not by chance and is real. Unfortunately, the calculation of the LSC by DXA centers is commonly not performed. Therefore, a center that has not calculated this value cannot accurately tell if your bone density differences are real.

GAIN, LOSS, OR NO CHANGE?

Although everyone wants to see a big increase in his or her bone density, don't be discouraged if your bone density is stable. The response to therapy is defined as either no change (stable bone density) or a significant increase. Since loss is expected without treatment, no change is *good*. Small changes are usually not significant. This is also good because it means that your bone mass is stable. Here are several examples:

Increase in BMD

The total hip BMD increased significantly after two years of therapy.

DXA Results Summary:

Scan Date	Age	BMD (g/cm²)	T-Score	BMD Change vs Baseline	vs Previous
09/08/2010	56	0.908	-0.3	3.9%*	3.9%*
08/11/2008	54	0.874	-0.6		

* Denotes significant change at the 95% confidence level, LSC is 0.010 g/cm²

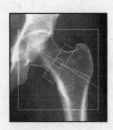
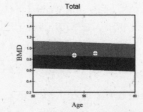

Reference curve and scores matched to White Female

Hologic

Tim Gunther, gunthergraphics.biz

Stable BMD

In both of these examples, the bone density is stable. The hip example uses the mean (or average) of both total hips, which shows a small increase that is not statistically different from the baseline scan.

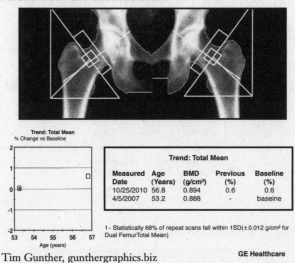

Trend: Total Mean
% Change vs Baseline

Trend: Total Mean				
Measured Date	Age (Years)	BMD (g/cm²)	Previous (%)	Baseline (%)
10/25/2010	56.8	0.894	0.6	0.6
4/5/2007	53.2	0.888	-	baseine

1 - Statistically 68% of repeat scans fall within 1SD(± 0.012 g/cm² for Dual FemurTotal Mean)

Tim Gunther, gunthergraphics.biz

GE Healthcare

The example of the lumbar spine shows a lower BMD. However, this is *not* statistically significant (the decrease of 0.014 g/cm² did not exceed the variability of the machine, which is 0.018 g/cm²). Although the number is lower, it is not actually different.

DXA Results Summary:

Scan Date	Age	BMD (g/cm²)	T-Score	BMD Change vs Baseline	vs Previous
09/08/2010	56	0.884	-1.5	-1.6%	-1.6%
08/11/2008	54	0.898	-1.4		

* Denotes significant change at the 95% confidence level, LSC is 0.018 g/cm²

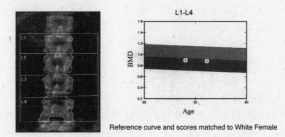

Reference curve and scores matched to White Female

Tim Gunther, gunthergraphics.biz

Hologic

Decrease

This hip example has two follow-up scans. On the first follow-up a significant decrease (0.077 g/cm² or 10.8 percent loss) was observed over about three years. With treatment, a one-year follow-up showed stable bone density, no change.

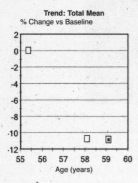

Trend: Total Mean

Measured Date	Age (Years)	BMD (g/cm²)	Previous (%)	Baseline (%)
3/4/2011	59.1	0.637	-0.1	-10.9*
3/4/2010	58.1	0.638	-10.8*	-10.8*
6/8/2007	55.3	0.715	-	baseline

* - Indicates significant change based on 95% confidence interval
1 - Statistically 68% of repeat scans fall within 1SD(± 0.012 g/cm² for Dual FemurTotal Mean)

GE Healthcare

If a significant loss occurs while on therapy, a further evaluation should be conducted to look for previously unrecognized problems. Something new that was not present initially may have occurred to cause bone loss. You should also review with your doctor that you are properly taking your prescribed medicines.

If you are not taking medicines and have significant bone loss, your risk of fracture increases. Higher levels of bone turnover increase risk of fracture independent of bone density. If losses exceed expected age-related changes, an evaluation should be done to look for other causes beyond age. If you are not taking osteoporosis medicine, a reassessment of risk using FRAX should also be done.

DYNAMIC USE OF FRAX

FRAX helps determine the risk of fracture if you have low bone density with a T-score between -1.0 and -2.5 and have not taken osteoporosis medicines. The more risk factors, the greater the risk. For example, Karen had her first DXA at age sixty. On her two-year follow-up, her bone density was stable but her risk factors had dramatically changed.

At age sixty, Karen had low bone density. The lowest T-score of -2.1 was at the femoral neck region. Using FRAX, she had no positive responses for any of the risk factors. Her ten-year probability of major osteoporotic fractures was 9.4 percent and for hip fracture it was 1.4 percent. Her only medicine was a blood pressure pill. Otherwise, she had no other problems. She focused on exercise, calcium, and vitamin D, then returned for a two-year follow-up DXA.

The good news: her bone density was stable. The bad news: her eighty-six-year-old mother had fallen and fractured her hip. Although her bone density did not change, *her probability of fracture doubled* as a result of her parent sustaining a hip fracture. Her ten-year probability of major osteoporotic fractures had increased to 20 percent. A parent breaking a hip becomes a *very strong predictor* of future fracture.

The Bare Bones

- If you begin an osteoporosis medicine, a follow-up DXA is recommended in two years.
- If you are not on treatment, the follow-up DXA is dependent on the results of your first DXA and the expected change.
- Try to have your follow-up DXA on the same machine in order for a valid comparison.
- The actual change in bone mineral density (g/cm^2) is used for monitoring, *not* the T-score.
- No change or increase in bone mineral density represents a decrease in fracture risk.
- Beyond bone density, changes in your risk factor profile may also change your risk of fracture.

PART THREE

GENERAL MEASURES
FOR BONE HEALTH

Exercise: On Your Mark, Get Set, GO!

Regular exercise is your best solution for finding the Fountain of Youth. After all, age is just a number. Is eighty the new seventy? By the looks of people I see working out, it may be. Aging is inevitable, but exercise can stem or delay physical changes by the "use it or lose it" principle.

The late Dr. Fred Kasch, Professor Emeritus at San Diego State University and founder of the Adult Fitness Clinic, now known as SDSU's Center for Optimal Health and Performance, is my all-time fitness hero. A pioneer in the fitness field and a regular exerciser long before there were health clubs, Dr. Kasch jogged into his nineties. Pull-ups, to gauge his upper body strength, were part of his daily routine. He did them on a bar he had hung from a tree branch. He never used anything too fancy to perform his exercises. One of the first internationally recognized exercise physiologists, he was a pioneer, a man ahead of his time.

Dr. Kasch piloted a fitness research study of middle-aged men, following them for more than thirty-five years. Dr. Kasch found that physical declines that occur with aging and that were considered "inevitable" could be slowed with regular physical activity. The positive effects on various physiologic and musculoskeletal parameters were seen in the men who engaged in exercise programs of moderate or vigorous intensity. Important changes to the body seemed to begin at ninety minutes a week and continued up to three hundred minutes a week. The participants engaged in a variety of physical activities.

Dr. Kasch used to say, "There are many ways to Rome." In other words, many different exercise regimens will achieve the same goal of physical conditioning. You just need to do one!

Following Dr. Kasch's sage advice, what you will find in this chapter are general principles for exercise that will enhance your bone health. Use this information to individualize your own program. It is impossible to prescribe something for you without knowledge of your starting level and a personal assessment. If you are already a regular exerciser, it is time to review your activities and make changes. You may be actually losing ground because your body gets habituated to the same exercise routine. Bone likes a variety of stimuli, so you must mix it up.

BUILD: Optimize Bone Growth (Children to Young Adults)

Depending on your age, you may remember taking a physical fitness test in grade school. I will never forget it! A classmate caught the back of my sneaker during the run and I ended up sprawled on a cinder track. I still have cinders tattooed on my right knee to remind me of that day. That memorable test, which consisted of a variety of exercises, including pull-ups, sit-ups, a shuttle run, and a six-hundred-yard run, challenged kids to be physically fit. Time has not changed those goals. Exercise early in life provides lasting benefits by establishing lifelong habits of physical activity. Start early and never stop.

"Let's Move!"

First Lady Michelle Obama has promoted her "Let's Move!" initiative for raising a healthier generation of children. It addresses all the various factors of childhood obesity, an epidemic fed by fast food, sugary drinks, too much television and computer time, too many computer games, and too little exercise.

One disease that has not been mentioned in Mrs. Obama's public health message is osteoporosis. Here's the connection: It takes movement to stimulate the mesenchymal stem cells in the bone marrow to create osteoblasts, the bone-forming cells. Inactivity creates *fat cells* instead! Movement directs the stem cells to operate in the correct way. The fate of these stem cells depends on it. Here is another compelling but often-overlooked reason to move!

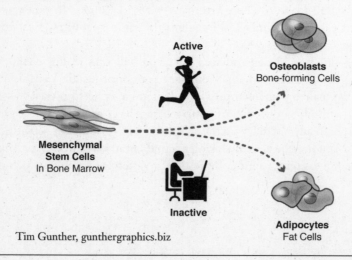

Tim Gunther, gunthergraphics.biz

Exercise can play an important role in building bone. Young bones respond better to exercise than adult bones, and impact exercise appears to produce the greatest bone mass. Weight-bearing exercises are the most effective. Therefore, running and jumping activities like volleyball, gymnastics, soccer, and basketball provide more impact and bone building than swimming or bicycling. Both impact and resistance exercises have been shown to increase bone mass by 3 to 5 percent and to alter bone geometry in girls and boys before adolescence.

Mechanical Strain

The "use it or lose it" principle of bone physiology is referred to as Wolff's Law. Bone microstructure is compromised by disuse and enhanced by exercise. One can find examples of this at either end of the spectrum. On the one hand, someone on bed rest will quickly lose bone along with muscle. This is the same phenomenon experienced by astronauts in space without the forces of gravity. On the other hand, a professional tennis player's racquet arm often has higher bone mass and larger muscles than his nonplaying arm.

The bone cells—osteocytes, osteoblasts, and osteoclasts—respond to physical signals. In response to increased mechanical load during exercise, the balance of bone turnover favors bone formation through increasing numbers and activity of bone-forming cells, called osteoblasts. This increases the strength of bone by adding new bone to resist the loading challenge. The mechanical signaling also influences the mesenchymal stem cells to make bone-forming cells instead of fat cells.

In the absence of mechanical strain, the bone-breakdown cells' activity is increased while formation of new osteoblasts is decreased.

Identifying the optimal amount of mechanical loading to create the right amount of strain has been the objective of many research studies. Too much loading will lead to bone failure—fracture. Too little loading accentuates bone breakdown. Like medicine that has a "therapeutic window," exercise has a "mechanical window." Animal data suggest that high strain followed by rest, rather than continuous strain, may be the most beneficial exercise pattern for bone formation.

The exercises that have high strain magnitude are bone building. Examples would be jumping for the lower body and racquet sports for the upper body, and repetitive activities such as running. Interval training that consists of repetitive bursts of high intensity work alternated with periods of rest or lower activity may enhance the bone effects of running. Any physical activities incorporating increased muscle activity may be beneficial. The best window of opportunity to maximize bone mass is during the preteen to teen years.

Jump at the Bell

Short interventions using jumping show the greatest gain in bone. Simple exercise like a daily jumping program of less than three minutes classroom time, using various jumping styles, makes a difference. The jumps create a strain environment that is defined by short bursts of high impact.

In a school program, students who participated in a ten-minute circuit of varied jumping activities three times per week over seven months gained more bone than those students who did not participate. Girls in early puberty at the start of the jumping intervention program enjoyed the biggest benefit. Other high impact jumping programs compared with healthy controls show greater gain in hip and spine bone mass in prepuberty.

Lesson from Racquet Players

The effect of age at which exercise is started during growing years was shown elegantly in a study of sixty-four former nationally ranked female racquet sports players. These adult women were divided into two groups according to the age at which they started playing tennis or squash. About half began before the start of their menstrual periods, while the other group started one year or more after beginning menstruation. The players were compared with peers who did not exercise and were the same age, height, and weight.

The three groups—"young starters," "old starters," and "controls,"—were evaluated with bone mass measurements of both arms. The results of the middle shaft of the upper arm (humerus) were the most striking and are illustrated to show the differences. The darker lines depict the side-to-side differences (see diagram on p. 105). Young starters had more than twice as large a difference in outer cortex of the bone than the old starters (20 percent versus 9 percent).

The older bone adapts to stress by increasing the amount of tissue lining the inner cavity of the bone. The young starters showed the best results for bone density and other measures of bone strength. This is because younger bone is more adaptable to stress than older bone.

Note that the age of "old starters" is not really old. Preteen bone may be the most responsive to exercise strain. This finding is consistent in multiple studies, suggesting that intense training can boost bone mass accrual beyond that associated with normal growth. The timing is critical, since these benefits are observed only in the preteen years.

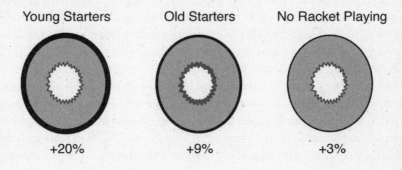

Women Racket Players
A comparison of middle of upper arm
Side to side difference of serving vs non-serving arm

Young Starters	Old Starters	No Racket Playing
+20%	+9%	+3%

Source: Kontulainen S et al. *Journal of Bone and Mineral Research*. 2002; 17:2281–2289. Adapted from figure 3.

Play an Hour a Day

Children and teens should perform sixty minutes or more of moderate-to-vigorous physical activity daily. The activity can be structured or unstructured as a part of play. As children grow up, their patterns of physical activity change. They transition into more organized sports and games and are able to sustain longer periods of physical activity. In addition to team sports, it is good to encourage a variety of activities that kids can carry into their adult lives.

But are children getting enough daily activity?

Dr. Philip Nader, a pediatrician at the University of California, San Diego, followed approximately one thousand kids wearing a device that kept track of the minutes of their moderate-to-vigorous activity. Kids at age nine did well, averaging about three hours a day. But by age fifteen, they averaged only fifty minutes a day during the week and barely more than thirty minutes a day on weekends! For a gender comparison: Girls crossed below the recommended sixty minutes per day at thirteen, boys at fourteen. The negative activities for bone health add up for this age group—not enough exercise, calcium, or vitamin D. As children grow older, parents need to encourage sustained and structured activity.

College and Young Adults

Leaving home for college is a huge transition. The challenge is to continue the healthy habits started earlier. Temptations abound and you have to adjust to different foods, schedules, and activities. The "Freshman 15" for me was twenty pounds! By the end of freshman year, I could not fit into any of the clothes I took to college. I bought two pairs of jeans to hold me over until summer when more sensible eating and exercise restarted—under my mother's watchful eye, I should add.

Whether physically active kids maintain their higher bone mass into their twenties is not well studied. Could I have blown my good bone health in just one year at college? The University of Saskatchewan's Pediatric Bone Mineral Accrual Study follow-up suggests that the skeletal benefits accrued by physically active children are maintained into young adulthood. Children who participated in this study returned as young adults (ages twenty-three to thirty). Comparison of the active to the inactive group showed bone mineral content at multiple sites was 8 to 15 percent higher for those in the active group.

Information is not available on whether intense physical activity in growing years, followed by reduced though not entirely stopped activity, decreases the risk of fractures later in life. Nevertheless, regular physical activity provides considerable health-related benefits throughout life.

PROTECT AND CORRECT:
Maintain Bone and Counteract Bone Loss (Adults)

Preserving bone and muscle health is a challenge with increasing age. Adults can benefit from exercise as well, but it may not be reflected in bone density changes. Studies show that the decline in bone density that happens during aging can be slowed with regular physical activity. To have a significant impact on bone density, the exercise must be of a high enough intensity to promote mechanical strain. In addition, the frequency and duration of the activity play a role. Based on accumulated evidence for all types of health outcomes, at least thirty to sixty minutes of moderate-intensity exercise on most days of the week are recommended for adults.

If you are already active and meet the minimum requirements of 150 minutes every week, turn it up a notch. You can gain additional and more extensive health and fitness benefits by increasing physical activity above this amount.

Physically active people have a lower risk of hip fracture than do inactive people. Leisure time activities like gardening and household work count, too. Research studies on physical activity to prevent hip fracture show that participating in 120 to 300 minutes a week of moderate-intensity activity reduces risk.

Walking

Walking is the most common physical activity, and it confers a multitude of benefits. Walking decreases risk of hip fractures. In the Nurses' Health Study, women who did no other exercise but walked for at least four hours a week had a 41 percent lower risk of hip fractures. However, walking may increase risk of wrist fractures due to falls. Walking exercises alone appear to be insufficient for positive effects at the spine.

As part of the Tasmania Older Adult Cohort Study, men and women aged fifty to eighty used pedometers and had their bone density measured by DXA. After an average of two and a half years, positive bone density effects were seen primarily at the hip. The strongest effect was for people over the age of sixty-five. The mean number of steps in the study was about 8,500 per day and 59,500 per week. That equals approximately 3.3 miles a day and 23 miles a week.

Walk Your Way to Fitness: 10,000 Steps a Day

Grab a pedometer and get going. Your goal is to walk 10,000 steps a day. Pick up the pace. Walking ten minutes at an energetic clip equals about 1,000 steps. The point is this: Everything you do is a form of physical activity. But unless you have an active job and are constantly moving throughout the day, you may not accumulate that many steps. You may have to add some dedicated walking time to reach 10,000 steps. If you are falling just short of your daily goal, you can walk in place while you watch television.

Here's a sample log:

15 steps:	Woke up, clipped on my pedometer, and headed to the bathroom
253 steps:	Got ready for work
350 steps:	Walked from my car to my office building
228 steps:	Went to a meeting and back, via bathroom
3,651 steps:	Took a half-hour walk on my lunch break
58 steps:	Walked down the hall to another office
232 steps:	Returned to my desk, via bathroom
425 steps:	Walked to a meeting and back
250 steps:	Visited coffee kiosk for mid-afternoon boost
152 steps:	Bathroom break
335 steps:	Walked back to my car in the parking lot

675 steps:	Walked through the grocery store to pick up dinner
288 steps:	At home to cook dinner
3,020 steps:	Dragged husband out for a 30-minute, after dinner walk to log steps
215 steps:	At home to get ready for bed

Here Are Some General Guidelines:

Exercise more days than not. Make an entry in your daily calendar for your exercise time—just as you would for scheduling a meeting or a date.

Vary your routine. Do a combination of cardiovascular exercises, stretching, weight training, and resistance work with cutting-edge tools like sport cords, superbands, and the TRX® suspension trainer™. Alternate days of cardio and muscle strengthening or focus on separate muscle groups, such as upper body one day, lower body the next.

Give your muscles a rest. Do two to three sets of eight to twelve repetitions with short rest in between. You should have at least forty-eight hours between workouts focused on the same muscle groups.

Keep challenging muscles. Change up your routine once your muscles become accustomed to the exercise or add more weight. Try different weight training techniques, such as kettlebells. On a treadmill, alternate between the flat level and an incline and use different speeds. When the exercises become "routine," which is usually every six to eight weeks, change again.

Do balance and core exercises. Keep your core muscles engaged to work on improving your balance. Walk heel-to-toe. Balance on one leg. Try a workout sitting on an exercise ball instead of sitting on a bench. This works on your focused muscle group plus balance at the same time. Lift your arm weights while standing on a BOSU® Balance Trainer (a half ball that can be used on either side, the dome or the platform), a core board, or a balance platform.

Postmenopausal women must push themselves even harder. With the loss of hormones, our bodies reset. The extra push is needed not only to decrease bone loss but also to ward off extra pounds. At least an hour a day—*that's sixty minutes of moderate-intensity exercise*—is the prescription.

Your exercise routine should not feel like drudgery. Use of a personal trainer may help to get a program started, to keep you on track, or to provide a "tune-up" for a new routine. Another option is using an accessory such as Wii Fit™. Designed by the video gaming company Nintendo®, it may help make exercise more enjoyable. Wii Fit programs incorporate games or offer just straightforward exercises while using the Wii Balance Board. Have fun!

Bone Estrogen Strength Training (BEST) Study

Change in bone density in adults engaged in an exercise program is difficult to demonstrate in research studies. Because so many factors contribute to bone density, it is difficult to tease out the exercise component. For example, suppose that I am going to recruit you for an exercise study but I don't want you to exercise—your job is to just be a couch potato. Do you think you would change your behavior or not?

One of the most quoted studies, the Bone Estrogen Training Study (BEST), was done in the mid-1990s. More than three hundred healthy postmenopausal women, aged forty to sixty-five, were randomly assigned either to a group that was instructed to exercise or to a group that was told not to exercise. About half were taking hormone therapy and all received 800 mg of calcium supplementation. The exercise intervention was a combination of aerobic, weight bearing, and weight lifting exercises three times a week. Strength training was done using free weights and machines.

After one year, the exercisers who were taking hormone therapy improved bone density at all regions of the hip, lumbar spine, and total body. The exercisers not on hormone therapy had significant bone changes only at the trochanter region of the hip.

BEST Exercise Program for Osteoporosis Prevention:

Six BEST Strength Training Exercises

- Wall squat or Smith squat
- One-arm military press
- Leg press
- Lateral pull-down
- Seated row
- Back extension

You can find BEST demonstration videos to see how these exercises are done at http://www.citracal.com/BEST

You may incorporate these BEST exercises, with cardio activity, balance training, and core strengthening, for example, to create a program for yourself.

REVITALIZE: Function and Prevent Falls (Seniors)

Exercise! It is never too late to start. The goal at this point is not focused on bone density but instead on decreasing risks of falls and fractures. Exercise can improve strength, balance, and mobility. Muscle mass tends to decline with the passing years; strength also declines. "Sarcopenia" is the term for this gradual decrease in muscle tissue. Some of these changes may be slowed with exercise. Also, vitamin D may have a role.

Although mechanical loading increases the bone density and structure in a healthy skeleton, exercise may not be as helpful and may even be risky for someone with a fragile skeleton. This is not meant to dissuade you from exercise. However, I want you to be safe and to protect your spine. With older age and low bone density, your spine may be vulnerable to fracture.

The precaution for exercise is "go slow" and start with professional instruction. Talk with your doctor about a referral to physical therapy for evaluation and training. You may also find resources in the community. Try calling different facilities (YMCA, senior, or community centers) to inquire whether they have a trainer who works with older individuals who have osteoporosis. The evaluation and training must target balance and fall prevention. Most fractures of the hip, shoulder, and wrist, and even some spine fractures are due to falls. Keep your doctor in the loop as well.

LOADS ON YOUR SPINE

Be cautious when you have osteoporosis in your spine or have already sustained a spine fracture. Simple movements of forward bending, such as getting up from a chair, can place a large force on your spine. This puts you at risk for fracture.

Learn proper movements to lessen the loads. If you have ever gone to "back school," the same types of principles apply. You want to maintain a neutral back and avoid bending forward. No abdominal crunches! The following figure shows the tremendous loads that are produced on the lower spine of the eleventh thoracic (T11) and second lumbar (L2) vertebral levels with common movements in comparison with relaxed standing.

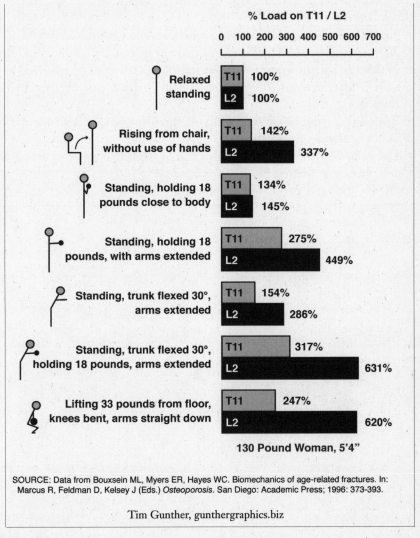

% Load on T11 / L2

Relaxed standing	T11 100%
	L2 100%
Rising from chair, without use of hands	T11 142%
	L2 337%
Standing, holding 18 pounds close to body	T11 134%
	L2 145%
Standing, holding 18 pounds, with arms extended	T11 275%
	L2 449%
Standing, trunk flexed 30°, arms extended	T11 154%
	L2 286%
Standing, trunk flexed 30°, holding 18 pounds, arms extended	T11 317%
	L2 631%
Lifting 33 pounds from floor, knees bent, arms straight down	T11 247%
	L2 620%

130 Pound Woman, 5'4"

SOURCE: Data from Bouxsein ML, Myers ER, Hayes WC. Biomechanics of age-related fractures. In: Marcus R, Feldman D, Kelsey J (Eds.) *Osteoporosis*. San Diego: Academic Press; 1996: 373-393.

Tim Gunther, gunthergraphics.biz

Think through your daily activities and modify them to decrease your chances of a spine fracture. When you are doing your leisure time activities, avoid those with heavier loads. For instance, when gardening, avoid lifting heavy bags of compost or soil. Stand straight, kneel, or sit to avoid forward bending. Ask someone else to tug on those stubborn weeds—doing so can generate a big load. Use a long-handled, lightweight trowel or hoe (do not use a shovel or spade) or use raised planters.

You can get up, strap on your pedometer, and go walk the dog now. Just be careful to avoid getting entangled in the leash or being pulled down!

The Bare Bones

- Young bones respond more to exercise than adult bones.
- Kids need to be physically active at least an hour a day.
- Adults can benefit from exercise as well, but it may not be reflected in bone density changes. Add core muscle and balance training to your routine.
- Brisk walking decreases risk of hip fractures but may increase the risk of falls and wrist fractures.
- Use good body mechanics to lower risk of spine fracture with exercise and physical activities. No forward bending!
- "If you don't use it, you lose it" is true.

Fall Prevention: Fall-Proof Yourself and Your Home

F alls are very common. If you are sixty-five or older, you have a one in three chance of falling this year, and these falls are not innocuous. Your life can change in a second when you fall off a ladder, trip on a sidewalk, or slip on a wet bathroom floor. Falls account for more than half of injury related hospitalizations. One in eight fractures seen in the emergency department is a hip fracture.

As a geriatrician, I see fall prevention as *the* most important factor in fracture prevention. No matter what your bone density may be, if you do not fall, your chance of having a nonspine fracture is small. More than 90 percent of hip fractures are a result of falls. Falling is a strong risk factor for fractures.

Rates of Falls in the US

The rate of falls and the severity of the resulting injuries increase dramatically with age. The highest rate of deaths attributed to falls is in the oldest age group, eighty-five and older. Based on these figures, you can see why persons aged sixty-five and older are targeted for fall prevention.

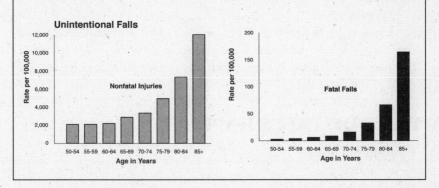

It is extremely important to prevent falls. While it may not be possible to completely prevent them, you certainly can lower the risk. The likelihood of "freak accidents" can be decreased with attention to fall-proofing yourself and your environment. Accidents do happen. My husband, who studied airplane mishaps in detail as a naval aviator, preaches "Situational Awareness." Take your time, don't rush, and keep alert to all your surroundings.

The biggest offender I see every day is cell phone use—walking and talking on your cell phone or, even worse, texting. You can't be alert to your surroundings while walking and using your cell phone. Concentrate on the task of walking. If you get a phone call, *stop* moving before you take the call. *Do not walk and text at the same time.*

Another lesson from airplane mishaps: Accidents occur as a result of a chain of events. If any link in the chain is broken, the accident will not occur. Your job is to lessen your risk of a fall by preventing events that would lead to an accident. Usually, there are modifiable risks in the chain of events leading up to the fall. Falls are not entirely random events.

YOUR STORIES...

Bruce, age seventy-six, was cutting the branches off a neighbor's tree because they were hanging over his side of the fence. He leaned too far to reach a branch and fell off the ladder, landing on his left side and breaking his left hip. He ended up in the intensive care unit because a tear in his spleen caused massive blood loss. Bruce's injuries and the repair of his hip put him in the hospital for two weeks. His full recovery, which allowed him to get back on his surfboard every morning, took an entire year.

Stay off ladders!

Ladders are dangerous. Take them out of your parents' garages so that they won't be tempted. I caught my eighty-plus-year-old father pulling out his ladder to hang Christmas decorations. Add staying off roofs to the list, too.

WHERE DO FALLS HAPPEN?

- Away from home?
- At work?
- On vacation?

Answer: More people are injured at home than anywhere else. Your home is a dangerous place. More fractures are seen during the winter, even in places without snow and ice. This is because most fractures actually occur indoors. Hip fractures are most likely to occur from a fall while standing or walking.

Interestingly, most fractures from falls occur during daylight hours. However, in my experience, nighttime is the most dangerous. Getting up to go to the bathroom during the night can be hazardous to your health.

Turn on the lights!

As you age, you need greater amounts of light. By sixty, you need about three times more light to see clearly than the amount you needed when you were in your twenties. Do not climb the stairs in the dark.

Stairs and steps are probably the most dangerous places in your home. A single step can be just as dangerous as a set of stairs. Always use a handrail. Do not leave objects on the stairs (I am guilty of this—leaving a stack of clothes or some books on the lower steps to take with me on my next trip up.)

Keep yourself safe while you move around your home:

- Get rid of scatter rugs and mats. This is one of my pet peeves. They are huge fall hazards. Toss them out, even the nonskid ones.
- Keep clutter off the floor.
- Immediately wipe up any spills on the floor. Keep an eye out for spills around your pets' water bowls, too.
- Wear well-fitting footgear while you are inside and outside. Get rid of your loose-fitting bathroom slippers and cheap plastic flip flops.

Outside, beware of sidewalks in your neighborhood! Sidewalks are a big hazard. They are often uneven or have cracks, holes, or a dangerous carpet of dead leaves and branches that could make you trip or slip.

BALANCE

Core muscle strength, along with strong thigh (quadriceps) muscles, are the keys to good balance. Even if you are physically fit, these muscle groups are not necessarily being engaged in your workouts. People are always amazed when they try a balance device such as a BOSU trainer and have difficulty. I will use the example of my strapping seventeen-year-old godson. He is a high school football player and the picture of health. I gave him this task: Stand on the BOSU, then squat. He fell over. He could not do it.

Core strength and balance ability are very deceiving. They look easy, but they are not. Add balance exercises to your regimen. Do what is appropriate for your level of function. Research studies show that it takes doing such exerscises three times a week to make a difference. You will know because you will have instant feedback. Your wobbling will improve with practice.

BE PREPARED

Make a plan in case you have a fall. Your homework is to practice getting up from the floor. Wait until you have someone around to help you. Then, go through a practice scenario. Get down on the floor and pretend a fall has happened. If you cannot get back up, discuss what your options are to get help. Make emergency plans. Being prepared will help you stay calm if you ever do fall.

If a Fall Happens...

If a fall cannot be avoided, toss anything you are carrying. Try to fall forward and to roll into the fall. Relax your muscles, if possible.

Once you have had a fall, the chances of another are even greater. Go systematically through the series of events just as though you were trying to find out why an airplane crashed. What can you change to prevent a fall from happening again?

Falls can also have psychological consequences. Fear of falling again and loss of confidence can set up a vicious cycle that leads to even less activity and poorer function. Professional help is needed. What I call "a touch of physical therapy" is not enough. Six to eight sessions with a physical therapist is the starting point. For the therapy to work, it needs to be consistently done week after week.

An evaluation of forty-four exercise research studies for falls with almost ten thousand subjects examined different features of the exercise programs. Three factors were found to be key for fall prevention exercise programs:

1. Balance training
2. "Exercise dose" over fifty hours
3. A walking program was not included

The greatest effects of exercise for reducing falls were obtained from programs that had these three components. The exercise dose of fifty hours was considered the minimum. It is equal to a twice-a-week program, over the course of twenty-five weeks. The third factor may have surprised you. But the risk of falls is greater while walking. However, because of the other benefits of walking, you should not exclude it from your regular exercise routine. The research results point to getting a more intensive program with appropriate medical supervision.

Other studies, not focused on exercise, showed robust decreases in falls when vitamin D is given as a supplement. Vitamin D may help improve your muscle strength. The simple measure of adding this vitamin may make a difference in lowering your risk of falls. The vitamin D level for optimal thigh (quadriceps) strength should be over 30 ng/ml, which is short for nanograms per milliliter. More on this topic is included in the section on vitamin D.

Falls have multiple causes. More than four hundred separate risk factors have been described. Many of them are potentially modifiable. The challenge is to identify the risks and remove them from the chain of events that could lead to a fall and an injury. Any one event taken out of the equation means that the fall will not happen.

The Bare Bones
- Falls are not entirely random events.
- Remove the hazards in your home.
- Light up your home.
- Include balance as part of your regular exercise program.

Nutrition: Take a Bite Out of Your Fracture Risk

The way to keep your health is to eat what you don't want, drink what you don't like, and do what you'd rather not.

—Mark Twain

You are what you eat—and drink. When you focus on nutrition, I want you to think about *both*. But in no way is it as bad as Mark Twain maintained! I promise, I am not going to mandate that you that munch on sardines or dig into tofu, unless, of course, you truly enjoy those foods.

There are no quick fixes, no special diets. Instead, healthy nutrition is a way of life. Eating smart, for your general health and for your bones, means a long-term approach. It is part of your healthy lifestyle. Since the effect of your nutrition is lifelong, evaluating a small slice of time does not provide the whole picture. As a result, differing opinions abound on the subject of dietary enhancement and bone health.

However, the value of calcium and vitamin D for bone health is well established. You will find thorough discussions of calcium and vitamin D in the next two sections.

GENERAL PRINCIPLE OF NUTRITION

As with most things in life, moderation is the key. Too little or too much may be harmful. This "u-shaped" relationship holds for most of nutrition and bone health. I like to refer to it as the *Goldilocks Principle*. You don't want too little or too much, but a "just right" amount. The challenge is knowing what that is.

Tim Gunther, gunthergraphics.biz

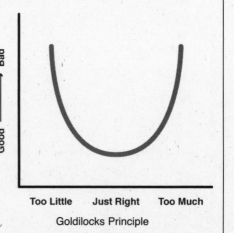

Goldilocks Principle

118

Protein

A steady supply of protein is essential for your bones and all cells in your body. Meat, poultry, fish, eggs, beans, nuts, soy, and dairy products are good sources of protein. You also will find items such as protein bars and protein powders stocked on the shelves of grocery and health food stores.

What kind of protein, and how much, sound like simple questions, but these are the basis of considerable debate. Proteins contain amino acids with sulfur that metabolizes to generate sulfate. The sulfate increases the acidity of the urine and causes greater amounts of calcium to be excreted in it. Both animal and plant sources of protein contribute to calcium loss in the urine. The proteins of plants can have either lower or higher amounts of amino acids containing sulfur than the proteins of animals. Most cereals, nuts, and seeds have higher concentrations than animal foods, while legumes have lower concentrations.

The amount of calcium loss in the urine is proportional to the amount of protein ingested. As the intake of dietary protein increases, the amount of calcium excreted in the urine increases. Also, some calcium is lost in the feces. The Recommended Daily Allowance (RDA) for calcium intake was set to cover the calcium losses associated with protein eaten in the average American diet.

Recent analyses of multiple studies (called meta-analysis) give a summary view of what has been published on this subject. The evidence shows that the effect of dietary protein on the skeleton appears to be favorable to a small extent and not detrimental. Regardless of the source of protein (animal or plant), the key is adequate calcium intake to cover protein-induced calcium losses.

As a geriatrician, I do not worry about too much protein intake; I worry more about deficits. Older individuals tend to decrease the protein in their diets. Cooking for one? Decreased enjoyment in eating? Limited resources? These could all be contributing causes.

Older men and women may benefit from a higher protein intake. Inadequate protein intake is common in patients who suffer a hip fracture. A low protein diet predisposes them to a greater rate of bone and muscle loss. The Framingham Study and the Rancho Bernardo Study both found that the greatest bone loss was associated with the lowest protein intake in older women. In the Rancho Bernardo Study, a high animal protein intake had a protective effect against bone loss. The greatest bone losses occurred in women with the highest vegetable protein intake. In a third study of older women, the Iowa Women's Health Study, those who had the highest animal protein intake had a decreased risk of hip fracture. In patients with a recent hip fracture, protein supplementation reduced the medical complication rate and recovery time.

A decline in caloric intake with age may be the appropriate adjustment for a reduction in energy expenditure. However, a reduction in protein intake may be detrimental for maintaining the integrity and function of bone and muscle. Increasing dietary protein to the normal intake (defined in the box below) is beneficial for bone health. But consider subtracting other foods so that the total number of calories is not increased.

Protein by the Numbers

Recommended Dietary Allowance for Protein

	Grams of protein needed each day	Grams per kilogram a day
Children ages 1 – 3	13	1.1
Children ages 4 – 8	19	0.95
Children ages 9 – 13	34	0.95
Girls ages 14 – 18	46	0.85
Boys ages 14 – 18	52	0.85
Pregnancy & Breastfeeding	71	1.1
Women ages 19 – 70+	46	0.8
Men ages 19 – 70+	56	0.8

The grams per day recommendations are the estimated requirement for a healthy person. To individualize your daily protein requirement use the grams per kilogram per day column and make a couple of calculations:

Step 1—Convert your weight from pounds to kilograms by dividing your weight in pounds by 2.2

Step 2—Multiply your weight in kilograms by the specific grams per kilogram listed in the far right column above according to your age and gender

Example: If you are a woman and weigh 140 pounds,

    Step 1   140 pounds/2.2 = 63.6 kilograms
    Step 2   63.6 kilograms × 0.8 = 50.8

51 grams is your recommended daily amount of protein

Repeat these steps for all members of your family.

SOURCE: Food and Nutrition Board, Institute of Medicine of the National Academies. *Dietary Reference Intakes for Energy, Carbohydrate. Fiber, Fat, Fatty Acids, Cholesterol, Protein, and Amino Acids (2002/2005).* Washington, DC: National Academies Press.

Adequate protein intake during childhood and adolescence is essential to support normal growth and skeletal development. The adolescent years are particularly important for providing adequate nutrition to maximize peak bone mass, though the specific role of protein and protein-diet interactions in the achievement of optimal peak bone mass is not clear.

The available evidence on protein suggests that protein has a biphasic or "U-shaped" effect on bone health. The upper and lower thresholds are not defined. You have to take into account overall diet, calcium intake, health status, and age to determine your individual needs. Dietary protein in the range of usual intakes is beneficial, not harmful, to bone health.

Carbohydrates and Fat

Invoking the Goldilocks Principle: Too little or too many calories and too much fat can negatively impact bone health. Fat is metabolically active, producing inflammation and other factors that may be influencing the bone. Obese children have a greater risk of fractures. And adolescent girls with more abdominal fat have lower measures of microstructure of bone. In other words, they develop poorer quality bone. In the Rancho Bernardo Study, older adults with obesity and high blood sugars had higher bone density at the hip but a higher risk of fracture. On the other end of the spectrum, being malnourished and underweight is also associated with bone loss and higher risk of fracture.

Vitamin ABCs

Vitamins are classified as either water-soluble or fat-soluble. Water-soluble vitamins B and C dissolve in water and are not stored. Instead, the unused amounts are excreted through your urine. Fat-soluble vitamins need dietary fat in order to be absorbed in the small intestines. The fat-soluble vitamins A, D, E, and K are stored in the liver and fat tissues.

Vitamin A

There are two basic types of vitamin A. *Retinol* is from animal products such as oily fish, liver, cheese, and eggs. *Beta-carotene* is found in fruit and vegetables that are orange, including carrots, sweet potato, apricots, and others such as tomatoes and spinach.

In Norway and Sweden, where there are high rates of herring and salmon consumption, researchers made the first association of high dietary intake of vitamin A with reduced bone mineral density and increased risk for hip fracture. Subsequently, other population studies have reported that either high intake of vitamin A or high serum concentration of retinol increased the risk of fracture in both men and women.

The risk of fracture increased with increasing amounts of retinol. Dietary intake of retinol greater than 1.5 mg a day is harmful for bone health. In the Rancho Bernardo Study, intakes slightly above the recommended amounts (seen predominantly in supplement users) were harmful for skeletal health. However, the majority of supplements now contain vitamin A as beta-carotene, which has no link to bone. (Caution to supplement users: beta-carotene supplementation *is* linked to an increased risk of lung cancer in former smokers.)

Vitamin B

B vitamins play an indirect role in bone health. Folate (or folic acid) and vitamins B12 and B6 help regulate homocysteine. High homocysteine levels, which you may have heard about in association with cardiovascular disease, are also associated with a significantly greater risk of fractures in women and men. A diet rich in B vitamins and a standard multivitamin can keep homocysteine levels in the normal range. Foods high in folic acid include green, leafy vegetables, and grain products fortified with folic acid.

Vitamin C

Nobel Prize-winning US chemist Linus Pauling made vitamin C popular, promoting it in the 1980s as a treatment for everything from the common cold to terminal cancer. Vitamin C, which continues to be the most used supplement today, may have a protective effect on bone health. It is essential for collagen formation and normal bone development. When we looked at vitamin C use in the Rancho Bernardo Study, the highest bone density was associated with 1,000 mg of supplemental vitamin C a day in older women. Other studies have shown less bone loss and lower fracture risk at the hip with vitamin C supplements.

Vitamin K

Vitamin K is best known for its role in helping blood clot properly, but it also activates at least three proteins involved in bone health. After observational studies suggested that vitamin K is associated with decreased risk of hip fractures, a flurry of further research resulted.

Vitamin K occurs as either phylloquinone (K1) or menaquinones (K2). The major dietary form of the vitamin is K1, which is found in dark green vegetables such as broccoli, kale, spinach, cabbage, asparagus, and dark green lettuce. (Chlorophyll is the substance in plants that provides both their green color and the vitamin K.) Gut bacteria makes K2 but they do not contribute appreciably to your vitamin K status. Menaquinones can also be found in fermented foods such as cheeses or in natto, a soybean product.

Natto is a popular food in Japan, where studies show decreased hip fracture risk. Also, many of the vitamin K intervention studies are from Japan. Japanese researchers have used menaquinone (MK-4) in doses considered to be medical intervention rather than nutritional supplementation.

Intervention studies using different K vitamins either in doses attainable in your diet or in supernormal doses have yielded conflicting results. Vitamin K1 supplementation in a dose attainable in the diet (500 micrograms) does not appear to confer any additional benefit for bone health at the spine or hip when taken with calcium and vitamin D.

The recommended intake for adult women (90 micrograms a day) and adult men (120 micrograms a day) is based on its function in blood. The amount needed for bone health is not clear. To meet the RDA for vitamin K, one serving of a dark green vegetable a day easily does it—two or three stalks of broccoli are all you need. Anyone taking blood thinners (Coumadin®) needs to be cautious about introducing more vitamin K into his or her diet because vitamin K decreases the effectiveness of Coumadin.

Minerals

Phosphorus

Phosphorus is a mineral essential for normal function of every cell in your body. The majority of your phosphorus is in bone. It makes up bone's major structural component in the form of a calcium phosphate salt called hydroxyapatite.

Phosphorus is a nutritional requirement for healthy bone. The good news is that phosphorus deficiency is rare. Phosphorus is abundant in most common foods, so no supplementation is needed. Phosphorus content of soft drinks has been implicated as a cause of low bone density. However, studies indicate that the displacement of calcium-rich milk is the actual culprit rather than the ingredients of soft drinks. The current RDA for adults is 700 mg and for preteens and teenagers it is 1,250 mg.

Magnesium

Although roughly more than half of the body's magnesium resides in the bone, its function is not entirely known. Magnesium is an important factor for many physiologic functions, especially for the cardiovascular system. Low dietary magnesium has been implicated as a risk factor for osteoporosis. The Framingham Study showed that low dietary magnesium was associated with low bone density. In general, magnesium's role in bone health has been poorly studied.

Magnesium is often combined with vitamin D and calcium as a supplement for bone health, but I have not found any convincing intervention data in the literature to support the use of magnesium as a supplement. In one three-year study, ninety-nine healthy postmenopausal women were randomly assigned to diet instruction alone, calcium and vitamin D supplement, or a multinutrient supplement that consisted of calcium, vitamin D, and assorted micronutrients, including 600 mg of magnesium. The dietary group was instructed to consume at least 800 mg of calcium a day with a goal of 1,450 mg, which was the calcium supplement dose for the two other groups. No differences were observed in bone mineral density at the hip, spine, and whole body at one, two, or three years. The addition of assorted micronutrients that included 600 mg of magnesium conferred no obvious skeletal effect beyond that of calcium and vitamin D alone.

The only individuals who may need supplementation are those with absorption problems such as celiac disease or inflammatory bowel disease; those on water pills such as Lasix® (furosemide), bumetanide, or torsemide; and those with a high daily caffeine intake (caffeine causes excess loss of magnesium in the urine). Supplementation should be discussed with your doctor in these cases.

The bottom line is that you should be getting enough magnesium in your diet. If not, nuts such as almonds and cashews are high in magnesium, as are spinach and soybeans. Three ounces of halibut tops the list of magnesium-containing foods with 90 mg. These are some of the same foods that are also good sources of either calcium or vitamin D. Adult men over thirty require 420 mg of magnesium per day, which is the highest for any age, and 320 mg per day are required for women.

Beverages

Alcohol

"Moderate" intake of alcohol appears to be positive for the bone, and for men and postmenopausal women it is even better than no alcohol consumption at all. More than two glasses of alcohol a day is harmful and is a risk factor for osteoporosis. The mechanisms involved in the benefits of moderate alcohol intake remain unclear and require further study. Beer is described as "good for bones" based on its silicon levels. But the conclusion was not based on an intervention trial, much to the disappointment of beer lovers. The link was based on the Framingham Study, which showed that higher silicon intake was associated with higher bone density.

Teas

As a beverage absent in calories and rich in antioxidants and other bioactive substances, the role of tea in health promotion has gained traction over the last decade. Tea contains large amounts of nutrients called flavonoids, particularly those called catechins. Green and black teas are a rich source of these catechins.

In countries that have large numbers of regular tea drinkers, studies have suggested that tea is good for the bones. In a British study, those who added milk to their tea had even higher bone density. However, not all studies have reported positive results for tea. The large Women's Health Initiative study found that the effect of regular tea drinking on bone density was small and did not alter the risk of fractures among older American women.

In animal observations, the bioactive components in tea seem to increase bone formation and decrease the actions of the osteoclasts. How this applies to humans is not known.

Learn more about soft drinks and coffee in the next section, which deals with calcium's role in bone health.

The Bare Bones

- Consider whole foods for bone and general health benefits instead of individual vitamins and minerals.
- A healthy diet consists of adequate fruits, vegetables, nuts, and protein.
- Protein supports bone as long as you have adequate calcium intake as well.
- Bone "super foods" include almonds, halibut, salmon, green leafy vegetables, and citrus.

Calcium: It Is Essential

Whenever there is mention of bone health or osteoporosis, the response I hear most often is, "Sure, I get my calcium." Almost everyone is clued in to the fact that calcium is essential for bones. However, this perception does not match the reality of what we are actually doing. The problem is that the majority of adults and children are not getting enough calcium each day.

So why are we doing such a poor job meeting our recommended calcium intake? One contributing factor is that many people do not know how much they or their family members need on a daily basis. Even if the target number is known, without a regular routine to ensure daily calcium, an adequate amount is not achieved. It is estimated that the average American diet provides about 600 to 700 mg of calcium a day.

Everyone Is Missing the Mark

Regardless of age, most Americans do not meet the recommended levels of daily calcium. Taking into account both dietary and supplement sources, Americans are falling short across the board. This figure presents national estimates of the percentage of individuals meeting recommended calcium intake from dietary and supplement sources. The data are based on a representative population group.

Overall, boys and men do better than women. However, for both boys and girls, the dramatic decline in calcium intake during the period of greatest bone building is especially troubling. Only 15 percent of girls and 23 percent of boys age nine to thirteen take in an adequate amount of calcium. And only 13 percent of girls fourteen to eighteen meet the requirement, while 42 percent of boys in this age group do. Just at the time of rapid bone growth, the essential building block of calcium is not being supplied in adequate amounts.

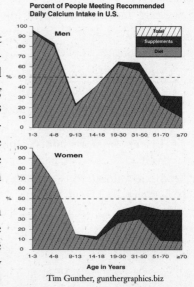

Percent of People Meeting Recommended Daily Calcium Intake in U.S.

Tim Gunther, gunthergraphics.biz

SOURCE: Bailey RL, Dodd KW, Goldman JA. Estimation of total usual calcium and vitamin D intakes in the United States. *The Journal of Nutrition*. 2010; 140:817–22.

DAILY CALCIUM RECOMMENDATIONS

Calcium provides many vital functions. The daily recommendations have been established primarily on the basis of bone health. By meeting the requirements of bone, the needs of other tissues will also be covered. This is because bone serves as a reservoir of calcium that helps to maintain normal blood levels of calcium.

Calcium by the Numbers: How Much Do You Need?

Recommended daily intakes of calcium are from your food, beverages, and supplements combined. If your diet includes the amount of calcium listed for you, no additional supplementation is needed. Pregnant and breastfeeding women should follow the recommendations for their age group.

Daily Recommended Dietary Allowance Calcium Intake		
Age in years	Amount in milligrams (mg/day)	Upper Level Intake (mg/day)
Infants 0 to 6 months	200	1000
Infants 6 to 12 months	260	1500
Children ages 1 to 3	700	2500
Children ages 4 to 8	1000	2500
Children ages 9 to 18	1300	3000
Adults ages 19 to 50	1000	2500
Men ages 51 to 70	1000	2000
Women ages 51 to 70	1200	2000
Adults ages 71 and older	1200	2000

These recommendations factor in the absorption of calcium. Preteens and teens have the highest requirements for calcium even though they also have a higher percentage of calcium absorption. The absorption of calcium also increases during pregnancy and breastfeeding to provide the extra calcium needed for the additional demands of the growing baby. In contrast, calcium absorption decreases with age, so the intake recommendation increases for all adults at age seventy-one and all women after reaching the average age of menopause. Also, keep in mind that adequate vitamin D is needed for optimal calcium absorption.

In the case of calcium, more is not always better. The upper limit of calcium intake is considered the safe upper boundary. Excess calcium ends up in your urine. When you consume too much over a long period, you are at risk for kidney stones and other problems.

SOURCE: Committee to Review Dietary Reference Intakes for Vitamin D and Calcium, Food and Nutrition Board, Institute of Medicine. *Dietary Reference Intakes for Calcium and Vitamin D.* Washington, DC: National Academy Press, 2010.

Calcium-Rich Foods

About three-quarters of calcium in the US diet comes from milk and dairy products. Common nondairy sources of calcium include almonds, beans, small bony fish like sardines, and a few green vegetables. Other foods fortified with calcium can make substantial contributions to your total calcium intake. Bakery products, such as bread, biscuits, and cakes may be made with calcium-fortified flour. Cereals, tofu, rice, and orange juice are other common fortified foods. You need to check labels carefully because not all of these products are fortified and the calcium content varies widely from brand to brand.

People who are lactose intolerant are unable to break down the lactose sugar in the milk and need to look for other sources of calcium. Many who are lactose intolerant are often able to tolerate other dairy products in small quantities. Also, "lactose-free" milk is widely available. Being lactose intolerant does not affect calcium absorption.

Calcium Daily Value Is 1,000 Milligrams

Reading the "Nutrition Facts" on food products requires some translation. The "Percent Daily Value" often shortened to "% DV" is given for the standard nutrients. Some nutrients have both the numerical quantity and the percent daily value specified. For calcium, only the % DV is given. To get the number of milligrams (mg) of calcium in one serving, you need to calculate it from the % DV.

Look at this example:

1% Milkfat Low Fat Milk

Nutrition Facts	Amount/serving	%DV*	Amount/serving	%DV*
Serving Size 1 cup (240ml)	Total Fat 2.5g	4%	Total Carb. 14g	5%
	Sat Fat 1.5g	8%	Fiber 0g	0%
	Trans Fat 0g	0%	Sugars 14g	
Servings about 8	Cholest. 15mg	5%	Protein 11g	21%
Calories 120	Sodium 150mg	6%		
Fat Cal. 20				

* Percent Daily Values (DV) are Vitamin A 10%•Vitamin C 4%•Calcium 35%•Iron 0%•Vitamin D 25%

The calcium daily value is 1,000 mg: a fact you must know because it is not on the label! The Percent DV on the milk label for 1% low fat milk is 35 percent, so you must multiply 1,000 mg times 35 percent to get 350 milligrams for one serving.

You can actually avoid any calculations by simply adding a "0" to the percent:

35 percent + 0 = 350 milligrams

Why don't the labels just specify the milligrams? Fortunately, there is a push to make labels more explicit so that consumers do not need to do any math.

Don't be lured by package claims of "Good Source of Calcium" without checking the exact amount per serving in the "Nutrition Facts" on the back or side of the product. Plus, the attention-grabbing claims that sound healthy may not translate into actually adding many milligrams of calcium to your daily intake because other nutrients in the food might modify the absorption or bioavailability of the calcium.

Also, the same types of food may have many different amounts of calcium depending on the brand. Cereals are a good example. If you pick up a couple of different brands of raisin bran, you will see a difference. When I checked the cereal aisle at the grocery store in early 2011, I found that a one-cup serving of the raisin bran cereals made by Kellogg and Post contain 2 percent of the daily value of calcium or only 20 mg. In contrast, the same one-cup serving size of Total® Raisin Bran contains 100 percent daily value or 1,000 mg of calcium.

Bioavailability

The low calcium content of common plant sources, including most vegetables, fruits, and cereal grains, makes it difficult to meet your calcium requirements exclusively from nondairy foods. Dark green leafy vegetables are presumed to be good sources of calcium. But the bioavailability of the calcium is what actually determines the amount available for absorption. In general, calcium absorption is inversely related to the oxalate content of the food. If oxalate content is high, absorption is low and vice versa.

Oxalates are natural compounds found primarily in plant-based foods. The role of oxalates in plants is not precisely known. Most vegetables have some oxalates. However, kale, broccoli, and bok choy are essentially free of oxalates. In contrast, spinach, beet greens, and chard have high concentrations of oxalates. Sweet potatoes and okra are intermediate. What does this mean? Spinach, although quite nutritious, is not a good source of calcium. Next time your recipe calls for spinach, try substituting kale.

Even though kale, broccoli, and bok choy are good bioavailable sources of calcium, keep in mind that vegetable sources do not have dense calcium content.

"I eat broccoli." That's what people tell me all the time to prove that they are getting plenty of calcium. Good, it is a nutritious food. However, one flow-eret of broccoli provides 5 mg and one stalk provides 15 mg. It takes a lot of broccoli to make a dent in your daily calcium requirements. You cannot just count on broccoli for calcium. It is not enough!

Bioavailable Calcium

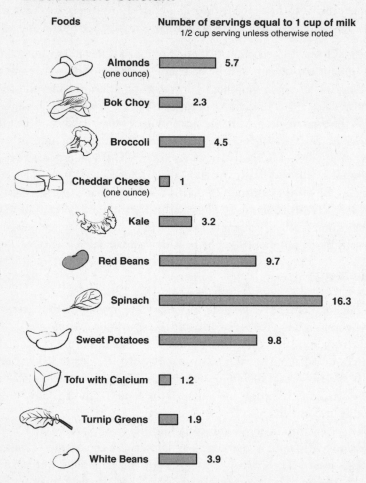

Foods	Number of servings equal to 1 cup of milk
	1/2 cup serving unless otherwise noted
Almonds (one ounce)	5.7
Bok Choy	2.3
Broccoli	4.5
Cheddar Cheese (one ounce)	1
Kale	3.2
Red Beans	9.7
Spinach	16.3
Sweet Potatoes	9.8
Tofu with Calcium	1.2
Turnip Greens	1.9
White Beans	3.9

Source: Weaver CM et al. *The American Journal of Clinical Nutrition*. 1999; 70 (supplement): 543S–548S. Data from table 2.

The calcium salts used to fortify foods usually have the same calcium absorption values as milk. The exception is calcium citrate malate, which is found in fortified drinks like orange juice and fruit punch. Its absorption is slightly higher. Therefore, those drinks are good substitutes for milk, but you need to watch the sugar content and make sure that you find foods containing the other key nutrients found in milk, such as protein and vitamin D.

Unfortunately, calcium added to soy milk is not readily available for absorption. Even if your brand is calcium-fortified, do not count that amount toward your daily requirements: soy drinkers, take note!

CALCIUM FOOD SOURCES

Food	Serving Size	Approximate Calcium Content (milligrams)
Dairy		
Cheeses Mozzarella, Muenster, Provolone, Swiss	1 ounce	200
Cottage cheese, low fat	½ cup	80
Milk, all types	1 cup	300–350
Yogurt, plain nonfat	1 cup	450
Yogurt, flavored	1 cup	300–350
Fish		
Halibut	3 ounces	95
Herring, pickled	3 ounces	65
Perch	3 ounces	69
Salmon, wild, filet	3 ounces	11
Sardines with bones	3 ounces	325
Trout	3 ounces	73
Tuna, canned	3 ounces	12
Vegetables and Legumes		
Bok choy	½ cup	130
Broccoli	½ cup	66
Kale	½ cup	94
Soybeans	½ cup	130
Turnip greens	½ cup	157
Black-eyed peas	½ cup	105
Black beans	½ cup	80
White beans	½ cup	77
Drinks		
Orange juice with calcium	1 cup	350
Orange juice	1 cup	27
Mineral water	1 cup	highly variable

Food	Serving Size	Approximate Calcium Content (milligrams)
Fruits and Nuts		
Almonds	1 ounce (24)	52
Figs, dried	2	62
Orange	1	52
Calcium-Fortified Foods		
Breads, check labels	1 slice	variable
Cereals	¾ to 1 cup	variable plus add milk
Tofu	3 ounces	variable

SOURCE: adapted from USDA National Nutrient Database for Standard Reference, Release 22 and Weaver CM et al. *The American Journal of Clinical Nutrition.* 1999;70(supplement):543S–548S.

Food Fight: Milk

Milk is in the middle of a nutrition battlefield. On one side is the public policy for milk or dairy consumption, which recommends three cups a day; on the other side are anti-milk groups who say that no amount of dairy is safe. Some claim that milk actually causes osteoporosis, which definitely turns conventional wisdom on its head. Research provides the data that *support* the conclusion that milk builds strong bones.

Studies of children with dairy-exclusion diets show lower bone acquisition during growth compared with those who drink milk. The outcomes of dairy-exclusion diets depend on whether other sources of calcium, vitamin D, protein, and other nutrients are replaced in sufficient quantities.

In observational studies, such as the Nurses Health Study, no link was observed between dairy intake and fractures. Other observational studies consistently show that lifetime milk consumption is associated with higher bone density. The majority of intervention studies show that higher amounts of dairy in the diet increase bone density.

Although the science behind milk and bone appears strong, the debate is far from settled. If you choose not to include milk and dairy products, be sure that you get sufficient calcium from other sources.

Caffeine

Although caffeine is regularly reported as harmful, the data are conflicting. Some studies show an increased loss of calcium by the kidney from moderate coffee intake while others studies show no effect. The reason for the differing results may be related to adequate calcium intake, since high caffeine intake is often a marker for low calcium intake.

In the Rancho Bernardo Study, lifetime caffeinated coffee drinking was associated with reduced bone density only when the coffee was not supplemented daily with milk. The negative effect of caffeine on calcium absorption was small enough to be offset by as little as one to two tablespoons of milk. After viewing the results of the Rancho Bernardo Study in 1994, I switched to lattes just to be sure! As with anything else, do not overindulge caffeine.

If you have sufficient calcium, your cup of coffee will not cause excessive losses of calcium. To quote Dr. Robert Heaney, an internationally recognized expert in calcium nutrition and bone biology at Creighton University: "The solution is not to decrease the caffeine intake of the Western world, but to provide adequate sources and intakes of calcium." That is good news for you coffee drinkers!

Soft Drinks

Soft drinks have been linked to lower bone mass. The caffeine and phosphoric acid content were initially thought to be the culprit. Further studies show that the association is due to displacing milk in the diet. Sugar-sweetened beverages including soft drinks have become a staple in the diets of children and teens. These nutrient-poor beverages displace milk just at the time when children and teens begin to have increased calcium needs for growing bones. Soft drinks may also add to weight problems.

Soft drinks are on the "hit" list for schools, and they are a focus of First Lady Michelle Obama's healthy eating for kids initiative. Data from Project EAT (Eating Among Teens) showed that those who consumed little or no milk gained significantly more weight than their peers who consumed milk.

Variations in genetics may also contribute to the association between milk consumption and bone density. A recent study of genes and low milk intake in teenage girls suggests that higher consumption of milk is needed for certain subgroups based on their vitamin D receptor gene type.

Promote the idea of putting on a "milk mustache" of low-fat milk and other low-calorie, nutrient-dense drinks to children and teens. Limit the availability of other beverages, including fruit juices, sport drinks, power drinks, and soft drinks.

Salt

High fat and high sugar foods are not the only culinary culprits for higher disease risk. Though we hear a lot about salt contributing to high blood pressure, heart attacks, and strokes, you may not realize that too much salt also increases calcium loss, which contributes to bone loss and osteoporosis. Sodium competes with calcium for reabsorption because sodium and calcium share the same transport system in the kidney. As a result, sodium minimizes even the effects of some good sources of calcium, such as processed cheeses.

Our table salt is sodium chloride or "NaCl" in chemical shorthand. Sodium is important for many biologic functions in our bodies. We cannot live without it. However, most of us use too much of it, and this pattern of overuse is hard to break because our taste buds have become accustomed to large quantities of salt in our foods.

The problem is not the salt shaker and those few grains you throw over your shoulder for good luck. The problem is the hidden sources of salt. Even though a food may not taste "salty," it may have plenty of salt. You may be good about the salt shaker but you need to be a label reader, too.

Unfortunately, labels have plenty of jargon: sodium-free, very low sodium, low sodium, reduced sodium, unsalted, no salt added, or without added salt. Who came up with these classifications that only make your head spin?

Ignore these labels and just go straight to the "Nutrition Facts." Look at this example from a bag of pretzels.

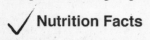

✓ Nutrition Facts

Pretzels

Nutrition Facts	
Serving Size 60g (14 Pretzels)	
Calories 230	
Calories from Fat 15	
	% Daily Value*
Total Fat 0g	0%
Saturated Fat 0g	0%
Cholesterol 0mg	0%
Sodium 1030mg	45%
Total Carbohydrate 50g	15%
Dietary Fiber 2g	8%
Protein 5g	10%

* Percent Daily Values (DV) •
Vitamin A 0% • Vitamin C 0% •
Folate 25% • Calcium 2% • Iron 15% •
Niacin 15%

Tim Gunther, gunthergraphics.biz

At least the "Nutrition Facts" give the amount of sodium in milligrams so that you don't have to do math! The current recommended daily value on nutrition food labels is "less than 2,400 milligrams." Calculations are based on that figure, which is about one teaspoon of salt. However, the report of the Dietary Guidelines for Americans, 2010, estimates that the average daily consumption is 3,400 mg a day for all Americans, ages two and over. The new guidelines reduce daily sodium intake to less than 2,300 mg. For persons who are fifty-one and older, and those of any age who are African American or have hypertension, diabetes, or chronic kidney disease, a further reduction of intake to 1,500 mg is recommended. The 1,500 mg guidelines apply to about half of the US population. About two-thirds of a teaspoon of table salt is equivalent to 1,500 mg of sodium. The highest concentrations of sodium are found in packaged foods, processed meats such as hot dogs and deli meats, canned soups and vegetables, and in many other products. It goes without saying that foods with visible salt are high in sodium—potato chips, corn chips, pretzels, nuts. Though you can get them all unsalted, I agree that without salt potato chips just do not taste the same. Despite the risks involved with overconsumption of sodium, you can eat these foods; just don't make a steady diet of them. The best approach is to substitute another food for the high salt variety. For instance, instead of using salt-laden ready-made rice mix, make your own rice without adding salt to the water.

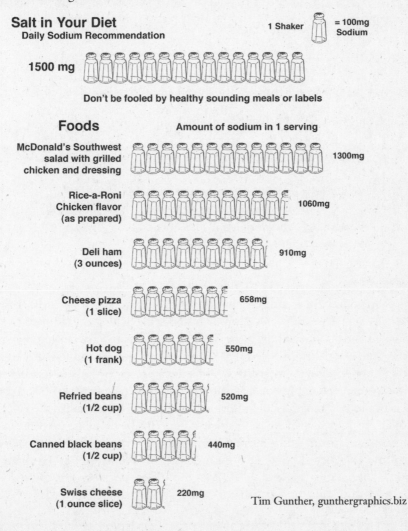

Salt in Your Diet
Daily Sodium Recommendation

1 Shaker = 100mg Sodium

1500 mg

Don't be fooled by healthy sounding meals or labels

Foods

Amount of sodium in 1 serving

Foods	Sodium
McDonald's Southwest salad with grilled chicken and dressing	1300mg
Rice-a-Roni Chicken flavor (as prepared)	1060mg
Deli ham (3 ounces)	910mg
Cheese pizza (1 slice)	658mg
Hot dog (1 frank)	550mg
Refried beans (1/2 cup)	520mg
Canned black beans (1/2 cup)	440mg
Swiss cheese (1 ounce slice)	220mg

Tim Gunther, gunthergraphics.biz

In fact, manufacturers are trying to come up with ways to decrease the salt in their products. For example, in 2010 the Campbell Soup Company decreased the sodium content in its Original V8 100% Vegetable Juice to 420 mg per eight-ounce glass; still too high, but at least it is moving in the right direction. Apparently, salt helps the consistency of certain foods, and food scientists have so far been unable to find acceptable, palatable substitutions.

Tips for Reducing Salt in Your Diet

The majority of sodium in the diet comes from processed or prepared foods. If you cut down on processed foods and use less salt in food preparation, you will be taking the right steps to help achieve the goal of 1,500 mg of salt a day.

- Read nutrition labels for sodium content.
- If you use canned foods, like beans and tuna, rinse them in water first.
- Substitute fresh or frozen vegetables for canned foods.
- Eat fresh poultry, fish, and lean meats instead of processed versions.
- Substitute herbs, spices, lemon, or vinegar for salt on foods.
- Make your own salad dressings.
- Use lemon juice and olive oil on vegetables.
- Try low-salt versions of sauces that are high in sodium, like soy or barbecue, and use in small amounts.
- Buy low-sodium chicken broth or soups.
- Select unsalted nuts and snacks.

When dining out, have your dressings and sauces served on the side. My favorite Chinese restaurant provides nutrition facts about everything on the menu. The sodium contained in some of the dishes is quite high, and that is before you drizzle soy sauce on your plate. Oh, so you're using the soy sauce with the green top or the label "low sodium"—no worries. Unfortunately, even the low-sodium soy sauce has plenty: 460 mg in one tablespoon. Maybe it does not seem so bad compared with the 1,200 mg of sodium for one tablespoon of the regular soy sauce.

Reducing your salt intake is generally a good thing, but don't go overboard. Taking away too much salt can cause problems with your body's water balance. During my residency training at the Emory University School of Medicine in Atlanta, Georgia, the now late Dr. B. Woodfin (Woody) Cobbs, a respected and well-loved cardiologist at the Emory Clinic, would order potato chips STAT (meaning bring immediately) to the bedside of patients who had been overzealous in restricting salt. However, usually it is a problem of too much rather than too little.

Writing about all this salty food is sending me to the cupboard craving something salty. The good news is that as you reduce the salt content in your diet, your taste buds become accustomed to less salt.

Supplements: Making Up the Difference

Dietary sources of calcium should be your primary way to meet your daily recommended intake. During the preteen and teenage growing years it is especially important to get those 1,300 mg a day. Studies suggest that supplemental calcium may not be as effective as calcium from dietary sources for individuals in this age group. If they rely on supplements, they may be missing many of the added benefits for the growing skeleton, such as protein, that other food sources provide.

If calcium supplements are substituted for dairy products to meet children's calcium needs, attention to other nutrients may be needed. Low calcium intake has been associated with low intake of magnesium and several vitamins, including riboflavin, B-6, B-12, and thiamine. Experts are mixed on supplements for kids. If you do use supplements, use the children's brands.

For adults, the sources do not seem to be as important. While diet is the recommended source of calcium, if you are not meeting your daily goals by diet alone, make it up with supplements. You have many options in terms of type and delivery. Tablets are the most common. Many of you do not like taking tablets. The calcium tablets combined with vitamin D are large tablets. Some can be dissolved in water. There are also other choices: soft chews, liquid, and even sprinkles.

Calcium carbonate is generally the most economical calcium supplement. Most calcium supplements should be taken with meals, although calcium citrate and calcium citrate malate can be taken anytime. The downside of calcium citrate is that the pills are larger and contain less calcium.

It is best to divide the dose of supplemental calcium to maximize absorption; take no more than 500 mg at one time.

Your Turn...

Step 1: *Diet*

Keep track of how much calcium you are getting in your diet. Do it daily for a typical week. An easy way is to write down everything you eat. Do not forget that protein bar or mineral water. Put a check next to the items that have some calcium content. To estimate the calcium, read the nutrition labels to determine the calcium based on serving size versus how much you are eating. For nonlabeled items like vegetables, estimate from the calcium food sources table (pages 131–32). Add each day's totals. Take an average of your total week.

Step 2: *Supplements*

Look at all the supplements you are taking. Add up all the calcium. For example, most multivitamins contain a small amount of calcium. Remember: start with identifying the serving size, which is not always one tablet. The number of tablets is the quantity that provides the amounts listed in "Supplement Facts."

Step 3: *Meeting your daily recommended dietary allowance?*

Write down your recommended daily calcium target number (refer to "Calcium By the Numbers"). Subtract your average daily dietary calcium and your average supplement use from the total.

Daily recommended target number _____ Example: 1200 mg

Subtract

Average dietary calcium _____ Example: 400 mg

Subtract

Supplemental calcium _____ Example: 500 mg

Equals

Difference _____ Example: 300 mg

What is your result? How did you do?

If you are at or close to zero, keep doing what you are doing. If you are not, make adjustments for too much or too little. In the example, only 300 mg more is needed. You can boost your dietary calcium by adding foods or make up the deficit with a calcium supplement.

Some ideas for increasing dietary calcium include the following.

Breakfast: Add yogurt to your breakfast routine

Snack: A handful of almonds

Lunch: Cheese on your salad or sandwich

Dinner: Beans or bok choy as a side dish

Step 4: *Check your family's calcium status*

Go back through the first three steps to examine how the rest of your family is doing with getting their daily calcium. Counsel and modify as needed.

Add Up Your Calcium From Diet and Supplements...

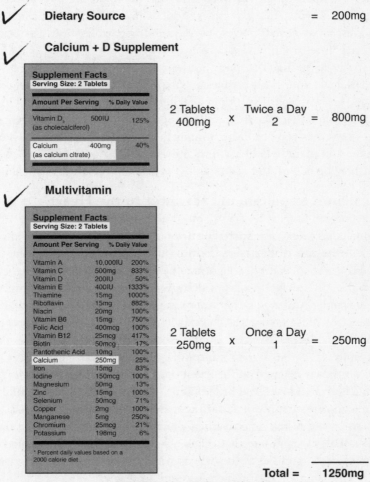

✓ Dietary Source		= 200mg

Calcium + D Supplement

Supplement Facts
Serving Size: 2 Tablets

Amount Per Serving		% Daily Value
Vitamin D₃ (as cholecalciferol)	500IU	125%
Calcium (as calcium citrate)	400mg	40%

$$\begin{array}{c} 2 \text{ Tablets} \\ 400mg \end{array} \times \begin{array}{c} \text{Twice a Day} \\ 2 \end{array} = 800mg$$

Multivitamin

Supplement Facts
Serving Size: 2 Tablets

Amount Per Serving		% Daily Value
Vitamin A	10,000IU	200%
Vitamin C	500mg	833%
Vitamin D	200IU	50%
Vitamin E	400IU	1333%
Thiamine	15mg	1000%
Riboflavin	15mg	882%
Niacin	20mg	100%
Vitamin B6	15mg	750%
Folic Acid	400mcg	100%
Vitamin B12	25mcg	417%
Biotin	50mcg	17%
Pantothenic Acid	10mg	100%
Calcium	250mg	25%
Iron	15mg	83%
Iodine	150mcg	100%
Magnesium	50mg	13%
Zinc	15mg	100%
Selenium	50mcg	71%
Copper	2mg	100%
Manganese	5mg	250%
Chromium	25mcg	21%
Potassium	198mg	6%

* Percent daily values based on a 2000 calorie diet

$$\begin{array}{c} 2 \text{ Tablets} \\ 250mg \end{array} \times \begin{array}{c} \text{Once a Day} \\ 1 \end{array} = 250mg$$

Total = 1250mg

Tim Gunther, gunthergraphics.biz

What If You Have Had Kidney Stones?

Many people with a history of kidney stones avoid calcium supplements. For most people that is not necessary. In fact, studies show that individuals who both use calcium supplements and have a history of kidney stones actually have a lower rate of new kidney stones than those not taking supplements. I recommend using calcium citrate for those of you with a history of kidney stones although definitive evidence is lacking for choosing one type of supplement over another.

The most common type of kidney stone is calcium oxalate. These stones typically form because of dehydration or a diet high in oxalate-containing foods. Therefore, drinking plenty of water every day is important, as is limiting high-oxalate foods in your diet. Examples of foods high in oxalates include spinach, beet leaves, swiss chard, chives, parsley, and vegetables that can be used as grains, such as amaranth and quinoa.

If you have not had one done, a twenty-four-hour urine collection for calcium to evaluate your risk of stones may be helpful. The urine collection is usually done after you have discontinued taking your calcium supplements and have limited your dietary intake to fewer than 800 mg for one to two weeks. The test will show whether you are losing too much calcium in your urine, which could predispose you to more kidney stones. Low dose of a "water pill" called thiazide diuretic may be helpful to lessen the loss of calcium. Talk with your doctor.

Are Calcium Supplements Harmful to the Heart?

A calcium controversy was stirred up again in 2010 concerning calcium supplements and the risk of heart attacks. Results of a meta-analysis done by New Zealand researchers and released online by the *British Medical Journal* created a media buzz and sparked widespread concern. The researchers found that 2.7 percent of subjects taking calcium supplements had heart attacks compared with 2.2 percent of those taking placebo tablets However, the study has been criticized for many design flaws.

In contrast, an Australian study (the Calcium Intake Fracture Outcome Study), which was released online about the same time in the *Journal of Bone and Mineral Research* and received little if any attention, showed no harmful effects. Calcium supplementation of 1,200 mg daily did not increase the risk of heart attacks or strokes in the older women who were followed for almost ten years. A further analysis suggested that calcium supplementation may reduce the risk of hospitalization and death in patients with pre-existing heart disease. More research will be undertaken to investigate this area.

The bottom line is that you should add up calcium from your dietary sources and take just enough calcium supplements to reach your recommended daily amount. For example, if your recommended calcium intake is 1,200 mg and your average dietary calcium intake is 700 mg, you will need 500 mg of calcium supplement, not 1,200 mg. In addition, make sure you are taking sufficient vitamin D. Vitamin D is essential for efficient absorption of calcium.

The Bare Bones
- Calcium recommendations for daily intake are based on your age.
- The richest sources of dietary calcium are dairy products. Kale, broccoli, and bok choy are examples of other bioavailable sources with lower calcium content.
- The interplay of salt and calcium is important for bone health. Limit your daily sodium.
- Increase your dietary calcium or add supplements to meet your daily recommended amount.

Vitamin D: Are You Getting Enough of the Sunshine Vitamin?

Vitamin D and calcium go hand-in-hand for promoting good bone health. While most people are attuned to calcium, vitamin D is another story. You probably know what your cholesterol is, or at least you have had it checked. But do you know what your vitamin D level is?

The majority of Americans have not had their vitamin D level checked. If you are among those who have not, you may have compelling reasons by the end of this chapter to have vitamin D included with your next blood tests. On the other hand, if you have had a recent vitamin D level, have your number handy while reading the chapter.

The evidence for bone health, based on calcium absorption and its skeletal effects, sets 30 ng/ml as the minimum level of vitamin D. I start my lectures on vitamin D with the number 30. Remember: 30 is key to your bone health. That guidance may change in the future, as new research emerges about the influence of vitamin D in other areas beyond bone and muscle health. For now, 30 is the number to keep in mind, and there is a very good chance your vitamin D is below this minimum level.

VITAMIN D BLOOD LEVELS

The barometer for your vitamin D status is a measurement of your blood level of "25-hydroxyvitamin D_3" (also written as "25(OH)D," which is descriptive of its structure). For vitamin D levels, this is what is actually measured in the laboratory, and it is what you may see written on your laboratory results. The "ng/ml" is just the unit of measurement most common in the US. In your reading, you may also come across another unit of measurement: nmol/L. To convert to ng/ml, divide this number by 2.5. (Example: 80 nmol/L ÷ 2.5 = 32 ng/ml)

Just as the cutoff for high cholesterol has changed, the definition of low vitamin D has been a moving target as well. There is controversy and plenty of debate over what is the correct minimum level of vitamin

142

D. In the scientific community, the debate revolves around the minimum level of 20 versus 30 ng/ml. The Institute of Medicine committee that updated the vitamin D dietary reference intakes in 2010 chose the level of 20 ng/ml.

However, other experts who have examined the same evidence conclude that 30 ng/ml is the minimum level based on calcium absorption, bone health, and muscle function. I share this opinion. In addition, what is established as public health policy may not apply to a particular individual's situation.

If identifying the *minimum* level of vitamin D seems difficult, pinpointing the *optimal* level is an even trickier subject. Vitamin D is used by practically every tissue in the body, and it is difficult to know what might work best for one area and what may not be enough for another. The Institute of Medicine committee suggests an upper level of 50 ng/ml. Using "reasonable extrapolations" from the data for maximum reduction of multiple diseases, other experts recommend an optimal vitamin D range of 40 to 60 ng/ml. Considering that the typical American's vitamin D level is quite a bit less than 30 ng/ml, this range is a lofty goal.

Laboratories typically give values between 30 and 70 ng/ml as the normal value range. Don't be alarmed if your laboratory lists different numbers. This variability just demonstrates the problem: lack of standardization of categories. These levels will continue to be a source of debate in the medical community, since more research is needed to fill in the knowledge gaps.

ARE YOU AT RISK FOR LOW VITAMIN D?

Yes, you are, and so is everyone else. Vitamin D deficiency is at epidemic proportions, despite the common use of vitamin D supplements. National data from the National Health and Nutrition Examination Survey (NHANES) show a marked decrease in vitamin D levels since the 1980s. Numerous factors play a role, such as your exposure to sunshine, body size, skin color, where you live, and your age.

In our modern era of healthcare, vitamin D deficiency was previously thought to be primarily a problem for older adults, particularly those confined to home or living in nursing homes. Recently, study after study has shown that low vitamin D is a worldwide problem, regardless of one's location, age, sex, or ethnicity. It is pervasive in the US, even in places with plenty of sunshine. Even among women taking prescription medicines for osteoporosis, who would be expected to have increased awareness of the importance of calcium and vitamin D, more than half in a study of more than 1,500 women from across North America had low vitamin D levels. It is not just a problem in women, but affects men, women, and children alike.

Clearly, what the average American is doing is not enough. Dr. Michael Holick, a leading vitamin D researcher based at Boston University School of Medicine, said, "It is inconceivable with all the advances in modern medicine that vitamin D deficiency should be a health concern in the United States."

ABC ... WHERE IS D?

Sunshine

The majority of vitamin D results from your skin being exposed to the sun. Actually, this exposure is the first step that sets in motion the chain of events that produce vitamin D. All you need is ten to fifteen minutes of sunlight two or three days a week. If you have a darker skin color, it will take longer. On average, it takes only fifteen minutes a day in the midday hours to get enough sunlight. Dr. Robert Heaney, a distinguished professor at Creighton University School of Medicine, estimates that the average person gets 2,000 IU of vitamin D from the sun each day (IU is a standardized unit of measurement short for International Units; one IU of vitamin D is equivalent to 0.025 micrograms). But—there is always the fine print—multiple factors determine whether sunlight will actually provide you with enough vitamin D.

You need to be outside in the middle of the day, and you need to have enough skin exposed—at least your face, arms, and hands. At noontime, two or three days a week, I used to shed my white coat and go up on the rooftop of our research building with my brown bag lunch to get my quick fifteen minutes of "vitamin D therapy." Beyond your vitamin D therapy time, you will need to prevent sunburn and potentially long-term skin damage from excessive sun exposure.

> *YOUR STORIES...*
>
> Sarah, age fifty-five, anesthesiologist in North Carolina:
>
> "I leave and come home in the dark. I was not taking any supplements. Even one of the orthopedic surgeons told me he had low vitamin D, too."
>
> Sarah does not see the "light of day." She leaves for work in the dark, works in operating rooms devoid of any natural light, and returns

home long after peak sun-exposure time. Her vitamin D level was quite low, 16 ng/ml, when it was first checked after Sarah experienced rapid bone loss.

Like Sarah, you may rarely be outside during peak ultraviolet light to have a chance to make vitamin D. Natural light inside the building would not have helped her either. Glass filters out too much of the ultraviolet light that is needed for production of vitamin D. You might feel better having a window, but you need to be outside to get the benefit of nature's vitamin D therapy.

A note of caution: Dermatologists warn anyone who has a skin type that burns easily or has a history of skin cancer that they should not have casual, unprotected sun exposure. If you are in that situation, use sun precautions and make sure you are getting vitamin D from other sources.

Peak ultraviolet light is needed to have a chance to make vitamin D. But wait! You might not need to rush outside just now.

What Time of Year Is It?

Time of year makes a difference since sunlight varies seasonally.

In Boston, Dr. Holick placed a photometer on the roof of Boston University Hospital to monitor the level of ultraviolet radiation. He measured adequate sunlight for making vitamin D during only four months of the year, from May to September. Dr. Holick also drew blood samples once a month from volunteers. Their vitamin D levels showed a seasonal pattern. The levels were highest at the end of the summer, then drifted down and were lowest at the end of winter.

Summer may be the only time you can count on sunshine as your source of vitamin D, and the effectiveness also depends on how much sunlight is available. Different weather patterns or atmospheric conditions may even sabotage that time of year.

Where Do You Live?

Location, location, location.

Okay, so sunshine is not a dependable source of vitamin D in Boston except during the four summer months out of the year. What about other parts of the country? Since San Diego has more apparent sun, you would not expect any problems with getting vitamin D there.

In 1993, Dr. Clifford Rosen, an endocrinologist and research scientist at Maine Medical Center, and I compared older women from San Diego with women from Maine over a period of one year, from one summer to the next. Dr. Rosen was based in Bangor, Maine, and expected to see vitamin D levels highest at the end of summer and lowest in the winter. We did not expect to see the same pattern in the San Diegans. Contrary to our predictions, the seasonal changes in vitamin D levels were identical for both groups.

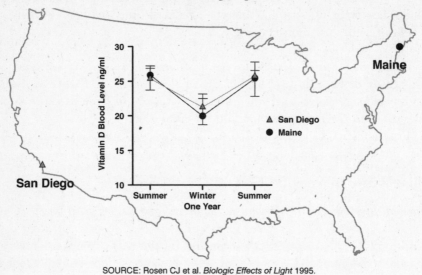

SOURCE: Rosen CJ et al. *Biologic Effects of Light* 1995.

Tim Gunther, gunthergraphics.biz

As you can see, the graph plotting the change in vitamin D levels for each group looked like superimposed Vs. The graph started at the first summer, the bottom of the "V" was the winter, and the second summer reverted to the same levels as the first summer. What struck me on rereading this paper is that none of the Maine or San Diego women had vitamin D levels above 30! The average summertime highs for both groups were 25 ng/ml. At the time this study was performed, the lower end of the normal reference range was 10 ng/ml. We have come a long way in our understanding of vitamin D and bone health since the early 1990s.

One more important point was made from this comparison. The seasonal changes in vitamin D and corresponding changes in higher parathyroid hormone translated into seasonal bone loss. This study demonstrated for the first time that wintertime bone loss was not exclusive to people living in northern latitudes. In addition, it might explain the observation that hip fractures are more common during winter months, even in places with no snow or ice. So I may be able to gloat about the sunny seventy-degree day in January, but San Diegans do not appear to be getting enough wintertime vitamin D, either.

Let us look at another state with sun: Florida. In the "Sunshine State," you'd think you would be more likely to have adequate sunlight throughout the year.

After a few reports had shown remarkably high occurrence of inadequate vitamin D levels in different parts of the country and the world, University of Miami endocrinologist Dr. Silvina Levis decided to perform a study of her patients in the Miami area. Dr. Levis and her associates recruited about two hundred men and women from the general medicine outpatient clinic. Vitamin D levels were checked at the end of winter and rechecked at the end of summer. The majority of vitamin D levels were lower than 30 ng/mg regardless of season.

Dr. Levis explained, "We thought that because of our southern, sunny location this would not be the case in Miami. Our results proved us wrong. We stay away from the sun, we use sunscreen, and we walk on the shady side of the street. Therefore, we have rates of low vitamin D that are pretty close to what has been found in locations farther away from the equator."

Low vitamin D occurs even in places with abundant sunshine.

Do You Use Sunscreen?

Dr. Levis mentioned sunscreen as a contributing factor for seeing more people with low vitamin D. You have probably been admonished by your dermatologist to wear sunscreen, wear a hat, and cover up. Sunscreens block the production of vitamin D because sunscreen does its job by blocking ultraviolet light. So, if you use sunscreen you have little chance of activating the vitamin D precursor that starts the cascade of events that results in the production of active vitamin D. Unfortunately, there is no sunscreen that lets in some of the "good stuff."

In some studies, sunscreen users tend to have higher vitamin D levels. It may be that sunscreen users end up with more overall exposure to the sun. Other studies, like the Maine versus San Diego study, showed opposite results. When we looked at sunscreen use among San Diego women, there were no differences in vitamin D levels during the summer. In winter, sunscreen users showed greater declines in vitamin D levels and increases in parathyroid hormone compared with the group that did not use sunscreen.

Dermatologists have been effective in delivering their message to use sunscreen and protective clothing. Sunscreen is just another reason you cannot count on sun for maintaining healthy vitamin D levels.

What Do You Wear?

The specialty sun protection clothing market has made its way into mainstream clothiers and stores. You may notice clothing with UPF ratings. Ultraviolet Protection Factor (UPF) is like the sun protective factor (SPF) used on sunscreen lotion bottles. However, clothing does not need to be specially made to block ultraviolet rays. Even normal daily clothing effectively blocks the ultraviolet radiation needed for producing vitamin D. Because clothing and sunscreen work so effectively, you will need to have another source of vitamin D.

What Is Your Skin Color?

The darker your skin, the longer you need to expose yourself to sunlight to produce adequate levels of vitamin D. Increased skin pigment (melanin) reduces the capacity of the skin to make vitamin D. The melanin in the skin acts as a natural sunscreen.

Lower vitamin D levels are observed in African Americans compared with Caucasians; Mexican Americans are in between. These studies have included children, adolescents, and younger and older adult men and women. Lower vitamin D levels are common in anyone with darker skin pigmentation.

However, African Americans have a much lower risk of osteoporosis and fractures. Reasons for this paradox are not entirely clear. It appears that the body adapts to low levels of vitamin D and bone loss does not seem to occur. It is thought that the kidney may compensate by not allowing as much calcium to end up in the urine.

Researchers are trying to explain this genetically programmed advantage. Because of the adaptations by bone and kidney, vitamin D may not be as important for maintenance of African Americans' bone health. However, the benefits of maintaining adequate vitamin D may have a role in other diseases.

Darker skin, regardless of your ethnic or racial background, predisposes you to vitamin D deficiency. If you have darker skin, longer sun exposure is needed to achieve adequate vitamin D levels. So, compared to fair-skinned individuals, you will need to pay attention to getting an even higher amount of daily vitamin D combined from all sources.

Low Vitamin D Levels in Girls

In a nationally representative sample of girls and young women, the likelihood of low vitamin D increased with age. The striking finding was that the majority of all girls, except young Caucasian girls, had low vitamin D. Nearly 100 percent of the African American teens and young women had inadequate levels. All children, and particularly those with darker skin color, urgently need to be targeted for supplementation.

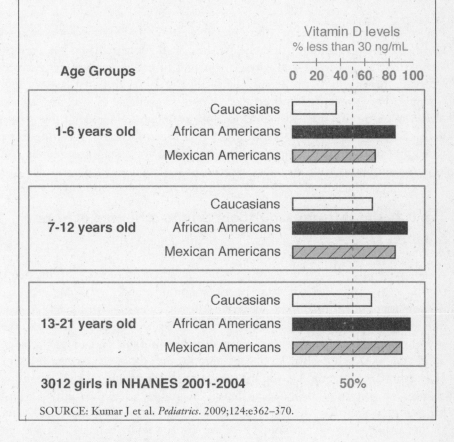

Vitamin D levels
% less than 30 ng/mL

Age Groups

		0 20 40 60 80 100

1-6 years old — Caucasians, African Americans, Mexican Americans

7-12 years old — Caucasians, African Americans, Mexican Americans

13-21 years old — Caucasians, African Americans, Mexican Americans

3012 girls in NHANES 2001-2004   **50%**

SOURCE: Kumar J et al. *Pediatrics*. 2009;124:e362–370.

Is It in Your Genes?

Beyond skin color, is there something else you inherited that may contribute to your vitamin D levels? Recent genetic research suggests that vitamin D genes may make a difference in how you respond to sunshine.

What Is Your Body Size?

One size does not fit all. The larger you are, the more vitamin D you need. Even though large or overweight people may not be at as a high a risk for fracture as thinner individuals they are at high risk for low vitamin D. Think about it as having to fill up a small car versus a large car at the gas station. The larger car is going to require more gallons than the small car. A larger person requires more vitamin D to get a "full tank."

What Is Your Age?

For years, it was thought that older people were the only group who required more vitamin D than everyone else because of their inability to get enough vitamin D through casual sunlight. As you age, your skin tends to get thinner, with a decrease in both the top skin layer (epidermis) and the fat layer of skin (dermis). This results in less precursor vitamin D available to start the cascade of vitamin D production. Even with adequate sunlight, older skin cannot produce enough vitamin D. Therefore, you need to compensate by getting more vitamin D from sources other than the sun. If you are older, the second strike against your ability to make active vitamin D is a decrease in the efficiency of your kidneys, which results in lower production of the active form of vitamin D.

What Is the Bottom Line about Sun as a Source of Your Vitamin D?

As you have just read, many factors modify the intensity of sunlight, including season of the year, weather, atmospheric conditions, and geographic location. The ability of ultraviolet rays to penetrate the top layer of skin to start the production of vitamin D is modified by skin pigmentation, aging, clothing, and the use of sunscreen. Therefore, it is quite difficult to count on sunlight to keep your vitamin D at a healthy level. So count out the sun as a source, at least for eight months of the year. During the summer months you might have a fighting chance, but you are probably inside during the midday when the sunlight is best for making vitamin D. Even if you are outside, use of sunscreen and many other factors are working against you. There are just too many barriers that prevent you from counting on casual sunlight as your main source of vitamin D.

What are you to do now? Where else are you getting vitamin D? Let us look at food sources.

FOOD

You may be thinking, "I am getting it in my food. I eat a healthy, balanced diet most of the time, so food must be my source of vitamin D." Well, probably not.

What food can you eat for vitamin D?

Interestingly, few foods naturally contain vitamin D. The main food sources of vitamin D are oily fish, such as salmon, mackerel, and sardines, and eel. Other foods, such as egg yolks and liver, contain only small amounts of vitamin D. While the Eskimos' diet of fatty fish compensated for their lack of sunlight exposure, the diets of most Americans are not adequate to supply the majority of our vitamin D needs.

Although salmon is one of the most consumed fish in the US, unfortunately, eating salmon does not guarantee that you are actually getting vitamin D. You need to pay attention to whether the salmon is farm-raised or wild. The nutrient-poor diets of farm-raised salmon translate into little available vitamin D. Also, compared with salmon caught in the wild, farm-raised salmon contain much lower quantities of the good omega-3 fatty acids.

You may have been given cod liver oil as a child or have seen pictures of kids being given a teaspoon filled with it. One teaspoon of cod liver oil contained about 400 IU of vitamin D, which was enough to prevent rickets. It was advertised as "Bottled Sunlight," rich in sunshine vitamin D. It is not used now because of its high content of vitamin A, which is detrimental to bone health—not to mention its intense, fishy smell and taste.

In the past, many more foods were fortified with vitamin D. For example, the Joseph Schlitz Brewing Company, producers of Schlitz, known as "The Beer That Made Milwaukee Famous," fortified their beer with vitamin D for three years from 1935 to 1938. A magazine ad page from 1936 proclaimed: "Keep Sunny Summer Health—Drink Schlitz All Winter."

Today, few foods are fortified with vitamin D. The most common fortified product is milk. An eight-ounce glass (one cup) of milk contains 100 IU of vitamin D_3. On your milk bottle or carton, the Percent Daily Value (DV) is listed for a one-cup serving as 25 percent vitamin D—meaning 25 percent of 400 IU RDA. A shortened calculation is to multiply % DV times 4 (for milk example, $25 \times 4 = 100$).

Other fortified foods include cereals, some brands of orange juice, and other dairy products. Generally, cheese and ice cream are not fortified but yogurt may be. *You must check the labels*. Take a look at the foods listed on the following table. There are not many available sources rich in vitamin D.

Vitamin D Food Sources		
Food	Serving Size	Approximate Content (IU)
Fish		
Halibut	3 ounces	200–300
Herring	3 ounces	96
Perch	3 ounces	49
Salmon, wild, filet	3 ounces	350–800
Sardines with bones	3 ounces	160
Trout	3 ounces	600
Tuna, canned	3 ounces	154
Other Natural Sources		
Egg	1 large	41
Liver, beef	3 ounces	42
Vitamin D-Fortified Foods (check labels)		
Bread	1 slice	variable
Cereals	¾ to 1 cup	variable plus add milk
Margarine	1 tablespoon	variable
Milk, all types	1 cup	100
Orange juice	1 cup	100
Yogurt, plain nonfat	1 cup	variable

So in reality, fortified foods are not an efficient way of raising or maintaining your vitamin D level. It is difficult to get enough vitamin D from your diet alone, even if you eat four to five servings of oily fish each week. The assumption has been that foods fortified with vitamin D will help you meet your daily requirements, but clearly, that is not the case. Data from a nationally representative sample (NHANES), collected in 2005 to 2006, showed that less than 10 percent of all adults age fifty-one to seventy were getting 400 IU of vitamin D from diet alone and less than one percent of those age seventy-one and older had diets containing 600 IU.

Sun is a negligible source, except during the summer. Food is not adding much, unless you drink a lot of milk or eat wild salmon for most of your meals. What is left to do? It boils down to supplements.

Dietary Reference Values for Vitamin D 2010

Daily Recommended Dietary Allowance Vitamin D Intake		
Age in Years	**Amount in International Units (IU/day)**	**Upper Level Intake (IU/day)**
Infants 0 to 6 months	400	1000
Infants 6 to 12 months	400	1500
Children ages 1 to 3	600	2500
Children ages 4 to 8	600	3000
Children ages 9 to 18	600	4000
Adults ages 19 to 50	600	4000
Adults ages 51 to 70	600	4000
Adults ages 71 and older	800	4000

Updated Dietary Reference Intakes (DRIs) for vitamin D were released by a committee of the Institute of Medicine in 2010. Despite the plethora of new evidence that has emerged since values were first set in 1997, the evidence supports vitamin D for bone health but not for other diseases or conditions. Even for bone health, there are few studies using supplementation above 800 IU per day. Note that these recommended values support a blood level of 20 ng/ml.

There are still many unanswered questions. Clinical trials using higher supplementation are currently being conducted, but it will be years before definitive results from these studies will be available.

The recommended dietary allowances are public health recommendations that serve as general guidance, and they are safe and reasonable. For individual care, assess your needs in the context of your personal health with your doctor.

SOURCE: Committee to Review Dietary Reference Intakes for Vitamin D and Calcium, Food and Nutrition Board, Institute of Medicine. *Dietary Reference Intakes for Calcium and Vitamin D.* Washington, DC: National Academy Press, 2010.

Supplements

How Much Vitamin D Do You Need?

The recommended values work as a whole for a public health message, but they may not necessarily meet an individual's specific needs. You can take 600 to 800 IU a day and still be under the minimum vitamin D level of 30 ng/ml.

The best approach is to know your starting vitamin D levels to determine the amount you will need to supplement. However, testing everyone is neither practical nor cost effective. A practical way to start is with 2,000 IU each day of supplemental vitamin D for adults. After three to four months of use, if you are at high risk for osteoporosis, have had fractures, have malabsorption, are overweight, or have other chronic diseases, then you may want to have your blood level checked. A good time for this is during the winter or early spring when your levels may be lowest.

Children

The American Academy of Pediatrics' latest recommendation, from 2008, is to give all breast-fed infants 400 IU of supplemental vitamin D. Infant formulas contain vitamin D in the amount of 400 IU per liter. This amount was incorporated in the latest update (2010) from the Institute of Medicine.

The recommendation for children is to increase vitamin D supplementation to 600 IU a day. The same amount is also recommended for preteens and teens. However, some research shows that vitamin D requirements increase with growth and larger body size. Therefore, vitamin D should be adjusted for body weight. Dr. Robert Heaney, distinguished professor at Creighton University School of Medicine, estimates that 75 IU of vitamin D per kilogram is needed from *all sources combined* to ensure adequate vitamin D. The problem is that there is no way to estimate the amount of vitamin D from sunlight exposure. As children and teenagers approach adult size, higher doses may be needed. Talk with your pediatrician about how to individualize your child's vitamin D intake.

Vitamin D is a basic requirement for the growing skeleton. Outside of bone health, it is not clear what long-term role vitamin D may play in the prevention of other diseases and in establishing lifelong health. Vitamin D is *essential* for the health of our children.

What kind of vitamin D are you taking?

Take a look at your multivitamin and calcium supplement bottles. Chances are you will need a magnifying glass or bifocals to read the small print. Turn your attention to the "Supplement Facts" on the bottle. The vitamin D could be identified as vitamin D, vitamin D_2, vitamin D_3, or by the less-obvious names "ergocalciferol" or "cholecalciferol." It may take some sleuthing. Vitamin D could be listed as "vitamin D" in the amount-per-serving table, but you will need to look in the ingredients list to determine if it is identified by type there. It could be identified as "ergocalciferol" or "cholecalciferol" in the ingredients list.

Ergocalciferol is vitamin D_2, which comes from plant sources. It is made by ultraviolet irradiation of ergosterol, which is a compound from yeast. Cholecalciferol is vitamin D_3, which is the vitamin D that our bodies naturally produce. It is produced from ultraviolet irradiation of the precursor of vitamin D (7-dehydrocholesterol) in the skin. For supplements, it is obtained from the lanolin of sheep's wool.

Conventional teaching says that D_2 is not absorbed as well as D_3. So it takes approximately one-third more vitamin D_2 to create the same increases in vitamin D levels that you would get from vitamin D_3. The major vitamin manufacturers took heed and many have reformulated their products to include vitamin D_3 rather than vitamin D_2. All vegetarian-only vitamins contain vitamin D_2. Those labeled "natural" tend to contain vitamin D_2, but not always. Interestingly, the only prescription vitamin D in the US is vitamin D_2. But there has been a movement to get it changed to vitamin D_3.

A few recent publications have shown that a 1,000 IU dose of vitamin D_2 daily is as effective as a 1,000 IU dose of vitamin D_3 in maintaining vitamin D levels. So whether you take a daily product with vitamin D_2 or D_3 may not matter. However, since the preponderance of research definitely favors vitamin D_3, I suggest that once you use up your current vitamin bottle you should change brands to one that uses cholecalciferol—vitamin D_3—because of its superior potency. In any case, it is your overall vitamin D *level* that is important, not the *amount* you are taking.

You do not need to take vitamin D every day. If it is more convenient to think about it once a week, then take your dose that way. You just need to make sure that the supplement you are taking is effective for maintaining a good vitamin D level. If you are starting out with a low vitamin D level, you need to have a follow-up in about four to six months to be sure that the extra vitamin D you are taking is sufficient to increase your level above the minimum level of 30 ng/ml.

Multivitamin supplements also contain vitamin D. The amounts of vitamin D range from 100 IU to 1,800 IU per tablet. There are differences not only between brands but also between categories: children's, prenatal, men's, women's, and over fifty. You need to pay close attention and read the labels carefully with each and every new purchase of supplements. Also, look closely at the serving size. You will need to figure out how many pills, chews, or liquid measures equate to the amount listed for vitamin D.

What is on your shelf? How much vitamin D are you taking?

You will need to take an inventory to figure out how much vitamin D you are getting. If you are taking vitamins and supplements, take the time to gather all your bottles and review the labels. Most likely your multivitamins and calcium are the only products that have some vitamin D. Multivitamins typically have 400 IU, but it could be more or less. Also, pay attention to the *Serving Size*. Is it one, two, three, or four tablets for which the content information is given?

Remember to check each time you buy a new bottle of supplements; you will need to recheck the supplement facts.

Add up your vitamin D...

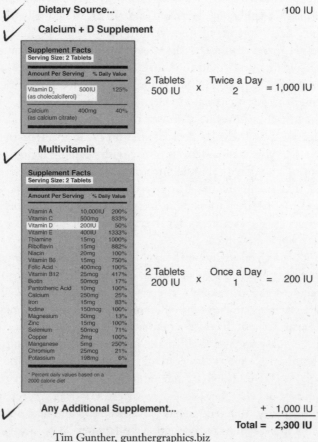

Tim Gunther, gunthergraphics.biz

Do you get extra vitamin D from diet or sun?

It is difficult to gauge your sun exposure. Beyond casual exposure, most people cannot count on a significant amount. Dietary enrichment of foods also accounts for only small amounts of vitamin D. You would basically need to eat fish three times a day to have enough from your diet, and few people follow an "Eskimo diet." Some brands of products such as yogurt or soy milk may have vitamin D added, but even then it is a small amount. To ensure a consistent source of vitamin D, you will need to supplement. For the "average adult," 2,000 IU each day should maintain a vitamin D level over 30 ng/ml.

What if your blood level is below 30?

Discuss with your doctor how to supplement vitamin D in order to raise your level to above 30 ng/ml. There are many different safe and inexpensive ways to achieve a higher level; if you ask ten doctors, you might get ten or more different approaches. Some of these approaches have been evaluated in research studies; others have not. The goal is first to *attain* optimal vitamin D levels, and, second, to prevent the level from dropping below 30 again.

Here are several common recommendations:

Vitamin D_2 50,000 IU weekly (available by doctor's prescription only)
Vitamin D_3, 50,000 IU weekly (available online or by special order at
your pharmacy)

Take one capsule once a week for eight weeks. That is equivalent to a base dose of about 7,000 IU per day. Recheck your blood level after eight weeks. If your blood level is still less than 30 ng/ml, take 50,000 IU of vitamin D_2 once a week for another eight weeks, then recheck blood levels.

When you reach the target blood level of 30 ng/ml, you have several options. You can keep using 50,000 IU of vitamin D_2, but take one every *other* week. Or you can switch to a lower daily dose of 2,000 IU. Note: Your daily dose will need to be individualized based on your requirements to maintain a level in the optimal range.

For D_2, the longest interval between taking two doses should be two weeks. Prescriptions sometimes call for taking D_2 once a month but the dose does not last that long. However, a once-monthly dose of D_3 does last the full month and can be given at that interval.

Daily Dosing

A general estimate is made to determine your additional daily vitamin D supplementation. After taking the daily dose for three to four months, recheck your vitamin D level.

Estimating Additional Vitamin D

Dr. Robert Heaney and his group at Creighton University studied responses to different doses of vitamin D to develop a prediction rule of thumb. Their subjects were 116 healthy men who were given vitamin D_3—cholecalciferol—for eight weeks during the winter. Note that these were healthy men, average age twenty-eight, who started the study with an average vitamin D level of 26.8 ng/ml.

Based on the observed vitamin D level responses to vitamin D supplementation, Dr. Heaney predicted that a daily dose of 400 IU would increase levels by 4 ng/ml. The 1,000 IU dose should increase levels by almost 10 ng/ml.

The "rule of thumb" is based on these observations, but it does not account for individual variation. For example, if you are overweight, you may need even more vitamin D. Since vitamin D is stored in fat, it will take more to fill up the storage area.

If you use the general rule of thumb that each additional 100 IU raises your blood levels 1 ng/ml, you can make a general estimate of what your additional daily needs are if your level is low. For example, if we go back to Sarah (see page 144), who had a starting vitamin D level of 16, she will need 14 x 100 = 1,400 *extra* units/day on average to raise her level to the minimum 30 ng/ml.

Can you take or get too much vitamin D?

Theoretically, yes. In all practicality, probably not. Only a few cases of toxicity have been reported. In medical school, we were taught to be careful with the vitamins A, D, E, and K because they are stored in fat or are so-called fat-soluble vitamins. This teaching has contributed to a reluctance to give "too much" vitamin D. Several previous studies have also questioned whether vitamin D causes kidney stones. However, doses of vitamin D that result in blood levels in the normal range do not cause kidney stones.

Actually, a large margin of safety exists between the normal levels of 30 to 70 ng/ml and toxicity, which occurs at levels of 200 ng/ml and higher. Toxic levels of vitamin D cause excessive calcium in the urine and blood. Symptoms of toxicity are related to the high blood calcium levels and may start with loss of appetite, nausea, and vomiting.

Think of jobs with sun exposure—outside workers, lifeguards, and the like. Typically, lifeguards have blood levels of 60 to 80 ng/ml. The skin has a built-in safeguard so that you can't reach toxic levels of vitamin D from overexposure to the sun. Though repeated and prolonged sun exposure will not result in toxic levels of vitamin D, your dermatologist will not be too happy with you.

However, unlike exposure to sunlight, you can reach toxic vitamin D levels from taking large quantities of supplements. A safe estimate for an upper intake level is daily doses of 10,000 IU a day, although the Institute of Medicine sets 4,000 IU a day as the adult upper level. Fortunately, you will not need to go that high to maintain optimal vitamin D levels. It turns out that there is a wide safety margin. But don't go overboard with your supplements. You can get too much of a good thing.

A study published in a 2010 issue of the *Journal of the American Medical Association* showed increased falls and fractures with vitamin D supplementation. This finding was the opposite of what was expected. Subjects in this randomized clinical trial (more than 2,200 Australian women age seventy or older) used either a dose of 500,000 IU of vitamin D_3 or a dummy placebo *once a year*. Study subjects were followed for three to five years.

Dr. Reinhold Vieth, vitamin D expert at the University of Toronto, explained that "the problems arose because of the long dosing interval, and not because of the cumulative dose, or the serum levels attained." In other words, it was not a toxicity problem. The effect of vitamin D_3 lasts two to three months. The interval of one year did not make biologic sense.

A word about laboratory testing

At the present time, two different methods (also called assays) are used to measure vitamin D levels in the blood. Both types should provide reliable and accurate results. There is no standardization of vitamin D laboratory testing. However, all laboratories have internal quality control measures in place. Just as with any other test, if your result is exceedingly high or low, you should have it redone.

WHY IS VITAMIN D IMPORTANT?

After all this information about vitamin D, why is it really necessary?

Calcium Balance

The main function of vitamin D is to preserve calcium balance. How well calcium is absorbed from the intestine is regulated by vitamin D. With adequate vitamin D, you absorb about 30 to 40 percent of the calcium that you take in from foods, drinks, or supplements. If your vitamin D level is low, the efficiency of calcium absorption drops to 10 to 15 percent. This comes at great cost to your bone health. Too little vitamin D results in a cascade of events that lead to increased fracture risk.

When not enough calcium is coming in, the body has a mechanism to get more calcium in order to keep everything running. The parathyroid's sole role is to regulate calcium in your body. Your parathyroid consists of four small glands that are located in your neck, usually on the backside of your thyroid, hence the name. Low calcium in the blood triggers the parathyroid gland to go into overdrive to produce more of its hormone, "parathyroid hormone." You may see it abbreviated as "PTH."

The increased amount of parathyroid hormone acts on the bone to release some of its calcium. This makes up for too little calcium being absorbed in the intestine, but it is at the cost of the bone. Bone is broken down faster than normal, and this causes a net bone loss. The accumulated effect of bone loss is weakening of bone structure and a much higher risk of fractures.

The goal is to have enough vitamin D to prevent the cascade of events that leads to bone loss, osteoporosis, and fractures. The level of vitamin D needed for calcium absorption defines the vitamin D level needed for bone health. The critical threshold level for vitamin D is 30 ng/ml, which allows you to absorb adequate calcium and prevent the overproduction of parathyroid hormone.

Parathyroid hormone levels move in the opposite direction from vitamin D. You can think of a teeter-totter, as one end goes up the other goes down. I also need to note that it is possible to have a low vitamin D level with a normal PTH. The lower your level, the more likely it is that your PTH is high. However, the expected response in PTH may be blunted by other factors, such as smoking or being overweight.

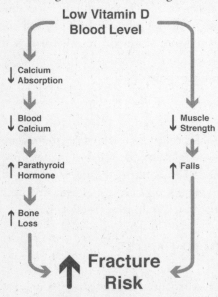

Tim Gunther, gunthergraphics.biz

For example, when Sarah had a vitamin D level of 16 ng/ml, her parathyroid hormone (PTH) level, at 65 pg/ml, was high (normal PTH values are 10 to 55 picograms per milliliter (pg/ml) but may vary between laboratories). She started taking vitamin D supplements. On a subsequent recheck, her vitamin D level had improved to a normal level, 47 ng/ml, and her PTH had decreased to 35 pg/ml, which was in the normal range as well. *By simply increasing your intake of vitamin D, you can steadily regain proper balance.*

Bone Density

Higher vitamin D levels are associated with higher bone density. When vitamin D versus bone density is plotted out, there is a steep curve up in bone density to a vitamin D level of 36 to 40 ng/ml. Above those levels, the bone density levels out to a plateau. Therefore, it is advantageous for your vitamin D level to be in the 30s for optimal bone density.

Fractures

It follows that if your bone density is lower then your fracture risk is higher. Clinical trials using vitamin D alone or in combination with calcium have been done to evaluate the risk of fracture. These were randomized, placebo-controlled studies, which means that by chance some subjects received the active ingredient, in this case vitamin D, or sometimes vitamin D with calcium. Others got an identical imitation pill called a "placebo" that did not contain vitamin D.

The data from individual studies were combined and redone in a new analysis, called a "meta-analysis." Multiple meta-analyses have been done to evaluate the effective dose for fracture reduction. The investigators found that only daily vitamin D doses of 700 to 800 IU were effective in decreasing the risk of fractures. There was an approximately one-quarter reduction of risk for hip fractures and any nonvertebral fracture. No benefit was observed in trials that used lower daily doses.

Rickets and Osteomalacia

The classic vitamin D deficiency disease in children is rickets, which results in malformed bones. When the same process happens in adults, the condition is called osteomalacia. Osteomalacia means soft bones. That is literally what happens. Very low vitamin D levels result in an inadequate supply of calcium and phosphorus, which are necessary to make the bones solid through a process called mineralization. If new bone does not mineralize, it is soft and rubbery.

In children, depending on their age, a variety of deformities of the bone may occur. These deformities are accentuated by the effects of gravity. A classic picture of rickets shows a child of diminutive height with bowed legs and a prominent head. Unfortunately, this disease still happens, not just in developing countries but in the US as well.

In adults, no outward signs of osteomalacia are usually seen. Instead, bone and muscle pain, as well as tenderness, are common. Because the pain can be dull and constant, it may be misdiagnosed as fibromyalgia, a disorder characterized by widespread musculoskeletal pain with localized tenderness and fatigue. Anyone with persistent and nonspecific musculoskeletal pain who has not responded to usual care should have his or her vitamin D level measured. The risk of fracture with osteomalacia is high. If a fracture does occur, osteoporosis may commonly be diagnosed instead of the real problem: osteomalacia as a result of vitamin D deficiency.

In addition to low levels of vitamin D that are typically less than 15 ng/ml, osteomalacia is often accompanied by other abnormal test results: low blood calcium and phosphorus and increased parathyroid hormone and alkaline phosphatase. Alkaline phosphatase is an enzyme that reflects both liver and bone activity. In this case, alkaline phosphatase levels are often high because the bone-building cells, osteoblasts, are working overtime. Early in the disease process there may be enough compensation so that some of the blood studies may still show results in the normal or close to normal range.

Don't Confuse Osteomalacia with Osteoporosis

Academy Award-winning actress Gwyneth Paltrow posted a story in her website newsletter *GOOP* entitled "Vitamin D."

The British press picked up her story and went to town with the information as only the Fleet Street reporters can do, penning headlines like "Diet Fan Gwyneth Paltrow Has Bone Disease" and "Gwyneth Paltrow: I'm Suffering from Brittle Bone Disease." In her online newsletter, she revealed that she'd had a "tibial plateau fracture a few years ago." (The tibia is your shinbone. Fracture of the tibial plateau occurs in the wide part of the tibia just below your knee). Because of the fracture, she'd had a bone density scan that showed she had the "beginning stages of osteopenia." That result led her doctors to test her vitamin D. She was told that it was the "lowest they had ever seen."

Based on her post, the Fleet Street reporters diagnosed her with osteoporosis.

They jumped to the wrong conclusion.

She most likely had "osteomalacia."

Her fracture of the tibial plateau is not a classic "osteoporosis" fracture. Instead it represents an insufficiency fracture, which means that the bone in this high stress area was not able to maintain its weight-bearing load.

With osteomalacia, the amount of bone is usually normal but the amount of mineral is too low. The bone mineral density measured by DXA will be low, not because of too little bone like in osteoporosis, but due to poor mineralization of the bone. Once vitamin D is increased and calcium is absorbed, the bone will become mineralized again. The next time Gwyneth has a DXA scan, it is likely to show a large improvement in her bone mineral density.

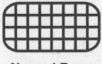 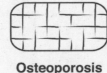 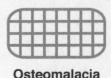

Normal Bone　　　**Osteoporosis**　　　**Osteomalacia**

Tim Gunther, gunthergraphics.biz

The take-home message is this: Just because you have low bone mass and have experienced a fracture does not mean it is due to osteoporosis. You need to think about other causes. In Gwyneth's case, she had vitamin D deficiency. True, her diet could have contributed to low vitamin D. However, it is more likely that the main factors were living in England without sufficient sunshine year round and not taking supplements.

Bottom line: Stay bone healthy with a sensible diet and *enough* vitamin D and calcium each day.

Muscle and Muscle Strength

Rickets and osteomalacia are associated with decreased muscle strength. Recently, it was recognized that people with low vitamin D levels have weaker muscles. This muscle weakness is a more subtle consequence of low vitamin D. Vitamin D acts directly on muscle. Treatment with vitamin D increases the size and number of individual muscle fibers that leads to improved physical performance.

Poor muscle function associated with low vitamin D is not just a problem for older adults; it is a problem for people of all ages. A group of almost one hundred young adolescent girls in England were instructed to hop as fast and as hard as possible. They hopped on a special platform that recorded their jumping power, jump height, and speed. Those with low vitamin D generated less power as well as less jump height and speed than those with higher vitamin D levels. Vitamin D is important along with exercise to keep your muscles strong.

Falls

Weaker muscles, particularly weaker quadriceps or thigh muscles predispose you to falling. Dr. Heike Bischoff-Ferrari, a leading researcher in the role of Vitamin D in aging and musculoskeletal health and head of clinical research at University Hospital in Zurich, Switzerland, showed that in a mere three months, supplementation of vitamin D made a large impact on the risk of falling in frail elderly women. She and her colleagues at the University of Basel, Switzerland, studied 122 elderly women residing in a nursing home. Over three months, half were given 800 IU of vitamin D plus 1,200 mg of calcium and the other half received only the 1,200 mg of calcium. For those on calcium plus vitamin D, vitamin D levels were increased and falls were reduced by half in comparison with the calcium only group. In addition, there were improvements in tests of muscle strength.

This was a major new insight and exciting news to me as a geriatrician. To think that by simply giving vitamin D to nursing home residents their rates of falls would decrease! What a boon for these patients' health.

In 2004, Dr. Bischoff-Ferrari published in the *Journal of the American Medical Association* a meta-analysis that assessed the overall effectiveness of vitamin D to prevent falls. This analysis included five randomized placebo-controlled studies (the most valid kind) with over 1,200 elderly men and women who were treated with vitamin D versus an imitation placebo pill. The risk of falling was reduced by 22 percent.

In 2006, Dr. Bischoff-Ferrari and her colleagues reported the results of their three-year clinical trial of *healthy* men and women ages sixty-five years and older. Half of the group received 700 IU of vitamin D plus 500 mg of calcium and the other half took imitation pills. Falls were reduced in all women by almost half. An even greater reduction in falls was observed in a subgroup of women who were less physically active. No effect was observed in men. In older women not considered to be at particularly high risk for falling, improving vitamin D resulted in a significant reduction in falls.

Improved muscle strength and lower risk of falling are added benefits of vitamin D. Unfortunately, this research has not been translated consistently into clinical practice. The most vulnerable individuals for falling and fracture are our seniors, particularly those residing in long-term care facilities or those who are homebound. Checking vitamin D levels and providing appropriate vitamin D supplementation is not consistently done in this high-risk group. Think of the health-care dollars that could be saved by decreasing falls and hip fractures with the simple use of vitamin D. Instead, because more testing has been done recently, some Medicare carriers are actually limiting the testing of vitamin D levels.

Other Diseases: Beyond Bone

Recently, there have been numerous reports about the role of low levels of vitamin D in contributing to other serious health problems beyond bone. Actually, this area has been evolving over about the past thirty years. Only now has it reached a critical mass based on new discoveries.

When I first arrived at the University of California, San Diego, I regularly passed by the office of Dr. Cedric Garland but noticed he was never there. Who was this mystery professor? "Oh, he is one of the Garland brothers," I was told. "He and his brother, Frank, are 'the vitamin D guys.'" They had shown an association of vitamin D with colon cancer. Their original paper was published in 1980 by the *International Journal of Epidemiology*. The opening sentence was: "It is proposed that vitamin D is a protective factor against colon cancer."

They had observed that when deaths from colon cancer in Caucasian men were plotted on a map of the US, there were many more dots in the northern states than in the southern ones. They examined a variety of different possibilities to explain this observation. They estimated the amount of sunlight reaching the ground for each state based on data from the US Weather Bureau and then overlaid the solar radiation information on the map with colon cancer deaths. Bingo! The highest colon cancer deaths occurred in places that had the lowest amounts of sunlight.

Twenty-five years later, their paper was republished along with recent cellular and molecular research that supported their original observation. A commentary in the same journal issue concluded, "The worms are at last wriggling out of the can that the Garlands opened 25 years ago."

Over the last few years, it has been more like a volcanic eruption of information. More diseases have been linked to low vitamin D including breast cancer, prostate cancer, ovarian cancer, non-Hodgkin's lymphoma, diabetes, multiple sclerosis, inflammatory bowel disease, rheumatoid arthritis, osteoarthritis, influenza, hypertension, heart failure, heart attacks, stroke, and even premenstrual syndrome (PMS). Wow, it seems like all the major diseases that are leading causes of death are in that list, and every time you turn around another is reported. Flu and influenza were the latest associated diseases reported. Could vitamin D be the next "panacea"?

Caution! For all these diseases and conditions, you need to keep in mind that these are still observations. The type of research study is key to determine what type of conclusions can be drawn from the data. There is strong cause and effect evidence for vitamin D and bone health based on clinical trials. For the most part, no clinical trials have been done for the other diseases. Therefore, so far, one cannot make the leap to cause and effect. Vitamin D and other diseases are still just "associations" without proven cause and effect.

It was thought that only the kidney was capable of producing active vitamin D. So far, researchers have found many other tissues, including cells in the breast, prostate, and colon that have the enzyme needed to produce active vitamin D. However, these tissues produce only local concentrations of active vitamin D. You may see the word "paracrine" used to describe this function, which means that the vitamin D acts locally and does not enter the blood stream. In contrast, active vitamin D produced by the kidney circulates in the blood to affect other organs and tissues and therefore is designated "endocrine."

In addition, vitamin D receptors seem to be ubiquitous and have been identified in more than forty tissues so far. Cells in these tissues may produce biologic responses. If enough active vitamin D is present, the cell "machinery" works smoothly. If there are inadequate amounts of vitamin D to attach to the receptors, the system breaks down. That is the basis of thinking for how low vitamin D could cause or contribute to the various diseases.

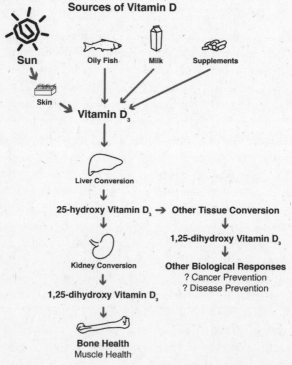

Tim Gunther, gunthergraphics.biz

It is amazing though to think that vitamin D may have such far-reaching effects. However, at the moment, some people come off sounding like "snake oil salesmen," making claims that vitamin D can prevent everything. The panacea of vitamin D effects may be likened to the early days of research into vitamin C. At the time, science was just discovering the many benefits of vitamin C, and some were overplayed while others turned out to be totally validated. The science is evolving. More research is needed to provide the cause and effect link. Stay tuned. It is an exciting time and a plethora of research is underway looking at practically every organ system and disease state.

THE NEXT STEP

As you have read, a multitude of factors can sabotage your ability to get enough vitamin D. Because of that, the amount of vitamin D required to maintain a level over 30 ng/ml will be different if you are young, petite, fair-skinned, and live in Arizona versus being older and residing in Detroit. In general, the average person taking an average supplemental dose of 2,000 IU daily will achieve an average blood level above 30 ng/ml. There is a lot of individual variability! Not everyone can be above average such as the children in Lake Wobegon, author Garrison Keillor's fictional Minnesota town in *A Prairie Home Companion*. Remember that average means that some people will be lower than the average and others will be higher.

Talk with your doctor about whether you are at high risk for low vitamin D and may need to check your vitamin D level (25-hydroxy or 25-OH vitamin D). If you are not at high risk and have not had your vitamin D level measured, you may take from 800 to 2,000 IU a day of supplemental vitamin D based on your individual circumstances. Many people observe that they feel "better" after increasing their vitamin D, even though they felt "well" with a low vitamin D level.

The general measures of regular exercise and adequate calcium and vitamin D are essential for bone and muscle health for everyone. However, if you are at high risk for fracture or already have osteoporosis, those general measures may not be enough to prevent fractures. You will need to consider adding specific therapies for prevention and treatment of osteoporosis. The next section will cover those options.

The Bare Bones

- Sun is the main source of vitamin D, but you can't rely on sunshine alone.
- In most parts of the country, only May, June, July, and August sun provide enough radiation to produce vitamin D.
- Sunscreen blocks the production of vitamin D.
- Few foods have naturally occurring vitamin D and few foods are enriched with vitamin D, making it difficult to get your daily requirements from dietary sources.
- If your vitamin D level is less than 30 ng/ml, calcium absorption drops to 10 to 15 percent.
- Vitamin D and calcium supplements decrease the risk of falls and the risk of fractures.
- Vitamin D supplements are nearly always necessary to maintain adequate levels of vitamin D (30 ng/ml and higher).
- In general, 2,000 IU of daily vitamin D maintains vitamin D levels over 30 ng/ml in adults.
- The only way to know your true status is to measure your vitamin D level.

PART FOUR

THERAPIES FOR PREVENTION AND TREATMENT OF OSTEOPOROSIS

Medicines for Treatment of Osteoporosis
Timeline of FDA Approval

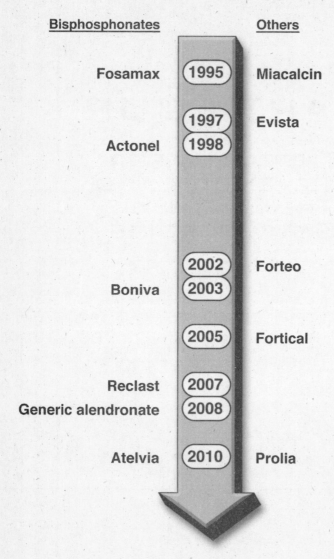

Bisphosphonates

Others

Bisphosphonates	Year	Others
Fosamax	1995	Miacalcin
	1997	Evista
Actonel	1998	
	2002	Forteo
Boniva	2003	
	2005	Fortical
Reclast	2007	
Generic alendronate	2008	
Atelvia	2010	Prolia

Tim Gunther, gunthergraphics.biz

FDA-Approved Medicines

Introduction

When lifestyle measures are not enough, medicines play an important role in the treatment of postmenopausal women and men with osteoporosis. Those individuals at high risk for fracture will benefit most from prescription medicine treatment. In general, you are considered to be at high risk if you have already had a fracture (including silent spine fractures), have low bone density with multiple risk factors, have bone density in the osteoporosis range (T-score below -2.5), or are losing bone rapidly. Assess your risk with your doctor to make sure prescription medicines are indicated. In addition, decrease any modifiable risks and assure adequate daily calcium and vitamin D with supplements as needed.

Matching your needs with the right available medicine is essential. The medicine you start with may not be the one you continue to use year after year. Always re-evaluate its use and need on an annual basis with your doctor. New research will continue to provide new information and offer new choices. Some of you may not be interested in prescription medicines at all. If you have low bone density, most likely your doctor will discuss medicines with you. Whether you are considering prescription medicines or alternative therapies, I encourage you to look at all the available evidence to ensure that the option you choose will actually decrease your risk of fractures.

HOW DO BONE MEDICINES WORK?

The medicines for osteoporosis either slow the breakdown of bone by interfering with the demolition cells (osteoclasts) or boost the formation of bone by turning on the bone-builder cells (osteoblasts). The medicines are divided into two categories depending on their target of action. The term "antiresorptives" refers to the medicines that target the cells responsible for bone breakdown. Most antiresorptives are in the bisphosphonate class of medicines. "Anabolics" is the name for those medicines that turn on the bone-builder cells that form new bone. Forteo® is the sole member of the anabolic group.

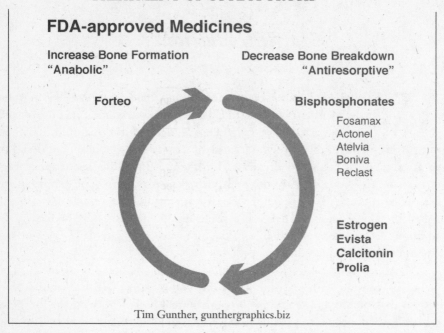

Tim Gunther, gunthergraphics.biz

A repeat bone density test after two years of treatment is indicated. Therefore, the typical improvement in bone density from clinical trial data at two years is given for each of the FDA-approved medicines in the next sections. If you and your doctor are worried about rapid bone loss, then you will need a repeat bone density sooner. Your repeat DXA should be done at the same facility that performed your baseline test in order to get an accurate comparison. Schedule a follow-up appointment with your doctor to go over the results. Your repeat bone density should show no change from the baseline results (stable) or increases at both your hip and spine. Stable is good and represents a treatment response. Keep in mind that small changes in bone density account for large decreases in fracture risk. If the numbers indicate a loss of bone density while on treatment, refer to the section on monitoring (page 311).

For medicines to work, you need to take them. If you expect to get the benefits shown in clinical trials for reducing risk of fracture, you need to follow the dosing regimen for the medicine as directed by your doctor. Too often, medicines are not taken as prescribed or the medicines are stopped altogether without consulting with the prescribing doctor. Keep an open dialogue with your doctor if you are having difficulty with the medicine or have doubt about taking it.

What Is a Randomized Clinical Trial?

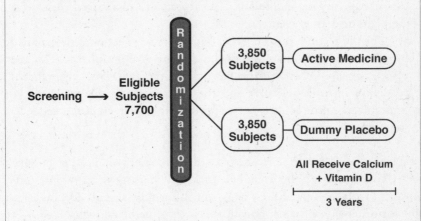

All FDA-approved medicines for treating osteoporosis have been proven to reduce the risk of spine fractures and sometimes other types of fractures in what is called a randomized, placebo-controlled clinical trial. These studies are referred to as the "pivotal fracture trials." This means that the FDA has participated in discussions with a sponsor regarding the design and conduct of the trial. In addition, the FDA assigns its own statisticians to review the data and it audits some of the study sites.

The diagram displays a typical design and the numbers of participants that are required in order to show differences in rate of fractures over three years. To qualify for entry into the study, prospective participants are carefully screened with questionnaires about their history, DXA scans, spine x-rays, and laboratory tests to see if they meet the entry criteria. If they meet the qualifying bone density or have a spine fracture and no conflicting factors that could influence response to therapy, they are eligible. Those who do not meet the entry criteria are excluded from participating in the study.

The eligible subjects are divided randomly into groups to receive the active study medicine or a look-alike dummy medicine called a placebo. In the osteoporosis studies, both the active and placebo groups received supplements of calcium and vitamin D. The participants, staff, researchers, monitors, and statisticians are all "blinded," meaning that no one knows the medicine assignment until the study is completed. The randomization process equalizes multiple features such as age, weight, and bone density so the groups are the same. Therefore, the differences measured at the end of the study will be due to the study medicine. During the study, the subject reports any illness or problem that occurs at each clinic visit. All subjects are monitored closely for safety, bone density changes, and fractures.

For the pivotal fracture trials, fracture risk reduction is determined by comparing fracture rates in the treated group with those in the placebo group. When statistical analysis of the data shows a significant reduction in spine fractures and the benefit-risk profile is felt to be favorable, the drug is likely to be approved for use in clinical practice by the FDA.

If you make a decision to start one of these medicines, you need to be sure that your risk of fracture is high enough to justify starting therapy. Fracture risk assessment with tools like FRAX helps quantify your risk and serves as a starting point for discussion of your individual risk. No medicine is risk free. Keep in mind that these FDA-approved medicines have all been through rigorous testing with thousands of people studied in a controlled setting. After approval, sometimes unforeseen problems appear that were not observed during the clinical trials. The FDA continues to monitor for these situations. In 2007, the FDA implemented an even stronger safety program. For some newer medicines, there are voluntary programs open to your participation to capture any problems that might arise.

Remember, treatment with medicine is not a panacea; it must be in combination with general measures of adequate calcium and vitamin D, nutrition, exercise, and fall prevention. You have to do your part in making healthy choices, exercising, and taking your medicine as prescribed.

OSTEOPOROSIS MEDICINES APPROVED FOR A RANGE OF OSTEOPOROSIS INDICATIONS

The medicines approved for osteoporosis by the FDA have specific indications for use. Treatment of postmenopausal osteoporosis is based on the effectiveness shown in decreasing risk of fractures in the pivotal fracture trial for each medicine. The fracture trials use the largest number of subjects in order to show fracture effectiveness. Additional indications are based on smaller studies that look at bone mineral density. The assumption is that equivalent bone density changes will confer the same fracture reduction benefit.

Medicine	Postmenopausal Osteoporosis		Steroid-Induced Osteoporosis		Men
	Treatment	Prevention	Treatment	Prevention	
Fosamax® or generic alendronate	✓	✓	✓		✓
Actonel®	✓	✓	✓	✓	✓
Atelvia®	✓				
Reclast®	✓	✓	✓	✓	✓
Prolia®	✓				
Estrogen		✓			
Forteo®	✓		✓		✓
Evista®	✓	✓			
Boniva®	✓	✓			
Calcitonin: Miacalcin® or Fortical®	✓				

Fosamax (and Generic Alendronate): The First Kid on the Block

The approval of Fosamax (alendronate) in the fall of 1995 marked a paradigm shift in our approach to the treatment of women with osteoporosis. Until then, our medicine cabinet held limited choices. The options were estrogen or daily shots of a hormone called calcitonin. If push came to shove, and neither of those medicines were appropriate, I would write a prescription for Didronel (etidronate) two weeks at a time in three-month cycles. This use was "off label," meaning Didronel was not approved by the FDA for the treatment of osteoporosis.

Back then, osteoporosis was not on the radar screen. Few women were treated for osteoporosis, even though they may have had broken bones or were stooped over due to spine fractures. Evaluation of bone health was not part of the routine care for postmenopausal women, let alone for anyone else.

At that time, the ability to measure bone density was new as well. The DXA machines were located primarily in academic or university settings. Most of them were used for research rather than for patient care. The World Health Organization (WHO) had just released the criteria for diagnosis of osteoporosis in 1994 and the concepts of T-score and Z-score were still foreign to most physicians.

The launch of Fosamax, the first bone-specific medicine by Merck, helped advance the field of bone health by leaps and bounds. Other medicines were soon to follow. We have come a long way, baby! Like anything else, the more you learn, the more you realize what you don't know. You can read summaries of the unknowns, the recent controversies, and where more research is needed in the section titled "Hot Topics: Cocktail Party Conversations" (see page 245).

Fosamax was the first kid on the block to move into the new area of bone-specific medicines. Fosamax remained on top as the market leader, even after other medicines entered the marketplace. In 2008, the patents for all pill doses of Fosamax expired, except for the liquid formulation and the one with vitamin D—"Fosamax plus D." Now multiple manufacturers produce generic alendronate. Since generics are less expensive than the branded medicine, generic alendronates account for the most prescriptions written for treatment of osteoporosis today.

SCIENTIFIC RATIONALE

Fosamax is a bisphosphonate. It reduces the breakdown of bone without a direct effect on bone formation by interfering with the activity of the bone breakdown cells, osteoclasts.

What Is a Bisphosphonate?

Bisphosphonates are synthetic compounds of the natural phosphorus that binds to the bone mineral. The name refers to the chemical structure of these phosphorus compounds: two phosphonate groups linked by a carbon atom. The side chains attached to the carbon atom differentiate the various bisphosphonates.

Bisphosphonates block the breakdown of the bone by physically interfering with bone breakdown cells, the osteoclasts. The active osteoclasts, shown with a convoluted bottom called a ruffled border, start the bone breakdown process by attaching to the bone mineral surface. Bisphosphonates work by binding to the bone mineral surface at the locations where bone is being broken down by osteoclasts. Osteoclasts eat the bisphosphonate (BP) along with other bone breakdown products.

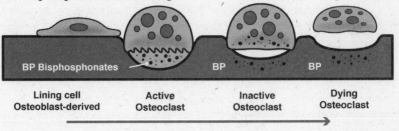

| Lining cell Osteoblast-derived | Active Osteoclast | Inactive Osteoclast | Dying Osteoclast |

SOURCE: adapted from Rodan G et al. *Current Medical Research and Opinion.* 2004;20:1291-1300.

Tim Gunther, gunthergraphics.biz

Once in the osteoclast, bisphosphonates (Fosamax, Actonel, Atelvia, Boniva, and Reclast) block key enzymes, and this disrupts the osteoclast's internal workings, which leads to the disappearance of its ruffled border as it becomes inactive. In this way, the bone breakdown is stopped. The bone forming cells, osteoblasts, proceed with new bone formation. The new mineralized bone covers the bisphosphonate. Ultimately, because of the coupling of the processes in bone remodeling, bone formation activity goes down as the result of the decrease in bone breakdown.

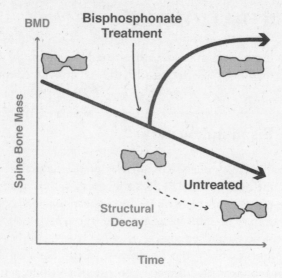

SOURCE: adapted from Seeman E. *Osteoporosis International.* 2009; 20:187-195.
Tim Gunther, gunthergraphics.biz

Remodeling pits that were excavated by osteoclasts before treatment are partially filled in during treatment and fewer remodeling pits are made. The net effect is an increase in bone mass and reduction in risk of fracture. Without treatment, bone loss continues with loss of microstructure.

Fosamax
(alendronate)
Category
Antiresorptive
Bisphosphonate
Manufacturer
Merck
Pivotal Fracture Trial
FIT
Fracture Reduction
Spine
Nonspine
Hip
Indications for Osteoporosis
Prevention postmenopausal women
Treatment postmenopausal women
Men
Steroid-induced treatment

Contraindications
Esophagus problems
Unable to sit or stand upright 30 minutes
Low blood calcium
Swallowing problems
Other Considerations
Stomach or digestive problems
Reduced kidney function
Possible Side Effects
Heartburn or chest pain
Swallowing difficulty
Stomach pain
Nausea
Change in bowel movements
Bone, joint, or muscle pain
Nonhealing sore in mouth or jaw
Atypical femur fracture
Doses
70 mg pill/week most common
35 mg pill/week prevention
Daily: 5 mg or 10 mg pill
Additional Information
Special dosing instructions
Fosamax plus D
Generic alendronate in 2008

EFFECTIVENESS

FIT: The Fracture Intervention Trial

This pivotal fracture study with about 6,500 postmenopausal women was planned for four years and set up as two separate studies, referred to as FIT1 and FIT2. Women were screened by bone density and spine x-rays at eleven universities. In FIT1, the women had low bone density and a spine fracture detected by x-ray. FIT2 participants had low bone density only.

Subjects either took Fosamax 5 mg or a placebo once a day. After two years, the dose was increased to 10 mg based on results of another study, which was investigating a range of doses. The following year that study also showed a robust decrease in spine fractures. Therefore, the FIT1 study was stopped to see if its high-risk participants experienced the same benefit after about three years of treatment. Fracture reduction was about 50 percent at the spine, wrist, and hip. The FIT2 study was continued as originally planned and concluded after four years.

In the FIT groups combined, fracture reduction with Fosamax was seen in women with osteoporosis at all sites:

Spine fractures by x-ray	48%
Painful spine fractures	45%
Nonspine fractures	27%
Hip fractures	53%

Other Studies

In addition to the studies for indications and different formulations, multiple other studies were performed with Fosamax. These thorough research investigations showed consistency of effect across age, both in men and women.

Ten Years of Experience

Fosamax has been studied longer than any other osteoporosis medicine in a controlled clinical trials setting. The original dose ranging study was continued for a total of ten years with around two hundred women. Treatment with 10 mg of Fosamax daily resulted in a continued gradual increase in bone density to an average of 14 percent. Bone density at the hip remained stable. The total hip bone density maintained at about 7 percent above baseline and the bone density at the femoral neck region maintained at over 5 percent above baseline. Bone turnover markers remained in the premenopausal range. No issues of safety or tolerability were seen with this length of treatment in this study population.

FLEX: Fracture Intervention Trial Long-Term Extension

The original participants in FIT who were taking actual Fosamax during the study were recruited to continue in a five-year extension of the study, called FLEX. A total of 1,100 women were reassigned by chance into three groups: placebo, Fosamax 5 mg, or Fosamax 10 mg. The purpose of the study was to see if continued treatment is required once you have already increased your bone density and decreased your risk of a fracture. If so, the researchers asked, what is the optimal dose? Those women taking 5 or 10 mg daily, by the end of the study, had used Fosamax for a total of ten years.

The study was designed to look primarily at BMD changes; because of the smaller group size, fractures were collected as adverse events. Those who switched to the placebo (the same as stopping your medicine) lost all or almost all of what they had gained in bone density over the first five years. The two groups of subjects that continued to receive Fosamax doses showed stable bone density at the hip sites. At the spine, bone density was maintained with a small increase in the placebo group, and those on Fosamax gained over five percent. At the spine, the average difference between groups was almost four percent at the end of FLEX.

Bone turnover markers showed that those continuing Fosamax maintained stable lower levels of bone turnover. Those who were no longer taking Fosamax showed a gradual rise in markers over five years. Their marker levels ended up close to the baseline measured ten years earlier. This correlated with a slow decline in bone density after stopping Fosamax. The bone density and bone marker changes showed some residual effect for at least five years after subjects had ended a five-year course of therapy. In addition, no difference in the number of fractures was seen between the group that had stopped taking Fosamax and the groups that had continued to take Fosamax.

So, should you continue Fosamax beyond five years? Well, it depends. If you are not at high risk for spine fractures and have a good response with Fosamax after five years of therapy, a "holiday" period of up to five years without therapy may be reasonable. Women who have had a spine fracture or are at high risk for one should continue treatment after five years. Reevaluate its use with your doctor every year.

SAFETY

The common adverse effects of Fosamax are different digestive complaints, including heartburn, stomach pain, and diarrhea. In the trials, the same number of subjects reported these problems in both the Fosamax and placebo groups.

Note that the generic alendronates are not made in the same way as branded Fosamax tablets, which were pressed, then coated. Therefore, the generic alendronate may tend to dissolve before reaching the stomach. Alendronate becomes an acid when it dissolves, which is fine for your stomach, but contact in your mouth or with the esophagus could lead to irritation. Be sure to drink a full glass of water to ensure the passage of the pill into the stomach.

Contact your doctor if you have heartburn or worsening heartburn while taking alendronate.

Postmarketing reports of muscle and joint pain that can be severe and non-healing sores in your mouth or jawbone (called osteonecrosis of the jaw) led the FDA to issue a warning for all bisphosphonates.

In 2010, investigation of atypical femur fractures that occur below the hip in patients on bisphosphonates was conducted by the FDA. These fractures have characteristics that are distinct from typical osteoporotic fractures. In light of the number of people treated with bisphosphonates and the few reports of these atypical fractures, their occurrence was considered rare. However, neither the actual cause of the fractures nor which individuals are at risk is known. In response to this observation, the FDA now requires that a "Medication Guide" be given to you when you pick up your prescription and additional labeling warns about these atypical fractures. The majority of patients on bisphosphonates who experienced these atypical fractures had dull aching pain in their thigh prior to fracture. Therefore, if you develop pain in your thigh or groin while taking any brand of bisphosphonates contact your doctor to have your symptom evaluated.

Bone biopsy in women who took Fosamax for ten years showed normal microstructure and mineralization. After ten years, only a small amount of Fosamax was in the bone—an estimated 70 mg.

EASE OF USE

Special instructions must be followed to ensure that the tablet reaches your stomach and that the medicine is absorbed well.

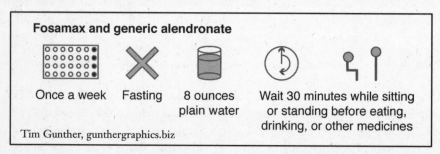

Fosamax and generic alendronate

Once a week   Fasting   8 ounces plain water   Wait 30 minutes while sitting or standing before eating, drinking, or other medicines

Tim Gunther, gunthergraphics.biz

In the morning before you have anything to eat or drink, take Fosamax with a full glass of plain water. You must sit upright or stand for half an hour before eating, drinking, or taking any other medicines whatsoever.

It takes some planning but you can easily incorporate this regimen into your once-a-week schedule. Pick one day in the week that works best for you to have a more leisurely morning. Take your pill, then go for at least a thirty-minute walk. Return home and get on with your day.

What if you miss a dose? Do not take it when you think about it later in the day. You always need to wait until the next morning to take your pill. Do not take two tablets on the same day. Do not worry about missing a week; just don't make it a habit. You have to take the medicine for it to work.

Extra Tips for Taking Fosamax (and any Bisphosphonate Pills)

Make one change at a time. Everything you do to optimize your bone health should be taken one step at a time. If you decide you need calcium supplements to boost your daily calcium to the required level, do not start calcium and your prescription medicine at the same time. Calcium can be the cause of many digestive symptoms. If you start everything all at once and develop constipation, for instance, you will not be able to pinpoint the cause. By making one addition at a time, you will have a better idea, if a symptom arises, what might have been the culprit and what needs to be modified.

Limit the amount of water to 6 to 8 ounces. Some of my patients thought more was better. They drank two or three full glasses, thinking it would lessen their chance for problems. However, water is a good laxative, and looser bowel movements or diarrhea sometimes resulted. If you have a tendency for reflux, the extra liquid may increase the chances of heartburn.

Consider taking a heartburn medicine the night before. If you have experienced a little bit of heartburn or indigestion on the day you take your pill, decreasing the acid in your stomach may help. The night before you take your pill, take a heartburn medicine such as Prilosec® or Prevacid® to see if decreasing acid production eliminates your symptoms. As an added bonus, the absorption of your medicine may be enhanced. Studies of the action of the medicines show a small improvement in absorption with a dose of heartburn medicine.

WHAT SHOULD I EXPECT?

Check back with your doctor after a month to let him know that you are taking the tablets in the prescribed way and that you have no side effects. If you do develop any side effects, contact your doctor in a timely fashion. Since each bisphosphonate is different, you may not have the same problem with another one.

In the pivotal fracture trial, after two years of treatment with Fosamax, the average bone mineral density increases were:

Lumbar spine:	7%
Total hip:	3.5%
Femoral neck:	3%
(neck region of hip)	

Changes observed on your first follow-up DXA at two years may differ; improvement in BMD or no change are both considered positive response to therapy.

FINAL NOTES

At least a dozen manufacturers supply generic alendronates. Pay close attention to each refill of your prescription. The generic pill may not be from the same manufacturer. Your pharmacy or healthcare plan may change supplier based on best costs. Each time, make sure you are tolerating the "new" tablet.

The prevention dose—35 mg once a week—is half of the treatment dose. Also, this is the dose tested and approved for premenopausal women or men taking long-term steroids.

One other formulation is also available. "Fosamax plus D" incorporates 70 mg of Fosamax with vitamin D_3 in the same tablet for once-a-week use. Fosamax plus D is available with two different doses of vitamin D_3, either 2,800 IU or 5,600 IU. It is a way to get branded Fosamax with a weekly dose of vitamin D. An oral solution of Fosamax was previously available but manufacturing of this product was stopped in early 2011.

The Bare Bones
- Generic alendronate is the most common prescription treatment for osteoporosis.
- Fosamax is effective in reducing all types of fractures.
- Although Fosamax was monitored for a ten-year period in clinical trials, rare adverse side effects have been observed in recent years.
- Once-a-week dosing regimen requires planning and forethought.

Actonel: Me, Too?

As number two on the scene in the bisphosphonate class, Actonel (risedronate) was placed in the position of always trying harder. Picture the classic Avis versus Hertz battle. Actonel is the "We Try Harder" product. The challenge is how do you differentiate yourself from number one? Is Actonel the same as Fosamax, or is it something different?

Actonel is different. Bisphosphonates share many common properties. However, the different chemical structure of each medicine in this class gives each one distinct properties.

Serendipity: From Water Softeners to Medicine for Bone Problems

How did Procter & Gamble (P&G), a household products company, maker of Tide®, Crest®, and Bounty®, end up in the pharmaceutical business? Their research scientists' discoveries took them down an unexpected path. In the 1960s, they were designing additives in an attempt to eliminate that pesky soap scum ring around your bathtub. These organic phosphorus compounds, diphosphonates, adhered to the calcium and magnesium in hard water. The name was corrected later to *bisphosphonates* to accurately reflect their chemical structure.

The physiologic properties of bisphosphonates led their research into the dental arena, where they had years of experience with Crest toothpaste. Their work on the prevention of cavities and tartar build-up provided the basis for experiments with bisphosphonates. The bisphosphonate blocked the formation of tartar by forming a surface film that protected the tooth enamel.

These studies on teeth provided much of the background for subsequent research on the phosphonates with hydroxyapatite, the major constituent of bone, which undergoes similar surface reactions as tooth enamel.

At the same time, Dr. Herbert Fleisch and his colleagues at the University of Berne in Switzerland were studying various phosphonates for use in blocking calcification. A chance meeting brought Dr. Fleisch and the researchers from P&G together. A merger of research pathways led to the discovery that bisphosphonates have a direct effect on calcium and bone metabolism. Their first paper was published in *Science* in 1969, which serves as the date of the beginning of bisphosphonate use for bone problems.

Animal experiments showed that bisphosphonates blocked bone loss by decreasing bone turnover. The first clinical trials were done in patients with Paget's disease, who have areas of increased bone turnover. The agent was etidronate (Didronel). It was effective also in lowering blood calcium and bone turnover in multiple myeloma (cancer of the bone) and other cancers.

Osteoporosis was studied subsequently in the first multicenter trial of postmenopausal women. This clinical trial was responsible indirectly for my career focus on osteoporosis. In conferences leading up to the start of the trial at Emory University, endocrinologist Dr. Nelson Watts taught me about "postmenopausal osteoporosis." That first exposure as a junior resident piqued my interest in bone health that has never stopped. Despite initial promising results, Didronel was never approved for treatment of osteoporosis in the United States.

Actonel was P&G's second medicine in the bisphosphonate class tested for osteoporosis. In 2009, the fortieth anniversary year of bisphosphonates, P&G sold Actonel and its prescription medicine enterprise to the Irish company Warner Chilcott.

SCIENTIFIC RATIONALE

Actonel is a bisphosphonate. Its mode of action is the same as Fosamax. It blocks the breakdown of the bone by interfering with the activity of osteoclasts. Actonel does not bind as strongly to the bone. When you stop Actonel, your bone will rev up its machinery back to full steam more quickly than after stopping Fosamax. It takes about twelve months to increase bone turnover after stopping Actonel in contrast to about two to three years for Fosamax.

Actonel
(risedronate)
Category
Antiresorptive
Bisphosphonate
Manufacturer
Warner Chilcott
(Procter & Gamble initially)
Pivotal Fracture Trial
VERT

Fracture Reduction

Spine

Nonspine

Hip

Indications for Osteoporosis

Prevention postmenopausal women

Treatment postmenopausal women

Men

Steroid-induced prevention

Steroid-induced treatment

Contraindications

Esophagus problems

Unable to sit or stand upright 30 minutes

Low blood calcium

Other Considerations

Stomach or digestive problems

Reduced kidney function

Possible Side Effects

Heartburn or chest pain

Swallowing difficulty

Stomach pain

Nausea

Change in bowel movements

Bone, joint, or muscle pain

Flu-like symptoms (monthly dose)

Nonhealing sore in mouth or jaw

Atypical femur fracture

Doses

35 mg pill/week most common OR

150 mg pill once a month

Daily: 5 mg pill

Additional Information

Special dosing instructions

Atelvia: delayed-release 35 mg tablet
          of risedronate taken after
          breakfast once a week

EFFECTIVENESS

In the laboratory experiments, Actonel looked more potent than Fosamax. However, for effectiveness in reducing the risk of fractures in postmenopausal women, the two drugs turned out to be similar at reducing spine fractures in part due to the doses chosen.

VERT: Vertebral Efficacy with Risedronate Therapy

The pivotal fracture trial was conducted in the United States, Canada, Europe, Australia, and New Zealand. It was designed and conducted as two separate studies: "North America" and "Multinational." As entry criteria for both studies, subjects were all postmenopausal women who had at least two spine fractures or one spine fracture with low spine bone density. However, it turns out on review of original x-rays that 20 percent of the women in the North American study did not have any spine fractures.

Two dosages of Actonel, 2.5 and 5 mg, were used versus a placebo group taking an identical looking "dummy" pill. Everyone took 1,000 mg of calcium daily. Those with low vitamin D received up to 500 IU each day. After one year, the 2.5 mg dose group was discontinued in the North American study and about 1,000 women completed the three years of study with the 5 mg pill versus placebo.

The North American fracture results at the end of three years for subjects using 5 mg daily of Actonel showed fracture reduction for:

Spine identified by x-ray   41%
Nonspine fractures   39%
Hip fractures   too few fractures to show any difference

HIP: Hip Intervention Program

In contrast to the previous osteoporosis fracture trials, which focused primarily on the spine, the objective of this study was to evaluate drug effectiveness for hip fracture reduction. Although spine fractures are the most common fractures after menopause, hip fractures are the most devastating. Because of the fewer number of hip fractures expected, a large number of women who were older and at higher risk of fracture were recruited to be part of the study. Over nine thousand women over age seventy were part of this Herculean effort to investigate the effect of Actonel on hip fractures.

Women in the seventy to seventy-nine age group were screened with a DXA for entry into the study. Women eighty and older were eligible based on risk factors alone. Only a small number of women who did not have risk factors had a DXA scan as part of their evaluation. At the end of two years, the results were surprising. The women eighty and older did not have a reduction in hip fractures. The younger group in their seventies had a 40 percent reduction in hip fractures. Putting all ages together, the overall reduction was 30 percent.

Why was a difference seen in the results between age groups? You would expect the older women to have even more benefit with treatment. However, it was not known whether the eighty-plus group actually had osteoporosis, since they did not have their bone density measured. Lesson: If you are going to receive treatment for osteoporosis, make sure you have it! You cannot use risk factors alone. If you are older, you need a bone density in addition to consideration of your risk factors, especially falls.

SAFETY

Digestive system complaints are reported for all bisphosphonates taken as pills. Nausea, heartburn, diarrhea, or constipation occurred in 10 to 13 percent of Actonel study subjects. However, there was no difference between the women taking the actual Actonel pills and those taking the inactive placebo pills.

The big question was whether Actonel was better tolerated than Fosamax in terms of digestive symptoms. In the Fosamax trials, fewer participants reported symptoms but women were not eligible if they had digestive problems. A lot of advertising dollars have been spent trying to convince you that one might be better tolerated than the other.

The reality is that you cannot predict whether you are going to have problems with one medicine versus the other. The important point is that the majority of patients have no problems with taking these medicines. They are all well tolerated. However, you need to be fastidious in following the dosing directions. Be aware of the possible side effects and contact your doctor if you have heartburn, worsening heartburn, or pain while taking Actonel.

The FDA issued a warning about muscle and joint pain that can be severe for all bisphosphonates (Actonel, Fosamax, Boniva, and Reclast) based on postmarketing reports. In addition, a warning about problems with nonhealing sores in the mouth or jawbone (osteonecrosis of jaw) was added to all bisphosphonate labeling.

You will receive a "Medication Guide" with each prescription of Actonel or Atelvia. This applies to all bisphosphonates and is required by the FDA in response to concerns about rare femur fractures that may occur below the hip in individuals taking this type of medicine.

Safety with long-term use is a hot topic. Read more about this in the section titled "Hot Topics: Cocktail Party Conversations" (see page 245).

EASE OF USE

You now have a choice of taking your Actonel weekly or monthly. You can choose 35 mg of Actonel once a week or 150 mg once a month. In addition, with the 2010 release of a 35 mg, delayed-release formulation called Atelvia, you have another option.

Special instructions must be followed to ensure that the Actonel tablet reaches your stomach and that the medicine is absorbed.

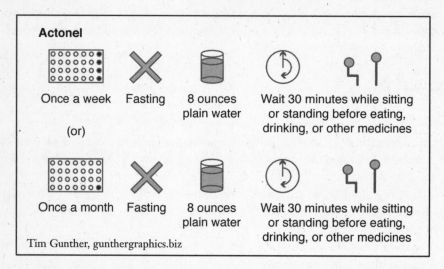

Tim Gunther, gunthergraphics.biz

In the morning, before you have anything to eat or drink, take Actonel with a full glass of water. Then you must sit or stand upright for half an hour before eating, drinking, or taking any other medicines whatsoever.

In contrast, the extended-release risedronate called Atelvia is taken right after breakfast with at least four ounces of water. Again, you must stay upright for at least thirty minutes.

If you forget to take your pill, do not take it later in the day. Always wait until the next morning to take your pill. For once-a-week dosage, do not take two tablets on the same day. For the once-a-month pill, take your forgotten pill only if it is more than one week before your next scheduled dose.

Atelvia delayed-release tablet

Once a week

Taken immediately following breakfast

4 ounces plain water

Sitting or standing for 30 minutes

Tim Gunther, gunthergraphics.biz

WHAT SHOULD I EXPECT?

Check back with your doctor after one month to let him know you are taking the tablets in the right way and that you have no side effects. If you do develop side effects, report them in a timely fashion. You may not have the same problem with one of the other bisphosphonates. Sometimes you have to do trial and error to see which one works best for you.

In the pivotal fracture trial, after two years of treatment with Actonel, the average bone mineral density increases were:

Lumbar Spine:	5%
Total hip:	3%
Femoral neck:	2%
(neck region of hip)	

Changes observed on your first follow-up DXA at two years may differ; improvement in BMD or no changes are both considered positive response to therapy.

FINAL NOTES

Two two-year extensions of the pivotal fracture trial with several hundred women showed continued effectiveness in increasing bone density by using Actonel for a total of seven years in a clinical trial setting. Side effects remained low and were similar to the placebo group.

The prevention dose is the same as the treatment dose (35 mg once a week). Also, Actonel is approved for both prevention and treatment of premenopausal women or men taking long-term steroids. Atelvia is approved for treatment of postmenopausal women with osteoporosis.

Procter & Gamble sold Actonel to the Irish company Warner and Chilcott in 2009. The patent on Actonel expires in 2014.

The Bare Bones

- Actonel is effective in reducing all types of fractures.
- Clinical trials were extended to a total of seven years to monitor bone density and safety.
- Actonel is available in a once-a-week *or* once-a-month dosing regimen.
- An extended formulation taken after breakfast once weekly is branded Atelvia.

Boniva: "The Sally Field Drug"

Prior to a few years ago, mention of the name Sally Field probably brought to mind fond memories of *Gidget*, the *Flying Nun*, or even Forrest Gump's mother. If you watch any television, you've probably seen her as the celebrity pitchwoman for an osteoporosis medicine. Academy Award-winning actress Sally Field's promotion of Boniva (ibandronate) has been extremely effective consumer marketing.

Prior to the release of the medicine, I sat on consultant boards with other experts, and the concern was that Boniva only showed effectiveness in reducing fracture risk at the spine. Although it was in the same class as Fosamax and Actonel, it did not show similar fracture effectiveness at the other common sites of osteoporotic fractures. Enter Madison Avenue. A television advertising campaign with Ms. Field, combined with eye-catching print ads, propelled its visibility. It was not long before women walked into their doctors' offices and asked about the "Sally Field drug."

With all due respect to the glitzy ad campaign, what made Boniva an attractive choice over Fosamax and Actonel was the fact that you took it just *once a month*. Only twelve tablets required all year made it the easy choice. Now that Actonel has a once-a-month product, Boniva no longer has a competitive dosing advantage.

SCIENTIFIC RATIONALE

Boniva is a bisphosphonate in the same class as Fosamax, Actonel, Atelvia, and Reclast. All bisphosphonates have a similar action. They attach to the bone and block its breakdown by interfering with the activity of osteoclasts.

Boniva (ibandronate)
Category
Antiresorptive
Bisphosphonate
Manufacturer
Genentech, part of the Roche Group
Pivotal Fracture Trial
BONE
Fracture Reduction
Spine only

Indications for Osteoporosis
Prevention postmenopausal women
Treatment postmenopausal women
Contraindications
Esophagus problems
Unable to sit or stand upright 60 minutes
Low blood calcium
Swallowing problems
Other Considerations
Stomach or digestive problems
Reduced kidney function
Possible Side Effects
Heartburn or chest pain
Swallowing difficulty
Stomach pain
Diarrhea
Back pain
Bone, joint, or muscle pain
Flu-like symptoms with first doses
Nonhealing sore in mouth or jaw
Atypical femur fracture
Doses
150 mg pill once a month
3 mg injection by vein every 3 months
Additional Information
Special dosing instructions
Note: 60 minute wait required after
   pill before eating or drinking

EFFECTIVENESS

BONE: Oral Ibandronate Osteoporosis Vertebral Fracture Trial in North America and Europe

About three thousand women with postmenopausal osteoporosis were divided equally among three groups: Boniva 2.5 mg pill every day, Boniva 20 mg pill intermittent dose, or dummy placebo pill. The intermittent dose of 20 mg every other day for twelve doses every three months provided a similar total dose to the daily 2.5 mg regimen. The goal was to see if Boniva given in a less frequent, intermittent dosing schedule would reduce the risk of fractures. The subjects were at high risk for spine fractures, since by x-ray all the women had at least one spine fracture and 40 percent had two or more spine fractures.

At the end of three years, women taking either form of Boniva had fracture reduction only at the spine:

Spine fractures on x-ray	52%
Painful spine fractures	49%
Nonspine fractures	no reduction
Hip fractures	no reduction

No reduction was seen in nonspine fractures, with a similar number of fractures occurring in each group. The number of fractures reported at individual nonspine sites, including the hip, wrist, leg, pelvis, and ribs, were the same for those taking Boniva and those taking placebo pills. Boniva is not as effective as the other bisphosphonates in lowering the risk of all types of fractures.

A further analysis performed after the initial analysis showed fracture benefit at nonspine sites in a smaller group of study subjects with lower hip bone density. Higher risk women, defined by a bone density T-score of -3.0 and lower at the femoral neck, had decreased risk of nonspine fracture. If you fit that bone density profile, Boniva will likely be an effective medicine for lowering your risk of fractures. For women with higher bone density, you may want to consider another choice of medicine.

OTHER STUDIES

MOBILE: Monthly Oral Ibandronate in Ladies

After the BONE study found that the intermittent dosing had similar fracture reduction at the spine, MOBILE investigated different dosing regimens. Four groups of four hundred postmenopausal women with osteoporosis were given either daily or different monthly doses of Boniva. After two years, women receiving Boniva 150 mg monthly had the largest bone density increases at the spine and hip.

It is important to note that the 150 mg dose is double the dose used in the BONE study, which showed fracture reduction at the spine. What is not known: Does higher bone density achieved with the higher dose translate into more effective lowering of fracture risk for nonspine and hip fractures?

DIVA Study (Dosing Intravenous Administration)

This clinical trial found that a shot into the vein, called an intravenous (IV) injection, of 2 mg of Boniva every two months and 3 mg of Boniva every three months is equivalent to the effectiveness and safety of a daily 2.5 mg dose. At two years, increases in lumbar spine bone density with intravenous administration were higher compared with the daily oral dose. The FDA approved the intravenous regimen of 3 mg every three months.

SAFETY

As with other bisphosphonates, about one in ten subjects complained of heartburn, but fewer complained of stomach pain, nausea, and vomiting. Similar numbers of study subjects reported these problems regardless of whether they were in Boniva or placebo groups. Contact your doctor if you have heartburn or worsening heartburn while taking Boniva.

The once-a-month dose is more likely to involve flu-like symptoms than more frequent dosing regimens. About one in eleven may experience this side effect, called an "acute phase reaction," which occurs within three days of taking Boniva.

Postmarketing reports of jawbone problems and muscle and joint pain that can be severe led the FDA to issue a warning for all bisphosphonates. In addition, you will receive a "Medication Guide" with each prescription or administration of Boniva. This applies to all bisphosphonates and is required by the FDA in response to concerns about rare femur fractures that may occur below the hip in individuals taking this class of medicines.

EASE OF USE

Boniva fits the bill. You only need to think about it once a month. *Don't forget!* Boniva literature encourages you to designate a "Boniva Day" to help you remember. Mark your calendar.

The special instructions below must be followed to ensure that the tablet reaches your stomach and the medicine is well absorbed.

Take the tablet with a full glass of water in the morning before you eat, drink, or take other medicines. You must wait *one hour, a full 60 minutes,* after taking the pill before you can eat or drink or take any other pill of any kind. You must remain upright during the whole hour. (Note: This is double the time of dosing regimen for Fosamax and Actonel.) Remember, this includes lying down to do your exercise stretches—don't do them until sixty minutes have passed. It is a good time for a nice, long, morning walk.

What if you miss a dose? Do not take it when you think about it later in the day. Wait until the morning of the next day. Take your forgotten pill only if it is more than seven days before your next scheduled dose.

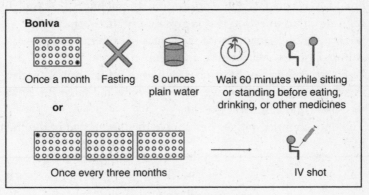

Tim Gunther, gunthergraphics.biz

WHAT SHOULD I EXPECT?

Check back with your doctor after your first dose to let him know that you are taking the tablets in the prescribed way and that you have not had any problems. If you do develop any side effects, you may not have the same problem with one of the other bisphosphonate pills. Talk with your doctor about your options.

In a clinical trial (MOBILE) after two years of treatment with Boniva 150 mg once a month, the average bone mineral density increases were:

Lumbar spine:	6%
Total hip:	4%
Femoral neck:	3%
(neck region of hip)	

Changes observed on your first follow-up DXA at two years may differ; improvement in BMD or no changes are both considered positive response to therapy.

FINAL NOTES

Boniva is approved for prevention and treatment of postmenopausal osteoporosis. It has no other indications. An intravenous formulation is reserved usually for women who are unable to stand or sit upright for sixty minutes, are unable to tolerate pills, or have esophageal or stomach problems.

Boniva's patent expires March 2012 unless legal challenges hold off generic equivalents awhile longer.

The Bare Bones

- Boniva is usually given as a once-a-month pill but is also available as an intravenous injection that is given every three months.
- Boniva is in the same class of medicines—bisphosphonates— as Fosamax, Actonel, Atelvia, and Reclast.
- Fracture effectiveness at spine is similar to other bisphosphonates.
- Fracture reduction at hip was observed only in a subgroup of women with low bone density at the hip.
- The once-monthly pill dose is double the dose tested in the fracture trial.

Reclast: Just Once a Year

Once a year! How can that be possible? The other medicines in the same class, bisphosphonates, were all tested in fracture trials with a once-a-day regimen, and Boniva stretched out the interval dosing to three months. How can a "relative" possibly be so different? If you think of your own relatives, you understand right away! You only need to take Reclast (zoledronic acid) intermittently because this medicine is thought to "recycle" in and out of bone. In a sense, the bone is on autopilot. Also, Reclast is given only by an infusion into your vein, which takes away any worries about absorption of medicine or digestive problems. Some people are not good about taking their medicine; this dosing method ensures that you get the medicine.

SCIENTIFIC RATIONALE

Reclast is a bisphosphonate. Its mode of action is the same as bisphosphonates in pill form. You may refer to the diagram in the Fosamax section to see its effect on the osteoclast activity. Reclast binds strongly to the bone and may later be released to recycle.

Reclast (zoledronic acid)
Category
Antiresorptive
Bisphosphonate
Manufacturer
Novartis
Pivotal Fracture Trial
HORIZON
Fracture Reduction
Spine
Nonspine
Hip
Indications for Osteoporosis
Treatment postmenopausal women
Prevention postmenopausal women
Men

Steroid-induced prevention

Steroid-induced treatment

Contraindications

Low blood calcium

Other Considerations

Reduced kidney function

Blood test for creatinine should be
   checked before each dose

Caution if aspirin-sensitive

Possible Side Effects

Fever, headache and flu-like symptoms
   within 3 days after dose

Nausea

Diarrhea

Bone, joint, or muscle pain

Nonhealing sore in mouth or jaw

Atypical femur fracture

Doses

5 mg given by infusion in your vein
   once a year

Prevention dose 5 mg every 2 years

Additional Information

Taking 2 acetaminophen (Tylenol®) before
   the infusion may decrease flu-like symptoms

Drink plenty of water the day before and
   2 glasses before dose

Zometa® is same medicine; don't take both

EFFECTIVENESS

HORIZON PFT: Health Outcomes and Reduced Incidence with Zoledronic Acid Once Yearly, Pivotal Fracture Trial

This pivotal fracture trial investigated once-yearly infusion of Reclast 5 mg in 7,700 postmenopausal women with osteoporosis. The criteria for entry in this study were designed to create a "real world" situation that included women who had taken similar medicines. Therefore, most of the women had been on osteoporosis treatment and one-fifth of the women also continued taking their regular osteoporosis medicines (not other bisphosphonates or Forteo) during the study. Their average age of seventy-three was a little older than the average age of subjects in other fracture trials. About two-thirds of all participants started the study with one or more spine fractures.

After three years, potent fracture reduction was seen for all sites:

Spine fractures by x-ray	70%
Painful spine fractures	77%
Nonspine fractures	25%
Hip fractures	41%

HORIZON Recurrent Fracture Trial: Health Outcomes and Reduced Incidence with Zoledronic Acid Once Yearly Recurrent Fracture Trial

The Horizon Recurrent Fracture Trial was completely different from any previous fracture study. All 2,100 men and women had a recent hip fracture. With the increased risk of another fracture, would these high-risk patients benefit from treatment? This study set out to prove what we have been "preaching"— treat to prevent the next fracture. Within ninety days of their hip fracture, participants received an infusion of either Reclast or placebo and the infusions were repeated at one-year intervals.

Rather than a set time frame, the end of this study occurred when a preset number of fractures occurred. The study lasted almost two years. Total fractures were reduced by 35 percent and painful spine fractures were reduced by about half. Spine x-rays were not done.

The exciting results of the study went beyond the fracture reduction, which was impressive in itself. The number of deaths was lower in the Reclast group; their death rate was 28 percent lower. This is a first for any study on bone, and it is an important result. Though the "why" has not been determined, the Reclast group had fewer deaths due to pneumonia and irregular heart rhythms. These observations suggest that Reclast may have immune or anti-inflammatory effects that explain the observed improved survival.

Reclast, given any time two to twelve weeks after hip fracture, showed effectiveness in decreasing risk of fracture and death. Therefore, this is the time interval after hip fracture for administration of Reclast to achieve results similar to this study.

SAFETY

Since all bisphosphonates are eliminated through the kidney, it is important to know your kidney function. A blood test for creatinine, which is a measure of your kidney function, should be checked before each annual dose is given. Be sure you stay well hydrated. You should drink plenty of water the day or two prior to your infusion. Drinking a couple glasses of water before your infusion is also recommended.

Since the medicine is given by vein, you do not need to worry about irritation of the esophagus or stomach. The infusion of Reclast can cause flu-like symptoms with fever and muscle aches within the first seventy-two hours after receiving the medicine. In the hip fracture study, two acetaminophen (Tylenol) were given to try to prevent those symptoms. Only one in fourteen subjects had fever. You may need a few additional doses of acetaminophen if you have any symptoms. Compared with the first infusion, there is usually a reduction in these side effects during subsequent infusions.

Like the other bisphosphonates, Reclast has an FDA warning about post-marketing reports of muscle and joint pain that can be severe and jawbone problems. The higher potency of this medicine may pose a greater risk for jawbone problems. However, cases of osteonecrosis of the jaw were not reported in the fracture trials. On review of the HORIZON PFT data, two possible cases were found: one woman on Reclast, the other on placebo.

You will be given a "Medication Guide" each time you receive Reclast. Atypical femur fractures that occur below the hip in patients on bisphosphonates are rare. Neither the cause nor the risk factors have been established. If you develop pain in your thigh or groin contact your doctor to have your symptom evaluated. The majority of patients had dull aching pain in their thigh prior to this type of fracture.

A type of irregular heart rhythm called atrial fibrillation happened more often in women taking Reclast in HORIZON PFT. On a close examination of these cases, it turns out that the numbers reporting atrial fibrillation were constant in the Reclast group, but fewer subjects in the placebo group reported the problem in the third year. When the comparison was done, it appeared that atrial fibrillation increased in the Reclast group, but the higher relative percentage was actually due to fewer cases in the placebo group.

EASE OF USE

You take care of everything in just one day a year, though the infusion requires some coordination and logistics. Your doctor may refer you to either an infusion center or the hospital to receive your medicine. The actual duration of the infusion is less than half an hour. You will be checked in and then an IV will be started. A small amount of liquid containing the medicine is given to you by vein over fifteen to thirty minutes. Count on an hour or so of total time.

Reclast

2011

2012

Once a year   Drink 2 glasses   Take 2 Tylenol   IV medicine
            of plain water   Acetominophen   given in vein

Tim Gunther, gunthergraphics.biz

WHAT SHOULD I EXPECT?

In the pivotal fracture trial, after two years of treatment with Reclast, the average bone mineral density increases were:

Lumbar spine:	6%
Total hip	4%
Femoral neck	3%
(neck region of hip)	

Changes observed on your first follow-up DXA at two years may differ; improvement in BMD or no change are both considered positive response to therapy.

FINAL NOTES

Reclast is also approved for prevention of osteoporosis. The dose is the same but the interval for use is extended to two years. Reclast is approved for treatment in men with osteoporosis and for prevention and treatment in men and women taking steroids.

Cancer patients are sometimes prescribed the same medicine in a lower dose under a different name, Zometa, which should not be taken with Reclast.

The Bare Bones
- Reclast is the only once-a-year treatment, and it is given by vein.
- Same class, bisphosphonates, as Fosamax, Actonel, Atelvia, and Boniva.
- Potent fracture reduction at all sites.
- Reduces deaths when given within two to twelve weeks after hip fracture.

Estrogens: Effects on Bone

In 2002, the results of the Women's Health Initiative (WHI) rocked our beliefs about estrogen. The use of the combination of estrogen and progesterone in the form of Prempro® showed more harm than good. The increased risk of breast cancer, heart attack, stroke, and blood clots outweighed the lower risk of colon cancer and reduction in fractures.

Overnight, estrogen went from the status of "favored child" to being disinherited. As a result, the use of estrogens changed dramatically.

For bone health, estrogen was moved to the prevention of postmenopausal osteoporosis category only. The additional caveat in the indications specifies that it is not a "first choice" for prevention. Estrogen should be considered only if you are unable to use other nonestrogen medicines.

Estrogen dropped out of the medicine chest as a mainstay of treatment for osteoporosis even though it is bone protective. Its other problems overshadowed its bone benefits. One outcome of the fallout from WHI was investigation of other doses and formulations of estrogens. We now know that quite low doses appear to prevent bone loss, but the effects of lower doses on breast cancer, heart disease, and stroke, are not known.

SCIENTIFIC RATIONALE

Estrogen therapy blocks the breakdown of bone by the osteoclasts. It also restores the estrogen support of bone remodeling that is lost with the transition to menopause. This form of therapy restores an approximate balance between breakdown of bone and formation of bone so that stable bone mass is maintained.

Estrogens (multiple brands)
Category
Antiresorptive
Estrogens
Manufacturer
Multiple
Pivotal Fracture Trial
(WHI)
Fracture Reduction
Spine

Nonspine

Hip

Indications for Osteoporosis

Prevention postmenopausal women

Contraindications

Genital bleeding

History of clotting problems in deep veins
of legs, lung, or eye

Recent heart attack or stroke

History of breast cancer

Other Considerations

Black box warning: risk of heart attack,
stroke, clotting in deep veins of legs,
lungs, or eyes; endometrial and
breast cancer; memory problems

Gallbladder disease

Elevated blood pressure

Abnormal liver function

High triglycerides

Possible Side Effects

Breakthrough bleeding

Breast tenderness

Ankle swelling (edema)

Joint pain

Headache

Dose

Multiple formulations and doses

Additional Information

Use with progesterone to protect
lining of womb (uterus)

Bone loss accelerates with stopping

EFFECTIVENESS

Although estrogen was used for years for the treatment of osteoporosis, there was no formal pivotal fracture trial to show its effectiveness. The evidence was observational and from smaller clinical trials. Women who took estrogen were observed to have fewer fractures when compared with women who did not take estrogen.

WHI: Women's Health Initiative

Fractures were assessed as one of the outcomes in two large estrogen trials, combination estrogen plus progesterone (Prempro) and estrogen alone (Premarin® 0.625 mg daily).

After an average of 5.6 years, women in the combination study had fewer fractures. One-third fewer hip fractures and clinical spine fractures were recorded in the Prempro users. In contrast to the bone-specific trials, spine x-rays were not taken and bone density DXA scans were done only in a small percentage of the participants at three of the forty study sites.

Below are the fracture reduction results after five years of use of a combination of estrogen and progesterone given as Pempro:

Painful spine fractures	35%
Hip fractures	33%
Wrist fractures	29%
All fractures	24%

In the estrogen-alone study, the fracture reduction was similar after an average of seven years of use.

SAFETY

The list of safety issues has grown over the years with the results of the WHI and other large clinical trials using estrogen. A "black box warning" in the package insert for estrogens includes multiple risks, which are highlighted in the summary box.

Are You at Risk for Clotting Problems?

Clotting problems are associated with using both estrogens and the "designer estrogen" Evista®. Do not overlook these potential problems. You may see several terms and abbreviations that refer to clotting problems. The general term for clotting problems is venous thromboembolism (VTE). A clot within a blood vessel is a thrombus. If a piece of the thrombus breaks off and travels to block a blood vessel, thereby cutting off the blood supply to the vessel's destination, that is an embolism. A clotting problem in the deep veins of the legs is called deep vein thrombosis (DVT). A pulmonary embolism (PE) occurs when a clot breaks off and travels to the lung, blocking part of its blood supply. This is a dangerous event.

Not everyone is at equal risk. It is important to understand your risk if you are considering using estrogens or Evista. Following are the general risk factors associated with clotting problems.

Racial Differences. In order of risk: African Americans, Caucasians, Hispanics, and Asians. African Americans are at highest risk, while Asians, at the other end of the spectrum, are at low risk. In addition, African Americans are more likely to suffer the more serious and life-threatening pulmonary embolism.

Age. Your risk increases with age. The older you are, the less likely estrogen is going to be a choice for you.

Family History. About 5 percent of Caucasian women of European ancestry have genetic mutations that make blood tend to clot more easily. (This trait may have evolved to help in surviving childbirth, but it may prove troublesome in later life.) DNA testing is the only way to know for sure whether you have this genetic mutation. Short of DNA testing, the best guide is family history. If someone in your family has had clots, you are at higher risk.

Lifestyle. Think cardiac risk factors: high blood pressure, high cholesterol, and obesity are also factors for increased risk of clotting. This is the main reason African Americans are thought to have higher rates. Some research suggests that using cholesterol-lowering medicines lowers your risk. If you have cardiac risk factors, choose a different type of medicine.

Pill versus Patch. Oral estrogen pills are processed by the liver, so factors that promote clotting may be increased. The patch and gels are absorbed through the skin and bypass the liver. Clotting problems are associated with pills, not patches or skin preparations.

EASE OF USE

Estrogens come in multiple forms and dosages. The lowest dose possible for symptom relief is recommended.

WHAT SHOULD I EXPECT?

Changes are dependent on the dosage of estrogen. You may repeat your bone density after two years of therapy, but don't expect much change if you are on the lower doses. Estrogen, as indicated for prevention, basically maintains your bone mass.

In a clinical trial using the lowest dose estradiol patch (Menostar® patch, which delivers 14 micrograms of estradiol a day) for two years, average bone mineral density changes were:

Lumbar spine:	2.6% improvement
Total hip:	stable no change
Femoral neck:	stable no change
(neck region of hip)	

Changes observed on your first follow-up DXA at two years may differ; improvement in BMD or no change are both considered positive response to therapy. Higher doses may yield better results, but you will want to take the lowest dose possible and avoid long-term use.

FINAL NOTES

Stopping your estrogen therapy will shift bone turnover to overdrive. When estrogen levels drop, the bone-loss machinery revs up just as though you are starting menopause. So-called *catch-up loss* occurs.

In the large observational National Osteoporosis Risk Assessment (NORA) study, women had an increased risk of fracture after stopping their estrogen therapy. This occurs because bone loss resumes at a faster rate when estrogen therapy is discontinued. High bone turnover is a risk factor for fractures. Plan ahead for measures that will decrease your risk. Consider another bone-active medicine to prevent the accelerated bone loss and higher risk of fracture.

The Bare Bones
- Estrogens may be useful in early menopause for control of hot flashes.
- Estrogens help preserve bone mass and lower fracture risk.
- Estrogens are indicated for prevention of osteoporosis, not for treatment.
- Use for short-term not long-term therapy is recommended, using the lowest dose required for control of your symptoms.

Evista:
The Designer Estrogen or "SERM"

You may have noticed that the long titles of clinical trials are often shortened by the use of acronyms. These shortened names, as with nicknames, are used many times without referencing or knowing the full name. Therefore, using an acronym that embodies information about the study is key. In an initial steering committee meeting for the Evista® (raloxifene) fracture trial, a contest to name the study was announced; a bottle of champagne was the prize.

I took a stab at the challenge with a couple of names. At that point, the study drug was known as raloxifene; the brand name was coined later. One of my submissions, ROSE, for Raloxifene Osteoporosis Study Effects, was the top vote getter. Yeah! I was imagining the ease of designing a logo and all the other uses of roses.

A few weeks later, my bubble was burst when the study name was announced as MORE, for the Multiple Outcomes of Raloxifene Evaluation. The reason for the selection turned out to be quite clear, when you consider what raloxifene is. Raloxifene/Evista is a Selective Estrogen Receptor Modulator—"SERM"—and can also be called an Estrogen Agonist/Antagonist—"EAA." It has a split personality. In some tissues, it works like estrogen; in others, it has the opposite effect. The potential of raloxifene/Evista for action at estrogen receptors throughout the body is immense and it effects *more* than just the bone.

Great name and reasoning, but I still thought I had won the contest—after all, my proposed name received the most number of votes. Eventually, I did receive the champagne—a nice bottle of Dom Pérignon®!

Evista: Given a Second Chance

Evista started its life as an anti-breast-cancer compound called keoxifene. It was developed as a medicine to compete with tamoxifen (brand name Nolvadex®, which was approved in 1977). Tamoxifen was the standard of care for postmenopausal women with breast cancer who had undergone lumpectomies; it was used following surgery to decrease the chances of breast cancer coming back. In preclinical testing, keoxifene was found to be no better than tamoxifen and the project was shelved.

Subsequently, studies of tamoxifen showed that it increased bone density. Tamoxifen has a split personality. In the breast, it behaved as an antiestrogen, and in the bone, it looked like an estrogen with positive effects. Eli Lilly and Company's scientists wondered, "Will our similar compound collecting dust on a shelf do that, too?".

Keoxifene was dusted off and rechristened "raloxifene," which we now know by its brand name, Evista. The investigation of Evista's bone effects was positive and the drug development of Evista proceeded.

During the pivotal fracture trial, women on Evista had a 90 percent lower risk of breast cancer. Investigator Dr. Steven Cummings, from the University of California, San Francisco, persuaded Eli Lilly and Company to continue a study with the same women to look further at the breast cancer benefit. In addition, another study compared Evista with tamoxifen in women at high risk for breast cancer. In 2007, ten years after its initial approval for treatment of postmenopausal osteoporosis, Evista received approval both for use in reducing the risk of invasive breast cancer in postmenopausal women with osteoporosis and for use by postmenopausal women at high risk for invasive breast cancer.

SCIENTIFIC RATIONALE

Evista is an antiresorptive, which puts it in the same category as bisphosphonates. It works by mimicking the action of estrogen on the bone to decrease the action of the bone breakdown cells, the osteoclasts. However, it is not as potent as estrogen itself. Evista has a modest effect on bone metabolism. The bone turnover markers decrease about 30 percent compared with the 60 to 70 percent decline observed with bisphosphonates.

Evista
(raloxifene)
Category
Antiresorptive
Selective Estrogen Receptor Modulator
    (SERM) also known as an
Estrogen Agonist/Antagonist (EAA)
Manufacturer
Eli Lilly and Company
Pivotal Fracture Trial
MORE
Fracture Reduction
Spine
Indications for Osteoporosis
Treatment postmenopausal women
Prevention postmenopausal women
Contraindications
Clotting problems in deep veins of legs,
    lung, or eye
Other Considerations
Black box warning: risk of clotting
Fatal strokes in women with or at risk
    for heart attack
Breast cancer survivor
Don't take if you are on estrogen therapy
Possible Side Effects
Hot flashes
Leg cramps
Ankle swelling (edema)
Joint pain
Flu symptoms
Dose
60 mg pill once a day
Additional Information
Lowers risk of invasive breast cancer
Stop three days before long plane flight or
    hospitalization to decrease the chance of
    clotting problems

EFFECTIVENESS

MORE: Multiple Outcomes of Raloxifene Evaluation

For the pivotal fracture trial, a total of 7,700 postmenopausal women were enrolled in a three-year trial. Approximately half of the women had spine fractures identified by x-ray at the beginning of the study, and the other half had bone density in the osteoporosis range. Two doses of Evista were used; a 60 mg group and a 120 mg group were compared with a placebo group. Ultimately, only the daily 60 mg dose was approved by the FDA. For this reason, all results discussed in this section are based on this dosing regime.

The fracture results after three years of treatment with Evista 60 mg a day showed spine effectiveness only:

Spine fractures by x-ray:	50% reduction in women with osteoporosis by bone density only
	30% reduction in women with spine fractures at baseline
Painful spine fractures:	41%
Nonspine fractures:	No reduction
Hip fractures:	No reduction

The placebo group in this study is instructive for the natural history of high-risk women with spine fractures. The study recruitment was done before the approval of Fosamax. At the time, the only choices were estrogen and calcitonin by injection. Even at that time, many women did not want to take estrogen. The placebo group received the standard of care at the time—calcium and vitamin D supplements along with the study pill. Because they had received a bone density test and were participating in an osteoporosis study, they increased their awareness about osteoporosis. They were doing everything possible to improve their bone health.

The majority of women did not know they had a fracture because their fractures had occurred without pain. The spine fractures were identified by x-rays at entry and at each annual study visit. Twenty-one percent of the placebo group fractured another spine level in that short three-year time frame: not good.

CORE: Continuing Outcomes Relevant to Evista Study

With continued use of Evista, the hope was that fracture reduction would be seen in nonspine sites including the hip. The additional four years did not show fracture protection beyond the spine. The numbers of nonspine fractures were similar in the Evista and placebo groups. However, it did demonstrate continued reduction of breast cancer.

Other Studies

Several other large studies investigated other potential health benefits of Evista. The Study of Tamoxifen and Raloxifene (STAR) trial showed that Evista was equivalent to Tamoxifen in lowering the risk of breast cancer in women at higher risk but with fewer side effects. The Raloxifene Use for the Heart (RUTH) trial investigated use of Evista in lowering heart attacks in women with heart disease or risk factors for heart disease. No significant differences were found between those on Evista versus those taking a placebo.

SAFETY

The most common adverse events among women taking Evista were leg cramps that usually decreased and stopped with continued use. Hot flashes and sweats occurred in one in ten women, but they were not severe enough to result in discontinuation of the study medicine. The lining of the uterus (endometrium) was not stimulated although more polyps were reported in the Evista groups.

The clotting risks of 1 to 2 percent are comparable to those associated with estrogen therapy. Refer to the preceding section on estrogen for more on your risk of clotting problems. In 2007, the FDA added a black box warning about blood clotting problems to Evista's label. After review of the recent studies CORE, STAR, and RUTH, the risk of blood clots in the leg, lung, or eye was increased in the Evista groups. The label change included the approval of the new indications for reduction of invasive breast cancer.

EASE OF USE

Evista is a pill taken once a day. There are no special instructions.

WHAT SHOULD I EXPECT?

A repeat bone density test after two years of use is indicated; however, don't expect much of a change. Based on the expected change, you could wait longer for your repeat bone density test.

In the pivotal fracture trial, after two years of treatment with Evista, the average bone mineral density increases were.

Lumbar spine:	2.5%
Total hip:	2%
Femoral neck:	2%
(neck region of hip)	

Changes observed on your first follow-up DXA at two years may differ; improvement in BMD or no change are both considered positive response to therapy.

FINAL NOTES

Small changes in bone density make a big difference in reducing risk of fracture at the spine.

If you have travel planned with a long car ride or plane trip, discontinue your pills three days beforehand to lessen risk of clotting problems in your legs. This recommendation also applies prior to any hospitalization or surgery.

The Bare Bones
- Evista is the only "designer estrogen" or SERM available for prevention and treatment of osteoporosis.
- Evista is taken once a day with no special regimen.
- Eight years of clinical trial experience shows reduction of spine fractures only.
- Evista also reduces the risk of invasive breast cancer.

Calcitonin—Miacalcin, Fortical: The Nasal Sprays

Calcitonin has been an option for a long time. Shots of calcitonin, which is a compound derived from salmon, hit the marketplace in 1986 for treatment of Paget's disease. However, it was not until the nasal formulation of Miacalcin was approved in 1995, just a few months earlier than Fosamax, that it was indicated for treatment of postmenopausal osteoporosis. The use of Miacalcin has never gained traction, due to lack of effectiveness. It was suggested that use of Miacalcin may improve bone quality but this was never proven. The indication is for treatment of postmenopausal osteoporosis in women more than five years after menopause, which is beyond the period of rapid loss.

In 2005, Fortical, a recombinant version of calcitonin, was approved by the FDA based on its equivalence to Miacalcin. In the FDA review of effectiveness from the work done on Miacalcin, it was concluded that the evidence supported increases in bone density only at the spine. As a result, a label change for Miacalcin reflects a "downgrade" from prevention of spine fractures to spine bone density changes.

Despite the lack of good evidence for fracture reduction, calcitonin continues to be prescribed because it is easy to use and there are few side effects. It is used more often in the nursing home setting and some areas of the country, reflecting regional variations of practice. For instance, in a study of nursing homes in North Carolina and Arizona, 14 percent of those treated with prescription medicines for osteoporosis were receiving Miacalcin.

SCIENTIFIC RATIONALE

Calcitonin is a natural hormone produced in the cells of your thyroid gland. It contributes to calcium regulation in the bone, kidney, and intestine. In bone, calcitonin blocks bone breakdown by decreasing the number and activity of osteoclasts. The decrease in bone breakdown markers is only 12 percent, a mild reduction in comparison to the potent bisphosphonates and Prolia.

Miacalcin
(calcitonin-salmon)
Category
Antiresorptive
Biologic hormone
Manufacturer
Novartis
Pivotal Fracture Trial
PROOF
Fracture Reduction
Increase spine bone density
No fracture reduction or effect on hip
    bone density
Indications for Osteoporosis
Treatment postmenopausal women
    five years after menopause
Contraindications
Allergy to calcitonin-salmon
Other Considerations
Lack of effectiveness
Possible Side Effects
Nasal irritation
(Nausea and irritation at injection site
    for shot)
Doses
Metered nasal spray 200 IU daily
Alternate nostrils each day
(available as injection 100 IU daily)
Additional Information
Generic available for nasal spray
Fortical approved based on equivalence
    to Miacalcin

EFFECTIVENESS

PROOF: Prevent Recurrence of Osteoporotic
Fractures Study

This fracture trial was not conducted in a standard randomized, double-blind fashion. The doctors who had patients in the study saw the results of the bone density tests. This led to a high dropout rate. At the end of five years, only about half of the 1,100 participants remained in the study.

A total of three doses of the Miacalcin nasal spray were used: 100 IU, 200 IU, and 400 IU. The fracture reduction was only seen in the 200 IU dose, which was chosen for the marketed dose of Miacalcin. However, because so many women who lost bone density did not finish the study, this observation may not be valid.

The fracture reduction after five years of use of Miacalcin 200 IU was:

Spine fractures by x-ray:	33%
Nonspine fractures:	no reduction
Hip fractures:	no reduction

SAFETY

The most common problems are related to the nasal spray local effects. About one in ten subjects experienced nasal irritation and nasal symptoms, such as crusting. To minimize the delivery effects, you should alternate the spray from nostril to nostril.

Nausea and mild abdominal discomfort with bloating or fullness may occur with the shot form of Miacalcin. These side effects may occur when you first start treatment, but they usually disappear with time. They may be minimized if Miacalcin is taken at bedtime.

EASE OF USE

Administering the nasal spray requires one spray once a day. Remember to alternate nostrils each day. Miacalcin shots are prescribed infrequently and require that you either learn how to give the shot to yourself or have someone else give you the daily shot under the skin.

WHAT SHOULD I EXPECT?

Expect to see very little variation in your bone density, since calcitonin has a minimal effect. It may take longer than two years to see a positive response (improvement or no change in BMD), if any. In the pivotal fracture trial, after two years of treatment with Miacalcin, the average bone mineral density changes were:

Lumbar spine:	1%
Total hip:	no change
Femoral neck:	no change
(neck region of hip)	

FINAL NOTES

If you have suffered a painful spine fracture, Miacalcin may be tried for pain control. This use is "off label." You will find a description in the section titled "Off Label Uses: What Else Is Being Treated?" (see page 242).

Since salmon is the source of Miacalcin, a potential exists for development of antibodies over time. Fortical was developed to provide a human calcitonin source as an option.

The Bare Bones
- Calcitonin has minimal effect on preventing the breakdown of bone.
- Calcitonin is not effective in reducing risk of fractures but may increase bone density in the spine.
- Calcitonin is easy to use but other options for treatment should be explored.

Forteo:
A Different Approach

Forteo brings to mind the children's nursery rhyme "Humpty Dumpty." Forteo (teriparatide) does something none of the other medicines can do: It puts back together connections that have broken. You can put Humpty Dumpty back together again with Forteo.

Forteo is an anabolic or bone formation agent. It is the only medicine that targets osteoblasts, the bone building cells. In contrast, all the other osteoporosis medicines' actions are directed at the osteoclasts, the bone breakdown cells.

SCIENTIFIC RATIONALE

Forteo is the first portion of the parathyroid hormone. Your own parathyroid hormone is produced by four small parathyroid glands that sit just behind the thyroid gland in your neck. Its sole purpose is control of your body's calcium. If you do not get enough calcium in what you eat or from a supplement, your parathyroid glands receive a warning signal: *calcium levels low*. They produce more parathyroid hormone, which causes calcium to be released from the bone, and over time this produces bone loss.

If too much parathyroid hormone causes bone loss, how does giving more parathyroid hormone in the form of Forteo help build bone? A high constant level of parathyroid hormone is what causes problems. Forteo produces a short burst of parathyroid hormone. The extra parathyroid hormone in the short burst generates bone formation by turning on osteoblasts independent of the bone remodeling cycle. It reverses remodeling imbalance and the resorption pits are overfilled in response. The osteoblasts increase in number from precursor cells, work harder, and live longer. In addition, Forteo speeds up the bone remodeling cycle. New bone is formed, connections are reestablished, and bone volume is increased by these actions.

Forteo
(teriparatide)
Category
Anabolic: bone formation
Biologic hormone
Manufacturer
Eli Lilly and Company
Pivotal Fracture Trial
Fracture Prevention Trial
Fracture Reduction
Spine
Nonspine
Indications for Osteoporosis
Treatment for postmenopausal women
   at high risk for fracture
Men
Steroid-induced treatment
Contraindications
Children and young adults
History of radiation therapy involving
   the skeleton
Cancer in bone
Other bone diseases
High blood calcium
Other Considerations
History of kidney stones
Possible Side Effects
Pain
Joint aches
Nausea
Leg cramps
Increase in blood calcium
Dose
Pen prefilled with 28 daily doses of
   20 micrograms
Automatic injection under the skin once
   a day; rotate sites on thigh or abdomen
Keep pen refrigerated
Additional Information
Black box warning risk of osteosarcoma
   in rats
Voluntary patient registry
Maximum lifetime use 2 years
Follow with other therapy to maintain gains

EFFECTIVENESS

Fracture Prevention Trial

The pivotal fracture trial enrolled over 1,600 postmenopausal women with spine fractures and lasted about twenty months. The women were at high risk for spine fractures, and almost two-thirds of the women had two or more spine fractures at entry. Two doses of Forteo, 20 and 40 micrograms, were tested in comparison with a placebo. Forteo was given as a once-a-day shot.

Few hip fractures occurred during this short study time. With less than two years of treatment with Forteo, fracture reduction was robust at the spine and nonspine:

Spine fractures by x-ray:	65%
Nonspine fractures:	53%
Hip fractures:	too few fractures

SAFETY

The Fracture Prevention Trial was planned as a three-year study. However, during the second year of the study, laboratory rats developed tumors of the bone called osteosarcoma. These animals received higher doses than those used in the fracture trial. However, the clinical trial was stopped to investigate the appearance of the bone tumor in the rats. After several years, Forteo was FDA-approved with a "black box warning" in the printed package insert about the occurrence of osteosarcoma in rats at higher doses.

Forteo is contraindicated in situations that would put someone at higher risk for development of osteosarcoma. Therefore, Forteo is not given to children or young adults who have not completed their growth. It should not be used by anyone with cancer in the bone, other bone diseases, or history of radiation therapy involving the skeleton. The radiation history excludes women who have had radiation treatment after breast surgery and men with prostate cancer who have received radiation or have cancer that has spread to their bones.

The median time of studying drug use in the Fracture Prevention Trial was nineteen months. The longest duration of medicine exposure was up to two years. Therefore, the use of Forteo is limited to twenty-four months total for your entire lifetime.

The most common adverse events are leg cramps, which usually go away with continued use. First doses may cause decrease in blood pressure, so you may want to take your dose at bedtime to start.

EASE OF USE

Forteo is a shot that you learn to give to give to yourself every day for twenty-four months. The idea of a shot is a big barrier for many who are considering this medicine but it shouldn't be. It is easy to learn how to administer the shot and the time is limited to two years, so you won't have to give yourself shots forever. Forteo is supplied in a pen syringe that holds enough medicine for twenty-eight days of use. The injection is "automatic," like pushing the top of a ballpoint pen. The needles are tiny, which makes the shots almost painless. A new needle is attached each day and you rotate sites of injection on your lower abdomen and upper legs. The syringe needs to be refrigerated. Do not leave it out after you use it. After disposing of the used needle in a "sharps" container, return the syringe to the refrigerator right away.

A handy tip is to write the end date on the syringe with a permanent maker. That way you will have your last day of use for the syringe. You will not have to keep track and count the number of days along the way.

If you go on a short vacation or trip, you may skip packing your Forteo because of the refrigeration logistics. Resume daily use on your return. For long trips, a travel pouch is included in your starter kit. Your doctor may need to write a letter for the TSA airport security explaining that you must carry needles on board in your hand baggage.

You should plan on taking the first couple of doses at bedtime because of the potential of having lower blood pressure upon standing. After the first week, take the medicine when it is convenient for you.

WHAT SHOULD I EXPECT?

You will be rechecking your bone density after you finish your two years of use. Your bone density changes may depend on whether you used another medicine before Forteo. The specific medicine you used prior to taking Forteo may make a difference, too.

In the pivotal fracture trial with Forteo, which was shorter than two years, the average bone mineral density increases after a median treatment of nineteen months were:

Lumbar spine:	9.7%
Total hip:	2.6%
Femoral neck	2.8%
(neck region of hip)	

Forteo increases bone density and bone size. Therefore, your repeat DXA may underestimate your actual gains. The density does not give you a measure of the microstructure changes that occurred while you were taking Forteo.

THE EFFECT OF FORTEO ON MICROSTRUCTURE

The bone formation effect of Forteo is shown in these images from bone biopsies of the iliac crest (pelvic bone) taken before and after a course of Forteo. This patient was a sixty-two-year-old woman with osteoporosis who enrolled in the Fracture Prevention Trial (Neer et al *NEJM* 2002). She received Forteo 20 microgams per day for twenty-two months. Her DXA lumbar spine BMD increased by 10.4 percent and her femoral neck BMD increased by 1.4 percent.

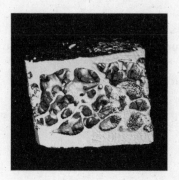

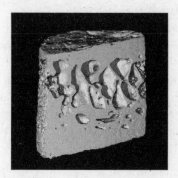

"before" Forteo treatment   "after" Forteo treatment

These improvements in bone microstructure and increases in bone size are only seen with Forteo. Its different mechanism of action stimulates the bone-forming cells, osteoblasts, to cause these dramatic changes.

FINAL NOTES

Forteo is intended for postmenopausal women with a high risk for fracture. The lumbar spine response is robust and builds bone. If your spine bone density is low or you have already had spine fractures, this medicine is a good choice to reduce your risk of spine fractures.

The biggest dilemma with Forteo is what to take when you have reached the two-year limit of your course of treatment. When Forteo is stopped after two years of use, bone density rapidly decreases. Therefore, you will need to select another osteoporosis medicine to maintain the gains you made while using Forteo. Before your prescription runs out, make plans with your doctor to make the next choice in your treatment plan.

Forteo is also approved for the treatment of steroid-induced osteoporosis. Although this trial lasted for three years, all uses of Forteo are approved by the FDA for two years only.

As part of the FDA's safety program, a monitoring system is in place for surveillance of osteosarcoma. So far, almost ten years after approval, no excess risk of osteosarcoma has emerged.

The Bare Bones

- Forteo is the only bone formation medicine available.
- Forteo is taken as a shot you give yourself under the skin once a day.
- Forteo is limited to a total lifetime use of two years.
- Another osteoporosis medicine should be started after two years of use to preserve bone gained while on Forteo.

Prolia: In a Class of Its Own

Watching the Academy Awards, you can feel the excitement mixed with tension build until the moment the envelope is unsealed and the results are revealed. The same palpable atmosphere was the experience of waiting for the Prolia (denosumab) results to be presented at an international bone research meeting in 2008. We were all atwitter with speculation about the findings of this novel drug's pivotal fracture trial.

The medicine was the result of an exciting discovery in bone biology made in 1995 when scientists first learned how the bone cells talked to one another. The bone cycle is a well-choreographed dance of the osteoclasts and osteoblasts working together. It was not clear what the cells used for signals to communicate with one another. Researchers found that the osteoblasts were the conductors of the dance. The osteoblasts sent signals to the osteoclasts via messengers. Prolia latches on to the messengers, so they cannot deliver their message.

SCIENTIFIC RATIONALE

Prolia is targeted at the osteoclasts. Therefore, it is an antiresorptive, which is the same category as bisphosphonates. However, Prolia is in a class of its own; it is designated a "monoclonal antibody." Prolia is a molecule that binds to the messenger between osteoblasts and osteoclasts.

The messenger's job is to kick-start the development of osteoclasts and tell them that it's time to work. Prolia treatment reduces the number of osteoclasts that are made, function, or survive. You can think of Prolia as birth control for osteoclasts. The shorthand scientific name for this action is called RANKL inhibition; RANKL is the messenger that communicates between the osteoblasts and the osteoclasts.

Prolia is potent and decreases bone turnover markers by about 80 percent within days. Since Prolia does not bind to the bone, it does not linger in the body once treatment is stopped. This is an advantage if you are worried about a medicine staying in your bones. But the downside is that you will start losing bone, and stopping Prolia may even cause bone loss more quickly.

Prolia
(denosumab)
Category
Antiresorptive
Biologic monoclonal antibody
RANKL inhibitor
Manufacturer
Amgen
Pivotal Fracture Trial
FREEDOM
Fracture Reduction
Spine
Nonspine
Hip
Indications for Osteoporosis
Treatment for postmenopausal women
    at high risk for fracture
Contraindications
Low blood calcium
Other Considerations
Caution if immune system is weakened
    by medicines or illnesses
Decrease in bone turnover
Possible Side Effects
Serious infections
Skin reactions and infections
Pain in back, muscles, arms, and legs
Bladder infection
Nonhealing sore in mouth or jaw
Doses
Shot administered in your doctor's office
Prefilled 60 mg dose given under the skin
    once every six months
Additional Information
Voluntary patient support program
Stopping leads to increase in bone
    turnover and bone loss

EFFECTIVENESS

FREEDOM: Fracture Reduction Evaluation of Denosumab in Osteoporosis Every Six Months

The pivotal fracture trial enrolled 7,800 postmenopausal women in a three-year trial. In contrast to other trials, subjects in this study ranged in age from sixty to ninety years old. However, fewer women had spine fractures at the beginning of the study. Approximately one-quarter of subjects were enrolled based on having a spine fracture and low bone density, while the others had bone density in the osteoporosis range.

Subjects received a shot of Prolia or placebo solution under the skin once every six months for three years. A total of six shots were given to each study participant over the course of the study.

After three years, Prolia reduced fracture at all sites:

Spine fractures by x-ray	68%
Painful spine fractures	69%
Nonspine fractures	20%
Hip fractures	41%

SAFETY

The reporting of side effects for Prolia is confusing because the FDA made a change to highlight problems even though the drug may not cause them. The top five adverse events reported were back pain, pain in arms or legs, muscle pain, high cholesterol, and bladder infections. These were the most common in the Prolia group *and* in the placebo group. Numbers were similar in both groups, but they were a little bit higher in the Prolia group. For example, back pain in the Prolia group was 34.7 percent versus 34.6 percent in the placebo group.

However, more subjects who received Prolia had skin problems, like eczema and skin infections. Serious infections were more frequent with Prolia (4.1 percent) versus placebo (3.4 percent). Other possible side effects include low levels of calcium in your blood and jaw problems called osteonecrosis of the jaw.

The extension of FREEDOM and the other clinical trials will provide longer-term safety data. In addition, a voluntary patient program is in place to capture additional safety information.

EASE OF USE

How you take Prolia is different. You make a visit to your doctor's office to have the shot given to you twice a year—every six months. The shot is given under the skin with a small needle in the upper arm, abdomen, or thigh. Local reactions at the shot site are uncommon. You do not need to do anything special beforehand or afterward.

A program sponsored by Amgen called Prolia Plus is available to you. It helps with reminders for when your next shot of Prolia is due and it will also provide periodic educational materials.

What If You Miss a Dose?

Make arrangements with your doctor's office to get your shot as soon as possible. The effects on the bone-breakdown cells disappear quickly. You do not want a long gap after the six-month interval when your repeat shot is due.

WHAT SHOULD I EXPECT?

In the pivotal fracture trial, after two years of treatment with Prolia, the average bone mineral density increases were:

Lumbar spine:	8%
Total hip:	4%
Femoral neck:	3%
(neck region of hip)	

Changes observed on your first follow-up DXA at two years may differ; improvement in BMD or no change are both considered positive response to therapy.

FINAL NOTES

In 2007, the FDA initiated a safety program for all new medicine approvals. For Prolia, a voluntary program has been set up for physicians to participate in with their patients. Prior to receiving each dose of the medicine, your doctor will ask you questions about possible side effects.

Prolia is intended for postmenopausal women with high risk for fracture. It may be an option if you did not tolerate osteoporosis medicines in pill form or if you did not achieve positive results with other medicines. Those with reduced kidney function can also take this medicine safely.

Other clinical trials with Prolia are in progress or have already been completed. These research studies are investigating the use of denosumab for other individuals who are at high risk for fracture and for patients with different cancers who are at risk for their cancer spreading to the bone (metastases). A higher dose of denosumab, branded as Xgeva®, is FDA-approved for the prevention of skeletal-related events in patients with bone metastases from solid tumors, such as breast or prostate cancer.

You may be at risk for bone loss after stopping Prolia, similar to what happens with discontinuing estrogen. Before stopping this medicine, discuss with your doctor options to ensure that you maintain your gains.

The Bare Bones
- Prolia is the first osteoporosis medicine in the class of therapy called "monoclonal antibody."
- Prolia is indicated to treat high-risk postmenopausal women with osteoporosis.
- Prolia is given as a shot in your doctor's office every six months.
- Prolia is effective in lowering risk of fractures at all sites.

Combination Therapy:
Are Two Really Better Than One?

Does it make sense to use two medicines instead of just one? Using two medicines runs the risk of more side effects. The cost of two medicines needs to be factored in as well. A combination of two medicines that work by different mechanisms may make sense. Therefore, different combinations of medicines have been evaluated by measuring bone density and monitoring safety in clinical trials.

ANTIRESORPTIVE COMBINATIONS (TWO MEDICATIONS THAT DECREASE BONE BREAKDOWN)

Bisphosphonates Plus Estrogen

Fosamax plus estrogen, tested in the form of Premarin 0.625 mg, resulted in higher bone density than either medicine alone. At the end of two years, the combination increased bone density at the spine by more than two percent over and above the changes seen with Fosamax or estrogen alone. If you are already taking estrogen and add Fosamax, you can expect a small boost in your bone density, too. Actonel used in combination with estrogen in early postmenopausal women and added to an ongoing estrogen therapy regimen increased bone density more than a single drug. Combining estrogen with other bisphosphonates may also yield increased bone density benefit, but studies have not been done.

Bisphosphonates Plus Evista

The combination of Evista plus a bisphosphonate makes sense. If you are taking Evista for reducing your risk of breast cancer but you have a high risk of hip fracture, Evista may not be enough to reduce your fracture risk. Adding a bisphosphonate may be beneficial, although fracture risk has not been assessed. This combination increases bone density like a "light estrogen."

YOUR STORIES...

Janice, age sixty-two, checked her bone density after her eighty-six-year-old mother fell and broke her hip. Janice had T-scores of -3.2 at the spine and -2.8 at the hip. When her sister was diagnosed with breast cancer three years earlier, Janice started taking Evista, so she never thought she was at risk for osteoporosis.

After her DXA scan did show osteoporosis, her doctor ordered blood work, and she collected her urine for twenty-four hours. Her vitamin D level, at 18 ng/ml, was below the recommended minimum level of 30 ng/ml. Everything else was in the normal range.

What to do? Evista is still indicated for lowering her breast cancer risk, but it may not be enough to lower her risk of fracture. She and her doctor decided that the next step was to add a bisphosphonate, and generic alendronate was the preferred choice by her health plan.

However, she decided to wait and repeat a bone density in a year to see whether she continued to lose ground while taking Evista. In addition, she wanted time to "clean up" her habits, start back on an exercise program, pay attention to her daily calcium intake, and increase her vitamin D.

ONE ANTIRESORPTIVE AGENT PLUS BONE BUILDER, FORTEO

The effects on bone density have been studied when Forteo and some of the other medicines are given in combination either both at the same time or sequentially—one after the other. However, bone density measured by DXA does not tell the whole story. The three-dimensional microstructure changes expected with Forteo are not captured with two-dimensional DXA scans. They also may underestimate change because bone size increases with Forteo.

Combination results may depend on the bisphosphonate. Taking Forteo and bisphosphonates at the same time produces different responses depending on which bisphosphonate is being used. Fosamax blunts the response and appears to inhibit the bone-forming effects of Forteo therapy. Actonel combined with Forteo did not blunt Forteo's effect; however, it did not show an added effect either.

A study done with Reclast and Forteo suggests that bone density increases faster when these two medicines are combined than when either medicine is used alone. Although spine bone density was similar for combination versus Forteo alone, hip bone density was better with the combination.

For now, a combination of Forteo and a bisphosphonate is not recommended, and in the case of Fosamax, it is not helpful.

These observations may explain the responses when Forteo follows treatment with Fosamax or Actonel, which is common practice. Forteo therapy after Fosamax may show a smaller improvement in bone density rather than a robust increase at the spine. Forteo therapy after Actonel shows the expected bone density increases. Previous use of Actonel does not appear to decrease the response to Forteo.

Bisphosphonates given after Forteo therapy are beneficial. Immediate use of bisphosphonates after completing a twenty-four-month course of Forteo is needed to maintain the increases in bone density. If no treatment follows Forteo therapy, bone density gains are lost.

The dilemma for you may be choosing which medicine to take. Some of you may have switched to Forteo because of difficulty with a bisphosphonate or concern that it was not working.

Combination with estrogens or Evista does not appear to interfere with response to Forteo therapy. If you are already taking estrogen or Evista, you can add Forteo and expect a good response.

Forteo in Combination with Other Osteoporosis Medicines

The bone density response using Forteo at the same time as another osteoporosis drug varies depending on the individual medicine. The majority of combinations do not add to the benefit of Forteo used alone and, in the case of Fosamax, there is actually decreased response. Therefore, combining Forteo with bisphosphonates is not recommended at this time. The new data for Reclast suggest that combination with Forteo may yield benefit, and this combination may be an option for someone with a high risk of spine and hip fractures.

Forteo Plus...	Bone Density Response
Fosamax (generic alendronate)	Decreased
Actonel	No added benefit
Boniva	No data
Reclast	Faster increases Added benefit at hip
Estrogen	No added benefit
Evista	No added benefit

Reassess the Reason for Medicines

Before adding any medicine, make sure that you should still be taking your original medicine. Estrogens or Evista along with another osteoporosis medicine are the combinations that may be helpful if there are other indications for their use. Keep in mind that estrogens are recommended for short-term use. If you have been on estrogen for longer than five years, discuss its continued use with your doctor. In the case of Forteo, combination therapy does not necessarily mean added benefit and is not recommended at this time.

The Bare Bones
- Taking two osteoporosis medicines is not usually necessary.
- Using Evista or estrogen, if needed for other indications, may be useful.
- Do not take Forteo at the same time as a bisphosphonate.
- Do follow Forteo with another osteoporosis medicine to preserve bone gain.

Making a Choice:
How Do the Medicines Compare?

Everyone always wants to know how the medicines stack up against one another. The only accurate way to answer the question is to include all of the osteoporosis medicines in one gigantic study. The medicines would need to be evaluated in a "head-to-head" comparison focused on fractures in similar study participants. Any fracture comparison study would require more than sixty thousand subjects. It is unlikely that such a study will be done. At the present time, there are only several small studies that compare bone density changes using two different medicines at a time.

Hopefully you have come to this point reassured that your risk is high enough for you to benefit from prescription medicine. It is time to figure out "which medicine is right for me." Take your time to weigh the options. Starting treatment is not an emergency. Do not go into panic mode. You have time to make your decision—unless you are on high-dose steroids that cause rapid bone loss or you have had a recent fracture. During your education and investigation phase, the first step is to optimize your nutrition, exercise, and calcium and vitamin D.

Do not do everything at once. Take a graduated approach; go slow and add one thing at a time. In this way, if an issue arises, like a side effect, you will be able to pinpoint the most likely cause. Is your stomach upset from the new pill or from the calcium supplement? If you need calcium supplementation of your diet, make sure you are tolerating the calcium supplements first before adding an osteoporosis medicine. If your vitamin D is low, take the next two to three months to bring your levels up above 30 ng/ml. Some research suggests that you may be less likely to have muscle pains with bisphosphonates if your vitamin D levels are within normal range. Research in animals showed that jawbone problems are more likely with low vitamin D levels. *Take your time.*

Prevention and treatment involve many aspects. Minimize your risks by changing whatever is in your control. A prescription is an important part of therapy, but it's certainly not the only part. For example, the majority of serious injuries and fractures are a result of falls. Fall prevention is key. Work on improving your balance and muscle strength.

Compare and contrast to individualize your choices. The task for you and your doctor is to compare your potential choices by looking at the individual medicines and their clinical trial results. Effectiveness in reduction of fractures is of prime importance. Review the summary of the medicines' effectiveness in reducing the risk of fractures. Your history and individual situation will provide a guide for your best options. Your preferences for pills versus other forms of delivery, your history of an ulcer or blood clots, a family history of breast cancer, whether your spine bone density is lower than your hip bone density or vice versa; these are all types of considerations that will factor into your decision.

Reality check: What does your healthcare plan cover? You may want to use a particular medicine but find that your insurance does not cover it or that you have to start with another medicine first. Find out what your healthcare plan covers as its first tier. Most likely it will be generic alendronate, since it is the lowest in price. I did not include the costs of medicines, which are a big consideration, because the "retail" costs are not what you pay out of pocket. Your costs are dependent on your insurance coverage, reimbursement, and co-pays and thus would be impossible to predict. All pharmaceutical companies offer patient assistance programs that may be available to you depending on your financial circumstances. If you are having trouble affording your medicine, talk with your doctor about options.

YOUR STORIES...

Wendy, age sixty-seven, stopped estrogen after twenty years of use because of Women's Health Initiative (WHI) findings and her doctor's recommendations. She has no family history of osteoporosis or any medical problems. She is fit, works out, watches her diet, and doesn't smoke or drink. About two and a half years after stopping estrogen, she had an accident in her home. Her foot got tangled in a footstool, which caused her to fall. She caught herself with her right hand outstretched, breaking her right wrist and left foot. Her baseline bone density was measured at age sixty-five, about the time she stopped taking estrogen. Her follow-up bone density was done just after her fractures. She had lost bone density at both her spine and hip in the two and half year interval. This loss in bone density is shown as percent change in the last column of the following table.

    The bone density shows a significant decline at her hip and spine. This rapid loss is similar to early menopause with the loss of estrogen. Because she had stopped estrogen therapy, Wendy had both accelerated bone loss and an increased risk of fracture.

	Baseline		2 ½ Years Later		% Change	
	BMD	T-Score	BMD	T-Score	From baseline	Per year
Lumbar spine total	1.065	-1.1	0.925	-2.2	-13.1%	-5.3%
Hip neck region	0.779	-1.9	0.737	-2.2	-5.4%	-2.1%
Total hip	0.860	-1.3	0.811	-1.6	-5.7%	-2.3%

Her evaluation included a search for other causes of bone loss. No related problems were uncovered; her healthy lifestyle did not need any major modifications. She decided, in consultation with her doctor, to begin taking medicine to stop her bone loss. Her health plan covered alendronate (generic Fosamax), which she started once a week without any difficulty.

FDA-Approved Medicines for Treatment of Postmenopausal Osteoporosis: Comparison of Fracture Reduction

The goal of therapy is reducing your risk of breaking a bone. These medicines increase bone density, and even modest improvements translate into reduction of fractures. However, the sites of fracture reduction are not uniform. The following table summarizes the types of fracture that were reduced in the pivotal fracture trials of each medicine.

Medicine	Effective in Reducing Fracture Risk by Site		
	Spine	Nonspine	Hip
Fosamax	✓	✓	✓
Actonel and Atelvia	✓	✓	✓
Reclast	✓	✓	✓
Prolia	✓	✓	✓
Estrogen (prevention only)	✓	✓	✓
Forteo	✓	✓	
Evista	✓		
Boniva	✓		
Calcitonin: Miacalcin/Fortical	?		

Generic alendronate is not listed because the fracture trial used brand Fosamax. Generic alendronates had similar characteristics in short-term evaluations that showed the body handles the generic compound in the same manner as the brand.

You should note that estrogen is approved only for prevention of osteoporosis, although a reduction in fractures at all sites is observed with its use. For Boniva, only a subset of women who had T-scores of -3.0 or lower at the neck region of the hip showed fracture reduction at nonspine locations. Forteo is the only bone-formation medicine on the list. Its use is limited to a maximum of twenty-four months and should be followed with another osteoporosis medicine to maintain benefit. Calcitonin nasal sprays, Miacalcin or Fortical, increase spine bone mineral density but have uncertain fracture efficacy.

Thinking about your choices. The above summary of fracture efficacy is a guide for starting your process of selection and discussion with your doctor. Since the goal is preventing fractures, the top choices are medicines that decrease risk of fractures at all sites. For treatment of postmenopausal osteoporosis, Fosamax and Actonel are the top medicines in pill form that have effectiveness at all sites. Now that Actonel is available for once-a-month dosing or in the form of Atelvia, which can be taken after breakfast once weekly, it rivals Boniva's ease of use with better efficacy. Reclast is potent and long lasting and is given by vein. It is a choice if you are unable to take a pill or if you want to take medicine only once a year.

Given as an injection twice a year, Prolia is an alternative to oral medicines. It has quick on and off action and is not incorporated in the bone. Some people are choosing Prolia because they are fearful of bisphosphonates that stay in the bone. However, because of its potency, Prolia has the potential for similar side effects as bisphosphonates. You should consider Prolia if you are at high risk, have not had adequate results from other medicines, or are unable to take other osteoporosis medicines. Prolia is also an option for those who have reduced kidney function.

Forteo is a short-term choice for high-risk individuals that offers a way to build bone microstructure, particularly in the spine. If you have already sustained fractures in your spine or have low spine bone density with a high risk for fractures, Forteo is an excellent option. After completion of a two-year course of Forteo therapy, you need to follow up with one of the other osteoporosis medicines.

Evista may move up to your first choice if you have a family history of breast cancer. If you are at high risk of fracture, you may consider combining Evista with another medicine, since you do not get fracture reduction beyond the spine. Caution: If you are early postmenopausal with hot flashes and sweats, these may increase with Evista. You may want to delay using it until your menopausal symptoms improve, and choose something else in the interim.

Boniva is a second-tier option because fracture reduction was observed at the spine only. However, if you have a T-score at the neck region of the hip of -3.0 or lower, it could be a top-tier option, since this subgroup of women subjects had fracture at nonspine sites.

Calcitonin used to be reserved for individuals who could not take or tolerate medicines by mouth. Now that effective choices are available by injection or infusion, calcitonin has lost its role as the only nonpill option. With its lack of efficacy, calcitonin should no longer be part of the medicine chest for treatment of osteoporosis.

YOUR STORIES...

Julie, age sixty, had a difficult transition through menopause. It was not so much hot flashes and night sweats, but all the other changes in her life. When her last child left for college, she thought she would be rejoicing, but instead she became depressed. Eventually, she was started on an antidepressant, Lexapro; she also saw a therapist.

At her doctor's suggestion, she had a DXA scan. She was surprised that she was diagnosed with osteoporosis. Her bone density results showed a T-score of -2.8 at the lumbar spine and she was within the normal range at the hip. She discussed possible treatment options with her doctor and decided on the convenience of once-a-month Actonel.

YOUR STORIES...

Donna, age fifty-five, had a bone density done because of her family history of osteoporosis. Her mother had fractured her hip at age eighty-seven. Her mother also had had breast cancer in her early sixties.

Her bone density results T-scores were -1.1 at the lumbar spine, -0.7 at the total hip, and -0.6 at the neck region of the hip (femoral neck). Her calculated ten-year probability of a major osteoporotic fracture was 5.6 percent and for hip fracture it was 0.3 percent.

Her fracture risk was low. However, she was one year past menopause, so a higher rate of bone loss would be expected over the next several years. In order to protect her bone mass and decrease her risk of breast cancer, Evista was prescribed. It did not increase her hot flashes.

Other Considerations

A few situations warrant special attention in making your selection. History of some problems eliminates choices or makes others more advantageous.

History	Preferred	Avoid
Family history of breast cancer	**Evista** –decreases risk of invasive breast cancer –consider combination if high-risk for fracture	**Estrogen** –increases risk of breast cancer
Personal history of breast cancer	**Bisphosphonates or Prolia** (depending on risk) –may protect bone from cancer	**Estrogen** –increases risk of breast cancer **Evista** –cannot use after Tamoxifen **Forteo** –may increase risk of bone tumors after radiation
Personal or family history of blood clot problems	**Bisphosphonates** **Prolia** **Forteo**	**Estrogen** **Evista** –both increase risk of clotting
Painful spine fracture	**Forteo** –forms new bone and may reduce pain and speed healing	
Hip Fracture	**Reclast** –may improve survival	
Menopause with moderate to severe hot flashes and menopausal symptoms	**Estrogen** –use lowest dose to control symptoms	

Swallowing or esophagus problems	Forteo Reclast Prolia –all bypass the digestive system by shot or infusion	Bisphosphonate pills
Reduced kidney function	Prolia	Bisphosphonates

YOUR STORIES...

George, age sixty-eight, had been struggling with worsening of his emphysema. He had been on and off prednisone to control his recurrent flare-ups but now was taking prednisone 10 mg every day. It seemed that when he went to a lower dose his breathing got worse, which necessitated the use of oxygen at night. One night, he became entangled in his oxygen tubing, which caused him to fall. He hit his dresser on his way down and the blow to his chest caused severe pain and worsening of his breathing. He had his wife take him to the emergency room where he was diagnosed with a rib fracture and a spine fracture. The emergency room doctor told him he had osteoporosis.

George followed up with his primary care doctor, who referred him to a rheumatologist specializing in osteoporosis. George was told that he had severe osteoporosis and was at high risk for more fractures. He was prescribed Forteo to decrease his risk of another fracture and to counteract the bone loss from prednisone. Calcium and vitamin D were also added to his regimen. He was sent to physical therapy and pulmonary rehabilitation to reduce his risk of falling.

REVIEW EACH YEAR

Keep in mind that whichever medicine you choose to start with may not be the medicine you continue using "forever." A decision to start one medicine today does not commit you to taking that drug for the rest of your life. Each year, you and your doctor should re-evaluate your treatment options. It should include a review of your lifestyle habits and the medicines you're taking, not just for osteoporosis but for everything, including over-the-counter medicines, vitamins, and supplements.

You may want to consider some of these questions when talking with your doctor:

- Are you tolerating your medicine?
- Is it fitting easily into your lifestyle?
- Is the medicine working?
- Is there new information about the medicine you are using?
- Are there new options available that may be better?
- Are you doing "all the right things" in your lifestyle?

The Bare Bones
In choosing which medicine is right for you:
- Compare the effectiveness of reducing fractures.
- Consider the potential side effects.
- Individualize to meet your situation and circumstances.
- Keep your doctor in the loop about any changes in your condition or medicine use.

Off-Label Uses:
What Else is Being Treated?

Each medicine approved by the FDA has indications for its use spelled out clearly in the product information or "label." From clinical-trial observations or after widespread prescription use of a medicine, other beneficial effects may be observed. In some cases, further investigation has been done or information has become available from current but incomplete clinical trials. This leads to doctors prescribing the medicine in a non-FDA approved, or "off-label" capacity. Pharmaceutical companies are very, very careful not to mention any off-label uses. Big fines have been levied on those who have made that mistake. The most common off-label uses of osteoporosis medicines are for helping in pain relief and for fracture healing.

CALCITONIN:
ACUTE PAIN FROM SPINE FRACTURE

One use for calcitonin that may be worth trying is for relief of acute pain associated with a new spine fracture. Spine fracture with pain can be incapacitating. Use of calcitonin is one way to try to minimize the use of narcotic painkillers.

If you or your family member is older, you can talk with the doctor about using daily calcitonin for a short time. In studies, the use of narcotics decreases usually within three to four days. If calcitonin works, you will know usually within the first week. Response to calcitonin may be as high as 80 percent. It will not work for everyone, but it may be worth trying.

If you or your loved one needs some extra assistance during this time, talk with the doctor about ordering calcitonin as a daily injection for the acute pain. In this way, getting a home health nurse to make daily visits may be a possibility.

If the idea of a shot does not interest you or you do not need home health support, use the nasal spray. A double dose of nasal spray, two sprays a day, equivalent to a daily shot of 100 IU, may help.

Calcitonin is thought to provide pain relief by a direct effect on pain threshold centers in the brain. The analgesic effect of calcitonin is attributed to the increase in circulating endorphins, which are chemicals that can block sensations of pain and act as your body's own pain relievers.

FORTEO: FRACTURE HEALING

Repair of a fracture requires increased transient bone formation at the fracture site. Since Forteo increases bone formation, it may be a potential agent to boost fracture repair. Faster healing of fractures was observed in patients already on Forteo who had recently experienced a fracture and in patients who had switched to Forteo after a fracture.

To date, only one randomized clinical trial of Forteo and fracture healing has been conducted. The study evaluated one hundred postmenopausal women who had experienced wrist fractures that did not require surgery. Subjects were divided into three groups, two of which received doses of Forteo. The two Forteo groups received either the marketed 20 microgram dose or a 40 microgram dose daily for eight weeks. The third group received a placebo daily for eight weeks. The treatment was started within ten days of fracture, and x-rays were taken every two weeks. The study failed to show significant difference in healing time between the 40-microgram and placebo groups. However, the standard-dose group showed a statistically significant acceleration of healing.

The type of fracture may make a difference. Since Forteo has the largest impact on the spine, healing of spine and other bone sites rich in spongy trabecular bone like the pelvis and the ends of long bones may benefit. Some clinicians have reported success with pelvic fractures healing in half the time. In addition, pain associated with the fracture improved faster.

Other reports of success include the healing of fractures that had previously failed to heal and had showed little healing activity on a bone scan or other imaging. Stimulation of bone formation by Forteo led to consolidation of bone, where time, surgery with bone grafting, or revisions had failed. Among those in the orthopedic community, additional interest has developed in using Forteo for healing following fusion operations, especially in patients who are at high risk for poor healing due to other problems like diabetes or hardening of the arteries.

YOUR STORIES...

Rene, age seventy-one, was watering her garden when her telephone rang. She turned quickly, caught her foot on the garden hose, and landed square on her back with her bottom hitting first. She got up and walked into the house but had intense pain in her right groin. She called her daughter-in-law, who drove her to the emergency room.

Diagnosis: pelvic fracture. She was hospitalized. Her fracture did not require surgery but it did require watchful waiting and time to heal. Based on some recent success with other patients who had experienced pelvic fractures, her doctor started her on Forteo. Pain subsided within three weeks and Rene only experienced discomfort on days with longer physical therapy. Six weeks after her fracture, Rene was back out watering her garden, this time with her portable telephone clipped to her belt.

FORTEO: BACK PAIN

Observations made in clinical trials with Forteo and from reports by patients taking Forteo suggest that it may also lessen back pain. A combination of data from several clinical trials showed that Forteo reduced back pain by a third overall and by more than half in those with severe back pain. The analysis also looked at trials with estrogen and bisphosphonates. The risk of back pain was lower in Forteo-treated subjects compared with estrogen- or bisphosphonate-treated subjects. The finding suggests that Forteo may have different effects on back pain than other osteoporosis therapies.

One theory is that Forteo reduces back pain by reducing the occurrence of new spine fractures. How it may modulate pain from other causes is not clear. The two-year limit on treatment means that you cannot use it over the long term, but short-term therapy for reduction of back pain is being investigated in a clinical trial.

The Bare Bones

Caution with these uses: Off-label treatments are not approved by the FDA.

- Calcitonin may help reduce the use of pain medicines after a spine fracture.
- Forteo may help accelerate fracture healing.
- Forteo may stimulate bone and promote healing in fractures that are having difficulty mending.
- Forteo may have the added benefit of reducing back pain.

Hot Topics: Cocktail Party Conversations

After people ask me, "What do you do?" at a cocktail party or get-together, the next question never fails to be about bone health. "What do you think about..." Usually, I am quizzed about the latest related topic to hit the media.

There are no definitive answers to the hot topics. Drug safety and the consequences of long-term use of medicines are topics of debate both in the bone health community and in the media. More research is needed to find the answers. Because medicine is an ever-evolving field, today's knowledge will inevitably be supplanted by future findings. Here is what is known so far about the controversies in treatment of osteoporosis.

SHOULD YOU TAKE A "DRUG HOLIDAY"?

How long should you take osteoporosis medicine? The answer to this question is far from certain and the evidence is thin in this area. Many doctors are now proposing to their patients on bisphosphonates that they should take a drug holiday. What does "drug holiday" mean? If you have been on one or more of the bisphosphonates (Fosamax, Actonel, Atelvia, Boniva, or Reclast) for five or more years, should you consider stopping your medicine for a year or two and then resume your medicine?

Most of the clinical trials have treated subjects for only three or four years. Some trials have continued with extensions to their fracture trials. The longest experience in clinical trials has been the use of Fosamax for ten years. The extension of the Fracture Intervention Trial (FIT), called FLEX, tried to answer the question, "If you increase your bone density, should you continue to stay on medicine?" The FLEX results provide some guidance, but the answer is still not cut-and-dried.

If you have achieved a bone density at the femoral neck of better than -2.5 after five years of treatment and you are not at high risk for fractures, you may consider discontinuing your medicine. If your hip bone density is still low, or you have had a spine fracture or are at high risk for fracture, you should continue taking prescription medicine.

The next question is, "What happens if you stop your medicine?" Bone breakdown and bone loss will occur again. However, the timing depends on the individual medicine.

Once Fosamax has been stopped, bone turnover gradually revs back up within about five years. Actonel has a shorter time frame of two to three years. Data are absent for Boniva and Reclast, but similar effects are expected based on strength of binding to the bone. Boniva would be comparable to Actonel and Reclast would be comparable to Fosamax. An analysis of one dose of Reclast showed fracture-reduction benefit for about three years. More data on Reclast will be available in the near future.

For Fosamax, about 70 mg of medicine is retained in the skeleton after ten years of therapy with 10 mg a day or 70 mg a week. The sustained effect of bisphosphonates may be the result of recycling. In other words, bisphosphonates retained in the bone may be released at new sites of bone remodeling. The recycled bisphosphonate may bind again to bone surfaces. Upon stopping treatment, the release of Fosamax from remodeling is estimated to be approximately the same as taking a daily dose of 2.5 mg. This results in a gradual upward trend in bone turnover rather than a rapid increase.

In contrast, bone turnover resumes right away after stopping other osteoporosis medicines. Bone loss restarts quickly when stopping Evista, estrogens, Forteo, or Prolia because these medicines are not retained in the bone. Ending a course of treatment with estrogens, like the loss of estrogen in natural menopause, results in rapid bone turnover. During this time of rapid loss, you may also be at higher risk for fracture. After therapy with Forteo, additional treatment with another medicine is required to preserve gains. Discontinuation of Prolia results in a rapid rise of bone remodeling, a transient increase in bone turnover markers above the pretreatment level, and an associated rapid decline in bone density.

If you have been on bisphosphonates for five to ten years or more, talk with your doctor about a drug holiday. In general, if your bone density has increased above the osteoporosis threshold this may be an option. A holiday of two to three years for Fosamax and Reclast, and a shorter holiday of one to two years for Actonel or Boniva, may be a consideration. If you are still in the osteoporotic range and at high risk for fracture, you want to remain on the same medicine *or* use another medicine, not a bisphosphonate, for one to two years before continuing with the bisphosphonate. Although no data supporting the latter recommendation are available at this time, many experts are now suggesting this option.

If you are on medicines other than bisphosphonates, stopping your medicine may lead to rapid bone loss. To protect the gains you made while on therapy, you need to plan ahead before completing two years of Forteo or stopping Evista, estrogens, or Prolia.

If you stop treatment, another important question follows: When do you restart? Here is where bone markers may be helpful in addition to bone density. Checking a bone turnover marker may possibly indicate when the effect of the bisphosphonate is waning. However, be wary: this is a "data-free" zone. At this point, there is no evidence that fracture risk remains reduced when you have discontinued your medicine, even if bone markers are reduced and bone density is stable.

The scant data available to direct decisions relating to duration of treatment and drug holidays has given rise to lively debates and all types of advice. You and your doctor must weigh your risks and benefits in formulating a prudent plan of action.

JAWBONE PROBLEMS

For a while, it seemed that one could not open a newspaper or turn on a television without seeing an advertisement inquiring, "Do you take Fosamax and have jaw problems? Contact our law firm."

The term for these jawbone problems is "osteonecrosis of the jaw" or "ONJ" for short, which refers to the development of lesions of the jaw that do not heal within eight weeks. ONJ may begin after one has had a tooth pulled or has had an injury to the mouth that exposed the bone. Very rarely, there may be spontaneous occurrence without a dental cause. ONJ may result when a sore at the site of exposed bone worsens. When this happens, part of the bone may become dead tissue characterized by an angry-looking area of yellow or white bone with swelling and drainage of pus.

The first case reports of ONJ in 2003 were in cancer patients receiving intravenous bisphosphonate therapy. They received higher doses than are used for osteoporosis. When the same problem occurred in patients receiving oral bisphosphonate therapy for osteoporosis with no history of cancer or chemotherapy, a possible association was established between ONJ and bisphosphonate therapy.

A review of clinical trials using bisphosphonates showed no reported cases in any of their phases. The extension studies with Actonel and Fosamax for seven and ten years of use uncovered no cases. However, it is common for rare adverse drug effects to be uncovered during postmarketing surveillance.

Multiple groups assembled expert panels to characterize the problem and set up guidelines. In 2006, the FDA issued a broad, class-wide warning for all bisphosphonates, including pills and intravenous preparations.

In 2007, the leading bone researchers in a task force for the American Society for Bone and Mineral Research released their report. The estimated number of cases was one to ten cases of ONJ for every one hundred thousand persons receiving treatment. For cancer patients, the risk was greater at one in ten thousand. Cancer patients have a higher risk, particularly if they are receiving radiation to the mouth region or chemotherapy for head and neck cancer. Also, they may receive higher doses of the bisphosphonates. Regular dental visits are recommended for oral health maintenance.

Risks for Jawbone Problems (ONJ)

- Intravenous bisphosphonate users are at greater risk than those using oral bisphosphonates
- Cancer patients
- Oral surgery or removal of teeth
- Poor dental hygiene, failure to care for teeth
- Periodontal disease
- Poor-fitting dental appliance
- Use of drugs for two years or more
- Smoking
- Alcohol abuse
- Diabetes
- Steroid use

If you are planning on dental surgery, talk with both your dentist and your prescribing doctor. Multiple medical and dental organizations have issued guidelines and recommendations. It is not known if stopping the bisphosphonate will make a difference in lowering the risk of ONJ. One specialty dental organization, the Association of Oral and Maxillofacial Surgeons, recommends stopping your bisphosphonate three months before an elective procedure and waiting until three months after to restart.

You may see this condition referred to as bisphosphonate-induced ONJ. However, any potent medicine that decreases bone turnover has the potential to cause the problem, including Prolia or any bisphosphonate. Label updates for all bisphosphonates include the possibility of ONJ. Prolia's label also specifies a risk of ONJ. Since the bone turnover markers start trending up with Prolia before the next six-month dose, you could wait to have a dental procedure until bone markers increase if it is not an emergency.

What is the cause of ONJ? It is not known. One interesting study out of the UCLA School of Dentistry suggests that vitamin D deficiency may be the cause. The UCLA researchers gave Reclast to laboratory animals. Some animals had vitamin D deficiency and others were supplemented with vitamin D. In their experiment, only the animals with low vitamin D developed jaw problems.

Vitamin D has not been assessed systematically in people who developed ONJ. But it makes sense to be sure that you have an adequate vitamin D level before starting a course of treatment on any bisphosphonate or Prolia. In addition, you should have an oral examination before beginning therapy.

Nevertheless, a robust remodeling system is essential for maintaining bone health. The pressures on the mandible are the highest exerted in the body. The frequency with which the mandible is mechanically loaded may explain why these uncommon adverse events may occur at this skeletal site.

Some have speculated that ONJ is related to oversuppression of bone turnover, which refers to a rate of bone turnover that is so low that the bone can't maintain itself. However, levels of bone turnover markers achieved with therapy do not appear to be correlated with risk of ONJ. Some individuals recommend checking bone turnover markers; if they are low, do not proceed with your dental work. But this is only the opinion of some experts, and it is not proven.

Take care of your dental health with routine checkups and oral exams. Avoid trauma to the tissues in your mouth. Carefully weigh the risks of any elective dental procedure involving bone. If dental treatment is required, such as removal of several teeth, do one at a time.

DOES TREATMENT CAUSE FRACTURES? CASES OF "ATYPICAL FRACTURES"

On March 8, 2010, ABC *World News* reported that Fosamax causes fractures. Barely a minute went by before my cell phone started ringing. "Dr. Di," one friend said, "I just watched the evening news and I am in a panic. Should I stop my medicine?"

In the segment ABC *World News Investigates*, medical correspondent Dr. Richard Besser described fractures spontaneously occurring in the thighbone below the hip in women treated with Fosamax. The story was retold the following morning on *Good Morning America*. These broadcasts created a flurry of additional media stories on "atypical fractures" and Fosamax.

Cases of atypical femur fracture in women taking the bisphosphonate class of osteoporosis medicines that includes Fosamax (generic alendronate), Boniva, Actonel, and Reclast had been reported at previous bone meetings and in the literature starting in 2005. Why all the attention in March 2010? The March meeting of the American Academy of Orthopedic Surgeons had several presentations on bisphosphonate-associated fractures that caught the attention of reporters who investigated further and created major media stories.

The media buzz ultimately produced positive steps toward characterizing the problem in depth. In mid-October 2010, the FDA issued a safety communication regarding atypical femur fractures and required labeling changes for all bisphosphonates approved to treat osteoporosis (Fosamax, Actonel, Atelvia, Boniva, Reclast, and generic products). Labels for these medications are now required to indicate the possible risk of unusual fractures of the femur. Although atypical femur fractures have been reported in bisphosphonate-treated patients, the cause of atypical femur fractures has not been established and the risk has been estimated to be rare—less than one percent.

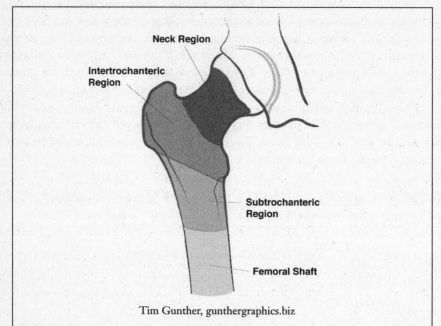

Tim Gunther, gunthergraphics.biz

What is an atypical femur fracture?

An atypical femur fracture is a fracture that occurs below the hip in the subtrochanteric region or in the shaft area of the thighbone, or femur. These fractures show characteristics that are not typical of osteoporotic fractures. Therefore, they are labeled "atypical femur fractures." The fracture may start as a stress fracture and progress to a completed fracture with little or no trauma.

The majority of patients who had atypical femur fractures experienced dull, aching pain of the thigh for months or even years prior to the fracture, and about one-quarter had involvement of the opposite femur as well. If you develop thigh or groin pain while taking bisphosphonates, contact your doctor to have your symptoms evaluated. Since changes may occur in both sides even though only one is symptomatic, both upper legs need to be looked at.

The large health plan in California, Kaiser Permanente, is one place to which the FDA went for numbers. Dr. Richard Dell, an orthopedic surgeon who spearheads a healthy bone program, has been systematically looking at fractures in Kaiser's northern and southern California operations. Kaiser treated more than fifteen thousand patients with fractures of the femur over three years (from 2007 to 2009). Of those, 135 were classified as "atypical femur fractures." About one-quarter had fractures in both femurs. A total of ninety-eight women sustained these fractures. Five individuals had never taken any bisphosphonates. In the others, the average duration of bisphosphonate use was six years. Dr. Dell estimated that more than three hundred thousand Kaiser patients have been treated with bisphosphonates, and that these medicines have helped prevent more than five thousand hip fractures in just three years, a period during which fewer than a hundred patients sustained an atypical fracture.

This topic is being discussed in every forum imaginable. For example, a debate at a large conference of endocrinologists pitted Dr. Joseph Lane, an orthopedic surgeon from New York's Hospital for Special Surgery against Dr. Juliet Compston, a bone scientist at the University of Cambridge. The participants typify the two disparate views. The orthopedic surgeons did not see this unique type of fracture until about 2000—five years after the FDA approved Fosamax. Since orthopedists see the individual patients who have the problem, they think it is not unusual or rare. Dr. Compston, who counts the numbers based on review of the clinical trials and the literature, thinks it is rare.

Clearly, more information is needed. What is known so far is that atypical femur fractures occurring in the thigh below the hip are statistically rare. A systematic accounting of cases is underway. Your chance of having an osteoporotic fracture is far greater than your chance of having an "atypical" one. At this time, it is not known who exactly may be at risk, whether a pre-existing problem is associated with developing this type of fracture, or how their occurrence may be a result of treatment.

ARE MEDICINES CAUSING "OVERSUPPRESSION"?

Underlying all of these topics is the question: Are antiresorptive medicines causing oversuppression? In other words, has bone remodeling been slowed down so much that it is harmful? You may have seen this problem referred to as "frozen bone." This means that bone remodeling is no longer occurring at a sufficient rate for the bone to repair itself. It is as though the construction workers have a work stoppage and aren't showing up for work. The building, after a time, falls into disrepair.

Reducing bone remodeling is how the antiresorptives work, and the effect varies from treatment to treatment. The bisphosphonates are more potent than Evista or calcitonin. The potency of the bisphosphonates differs. Fosamax binds to the bone more strongly than Actonel or Boniva. Reclast is potent and has a rapid and protracted effect, which is why it is given only once a year. Prolia has a rapid and greater effect than bisphosphonates on bone turnover, but it is short-lived and reversible.

The clinical trials are constructed carefully to follow safety protocols and to collect as much information as possible. Bone markers are the measure of bone remodeling. Biopsy of the bone is the only way to get a direct examination of the microstructure. All clinical trials collect a small number of biopsies from each study group to examine the effect of the medicines. Normal mineralization and structure must be demonstrated to get FDA approval. The longest clinical experience with Fosamax, at ten years, showed normal bone formation and bone structure. Normal mineralized bone is formed with all the osteoporosis medicines.

Concerns about oversuppression have been raised by case reports of individuals treated with bisphosphonates who fracture and have bone turnover below the normal premenopausal levels. These observations occurred in post-marketing of the medicines but not during clinical trials, which may mean that they are rare, that the duration of the studies was too short, or both. In addition, oversuppression has been discussed but not proven as a possible cause of both ONJ and atypical femur fractures. The mechanisms for these events have not been worked out. Whether there are certain predispositions or genetic characteristics that increase risk is being investigated.

Based on normal biopsies and the fracture reduction seen with treatment, the effect of reduced bone turnover appears to be beneficial rather than harmful. Monitoring will continue to address concerns about bone safety.

OTHER CONCERNS

Bisphosphonate therapy was implicated in an increased risk of irregular heart rhythm called atrial fibrillation. However, continued patient follow-up proved that it was related to heart problems and not to use of osteoporosis medicines. Early on, questions were also asked about the risk of esophageal cancer. In 2010, a systematic evaluation of esophageal cancer showed that risk did not go up with bisphosphonate medicines. After that report was published, a second paper found a small increase in risk with five years' use of bisphosphonates. While it is not unusual to have conflicting evidence, in this case, both reports used the United Kingdom patient population database. Nonetheless, it appears that, overall, esophageal cancer is a rare event.

NO MEDICINE IS 100 PERCENT PERFECT

All medicines have potential side effects. As with any medicine, you must weigh the benefits of treatment against the potential risks. Recommendations have evolved over time. Doctors once advised everyone with low bone density to take medicine to increase bone density; treatment is now focused on only those patients with a higher risk of fracture. If you have had a fracture, have multiple risks with low bone density, or have a bone density score lower than -2.5, the benefits of lowering your risk of fracture definitely outweigh the risks of side effects. Talk with your doctor to make sure treatment is appropriate, and reassess its continued use every year.

The Bare Bones
- If you have taken a bisphosphonate for five years or more, reassess its use with your doctor. A "holiday" from your medicine may be possible.
- Jawbone problems called osteonecrosis of the jaw are linked to use of bisphosphonates and Prolia but are very uncommon. Good dental hygiene lowers risk.
- Reports of femur fractures below the hip while taking bisphosphonates are rare occurrences. If you develop thigh or groin pain, contact your doctor.
- Medicines that work by decreasing bone turnover do not appear to interfere with normal repair of the bone.

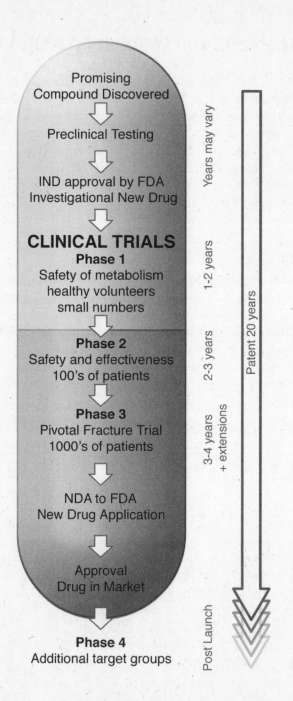

Promising
Compound Discovered

⬇

Preclinical Testing

⬇

IND approval by FDA
Investigational New Drug

⬇

CLINICAL TRIALS
Phase 1
Safety of metabolism
healthy volunteers
small numbers

⬇

Phase 2
Safety and effectiveness
100's of patients

⬇

Phase 3
Pivotal Fracture Trial
1000's of patients

⬇

NDA to FDA
New Drug Application

⬇

Approval
Drug in Market

⬇

Phase 4
Additional target groups

Years may vary

1-2 years

2-3 years

3-4 years
+ extensions

Post Launch

Patent 20 years

Tim Gunther, gunthergraphics.biz

Drugs in Development

Novel Medicines: What is in the Pipeline?

New medicines in development remind me of the "coming attractions" in the movie theatre. They promise something exciting in the future. And just as movie studios hope for blockbusters but cannot predict success ahead of time, so it is with drug development. Many new compounds hold promise, but there are plenty of surprises along the way. Until the FDA has deliberated, pharmaceutical companies never know which drug will actually reach the marketplace and become a hit. (See phases of development on page 254.)

New drugs in the pipeline for treatment of osteoporosis fall into two broad categories: those that are refinements of current medicines and those that are completely novel compounds. Refinement includes modifying the structure of the molecule, inventing a new delivery system, and using new combinations. Examples include an effervescent form of Fosamax that is similar to Alka-Seltzer®, calcitonin in a pill form, and different parathyroid hormone formulations.

FORTEO THAT IS NOT A SHOT

Since Forteo (teriparatide) is an effective medicine that has the drawback of requiring daily shots, other methods of taking the medicine are being investigated. These include nasal spray, topical preparation, tablet, patch, implantable chip, and a tablet that tricks your body into producing its own parathyroid hormone.

Skin applications. Multiple companies are working on delivery of Forteo through the skin. Various methods of skin application are under development. One of the most promising developments is a microneedle patch produced by Zosano Pharma. It is an adhesive patch about the size of a postage stamp that looks like fine sandpaper. It is made up of thirteen hundred miniscule titanium arrowhead-shaped needles that are coated with medicine. After the patch is applied to the skin, the medicine dissolves away from the needles. It is virtually bloodless and painless.

Almost two hundred postmenopausal women were recruited for a six-month study to test effectiveness and safety. Three different doses of generic

Forteo, called teriparatide, were tested in the patch form and compared with daily Forteo shots and a placebo patch. The patch, which was worn for a total of thirty minutes once a day, caused a small area of redness that resolved quickly.

The medicine from the patches reached the bloodstream faster than from the Forteo shots and achieved a shorter burst of medicine, which is how teriparatide works best. After six months of treatment, the highest dose patch tested, 40 micrograms, showed bone density increases at the spine equivalent to the Forteo shots. A larger trial is planned.

Microchip. The firm MicroChips is pursuing a device that is implanted under the skin like a pacemaker. The device is about the size of an Oreo® cookie and contains a battery, wireless antenna, and microchip with the generic version of Forteo. The medicine is released on command for a full year. In addition, the researchers are testing the device as a platform for transmitting health information, possibly even to your smartphone.

Make your own. Rather than focusing on a resource to deliver Forteo, an alternative approach is to give a medicine that stimulates the release of your own parathyroid hormone. This approach focuses on inhibiting the calcium-sensing ability of the parathyroid gland. An oral medicine would stimulate the parathyroid to release a pulse of parathyroid hormone. The most advanced compound in clinical trials was ronacaleret, but it showed insufficient effectiveness in the trials. Other similar compounds are in testing.

ALL NEW AND DIFFERENT

Advances in defining the molecules that regulate bone remodeling have led to the development of medicines that target those molecules. Investigational medicines with novel mechanisms of action may provide benefits beyond those of the current medicines.

Odanacatib. Of all the novel medicines, odanacatib, developed by Merck, is the farthest along in clinical trials. It decreases bone breakdown but at the same time does not decrease bone formation as much as other antiresorptive medicines. Odanacatib blocks an enzyme called cathepsin-K, which is produced by osteoclasts, the bone breakdown cells. Cathepsin-K helps to carve out the pits where bone remodeling happens. Odanacatib works by blocking this action. This leads to shallower bone breakdown pits and greater bone mass but preserves the function of the osteoclasts.

The results of early clinical trials showed increases in bone density with bone formation preserved to a greater degree than bisphosphonates. A large fracture study of women ages sixty-five and older is underway, using two formulations of odanacatib taken once weekly: a 50 mg tablet alone and a tablet combining 50 mg of Odanacatib with 5,600 IU of vitamin D_3.

Another cathepsin-K inhibitor compound called ONO-5334, produced by a Japanese company, Ono Pharmaceutical, is also in clinical trials.

REGULATORS OF BONE FORMATION

Since Forteo is the only available medicine for targeting osteoblasts, the bone building cells, the need in the osteoporosis "medicine cabinet" is for more bone formation medicines. Research on how cells communicate with one another led to the identification of a complex system of messengers, called the Wnt signaling pathway, which plays a central role in regulating the growth and activity of osteoblasts. Its discovery has opened the door for development of new compounds that target these messengers and may eventually yield new osteoporosis therapies. Approaches will either use factors that lead to new bone formation or try to block factors that decrease bone formation.

A protein called sclerostin, produced by bone cells (osteocytes), is one of the messengers that sends the signal to apply the brakes in making new osteoblasts. The blocking of sclerostin would allow the rate of bone formation to increase. Amgen is testing a protein that neutralizes the effects of sclerostin. The compound AMG 785 is in clinical trials. A shot given either monthly or every three months is being compared to daily Forteo and once-a-week Fosamax.

Other agents are in earlier stages of development.

The Bare Bones
- New medicines are in development that either refine the current medicines available or are something completely different.
- Finding ways to deliver Forteo other than by a shot is one of the active areas of research.
- The medicine farthest along in testing is Merck's odanacatib, which blocks a key enzyme produced by osteoclasts, the bone breakdown cells.
- Compounds are under development that promote bone formation by targeting messengers that allow the bone cells to communicate with one another.

Investigational SERMs:
A Promise of an Ideal Estrogen

An estrogen designed to prevent fractures, breast cancer, heart attack, stroke, and dementia would be perfect. If that's not enough, add the benefits of increasing your sex drive and maintaining your skin's youthful look. Sounds too good to be true, doesn't it? So far, it is.

SERMs, short for "selective estrogen receptor modulators," hold the promise of being such an ideal medicine. You may also see them referred to as estrogen agonist antagonists (EAAs). These designer drugs have a split personality. They mimic estrogen in some tissues and have the opposite effects in others. Evista was the first drug of this type approved for osteoporosis. Tamoxifen is in the same class, but it is used in patients with breast cancer. Because neither Evista nor tamoxifen is ideal, there is still room for "new and improved" versions.

Although multiple promising SERMs have entered clinical trials, only two medicines, lasofoxifene and bazedoxifene, have made it all the way to filing for FDA approval. However, neither had received FDA approval as of midyear 2011.

FABLYN®

Lasofoxifene was branded originally as Oporia®, then its name was changed to Fablyn. Fablyn was Pfizer's first foray into the bone arena.

Fablyn (lasofoxifene)
Category
Antiresorptive Selective Estrogen Receptor Modulator (SERM), also referred to as an Estrogen Agonist/Antagonist (EAA)
Manufacturer
Pfizer and Ligand Pharmaceuticals
Pivotal Fracture Trial
PEARL

Fracture Reduction
Spine
Nonspine
Indications for Osteoporosis
Not approved
Dose
0.5 mg pill once a day
Additional Information
Lowers risk of invasive breast cancer
Causes uterine polyps

EFFECTIVENESS

PEARL: Postmenopausal Evaluation and Risk-Reduction with Lasofoxifene

In a five-year global study, researchers evaluated the effects of Fablyn on fractures and breast cancer. More than 8,500 women with postmenopausal osteoporosis were given one of two doses of Fablyn or a placebo. The 0.5 mg dose of Fablyn lowered spine fractures by 42 percent and breast cancer by 81 percent. However, it also doubled the risk of blood clots.

Unlike Evista, Fablyn decreased nonspine fractures by 24 percent *and* reduced the risk for heart attacks and stroke by about a third. Nevertheless, the overall rates of death were higher in the Fablyn groups, which is one of the concerns for the FDA. On further review, only the study sites located in Central and South America showed an increase in lung cancer and deaths. Also, women taking Fablyn needed more procedures for problems like polyps in the uterus and incontinence. In the meantime, European Medicines Agency, the European equivalent to our FDA, approved Fablyn 0.5 mg a day for treatment of osteoporosis.

VIVIANT® AND APRELA®

Another SERM not yet approved by the FDA is bazedoxifene, which has the brand name Viviant. Bazedoxifene is also put into a combination tablet with the estrogen Premarin and is branded as Aprela. The pairing of a SERM and estrogen is categorized as a tissue selective estrogen complex (TSEC). The motivation for adding an estrogen to a SERM stems from the concept that the benefits of each will be achieved with better overall tolerability. Together they are different than either agent alone.

For example, the tendency of SERMs is to cause or worsen hot flashes. If an estrogen is added to a SERM, are hot flashes prevented or relieved? In the series of studies called SMART (Selective Estrogen Menopause and Response to Therapy), Aprela (bazedoxifene 20 mg combined with either Premarin 0.625 or 0.45 mg) was effective in decreasing hot flashes. The combination did not cause breast pain or thicken the lining of the uterus, which is common when estrogen is used alone. This combination also retained the positive features of a SERM. In addition, Aprela prevented bone loss in healthy postmenopausal women. Pairing of a SERM with estrogen in Aprela created a new approach for controlling hot flashes and preventing osteoporosis while protecting the uterus from estrogen stimulation. Although no effect was observed at the breast, long-term safety is not known.

Aprela
(bazedoxifene with Premarin)
Category
Antiresorptive
SERM plus estrogen is called a
tissue selective estrogen complex
(TSEC)
Manufacturer
Pfizer
(developed in collaboration by
Ligand Pharmaceuticals and Wyeth)
Phase III Trial
SMART
Indications
Not approved
Dose
Combination pill once a day
Additional Information
Controls hot flashes

Viviant (bazedoxifene alone) was evaluated for the prevention and treatment of postmenopausal osteoporosis in two large clinical trials. Participants were randomly assigned to take different doses of Viviant, Evista 60 mg, or placebo. This study design allowed direct comparison with the only FDA-approved SERM, Evista, and the study drug. The three-year pivotal fracture trial included approximately 7,500 women and tested 20 mg and 40 mg of Vivant. It was extended for two years without the Evista group for more complete safety information.

More than half of the women had spine fractures at the beginning of the study. The treatment effect was similar for those with and without spine fractures. Evista and the 40 mg dose of Viviant showed the same fracture reduction at the spine (42 percent). The 20 mg dose of Viviant also showed similar fracture reduction at the spine (37 percent). Nonspine fractures were not reduced by any of the medicines. Only an analysis of a higher risk subgroup showed a reduction of nonspine fractures compared with placebo or Evista. Similar to Evista, hot flashes were common side effects of Viviant in about one in ten women. The lining of the uterus (endometrium) did not have a tendency to thicken or develop polyps. Changes in cholesterol were favorable, including increases in good cholesterol. The numbers of strokes and heart attacks were similar in all groups, including the placebo group. Clotting in the legs (deep venous thrombosis) occurred more frequently with Viviant and Evista but was uncommon. The effect of Viviant on breast was neutral.

A two-year prevention study evaluated 10, 20, and 40 mg of Viviant in over 1,400 postmenopausal women with low bone mass (T-score between -1.0 and -2.5 at the femoral neck or lumbar spine). All doses of Viviant and Evista prevented bone loss and had modest gains of less than 2 percent. Bone markers decreased by about 20 percent in all Viviant groups compared to a 27 percent decrease in the Evista group. Overall, Viviant was tolerated well.

The 20 mg dose was approved in Europe in 2009; it is marketed as Conbriza®.

Viviant
(bazedoxifene)
Category
Antiresorptive
Selective Estrogen Receptor Modulator
  (SERM), also referred to as an
Estrogen Agonist/Antagonist (EAA)
Manufacturer
Pfizer
(developed in collaboration by
  Ligand Pharmaceuticals and Wyeth)
Pivotal Fracture Trial
Phase III trial for 3 years with
  2 year extension
Fracture Reduction
Spine
Nonspine

Indications for Osteoporosis
Not approved
Dose
20 or 40 mg pill once a day
Additional Information
Improves good cholesterol
Does not stimulate the uterine lining

APPROVAL FOR ANY NEW SERMS?

Ten years ago the buzz was designer estrogens. Every pharmaceutical company seemed to have one in development. It looked as if this class of medicines would be a hit for bone and other menopausal health benefits. In early trials, new drugs appeared to be superior to Evista. What a difference a few years make! Evista is still the only choice available. The medicines yet to be approved are all under the Pfizer umbrella, after their acquisition of Wyeth.

Will the FDA ever approve another designer estrogen? Aprela has the best chance. Its unique combination—bone-building effects plus its ability to reduce hot flashes—makes it different. Because it can prevent the undesirable side effects of estrogen in nonbone tissues, it may become a reasonable option for someone with severe menopausal symptoms. Stay tuned.

For now, the perfect SERM remains elusive. There is still room for improvement.

The Bare Bones

- Fablyn and Viviant, investigational SERMs, have completed pivotal fracture studies.
- Both Fablyn and Viviant decreased spine fractures; only Fablyn decreased nonspine fractures.
- Fablyn also decreased heart attacks and stroke, but rates of death were higher overall.
- Aprela, a combination of Viviant with estrogen, improved menopausal symptoms—hot flashes—and prevented bone loss.

Other Medicines: Available Elsewhere But Not in the United States

It must be human nature to want something we cannot have. Two bone health medicines fit into that category: strontium ranelate and tibolone. Some patients end up seeking sources for these medicines as alternatives to the current "medicine chest" of FDA-approved drugs for osteoporosis. Strontium ranelate (marketed as Protelos® or Osseor®) and tibolone (brand names Livial® or Xyvion) are available in many other parts of the world. Both have pivotal fracture studies, but neither has been approved for sale in the United States. Strontium ranelate does not even qualify for submissison to the FDA because no US study sites were used in the pivotal fracture trial.

TIBOLONE

The effects of tibolone are similar to combination estrogen and progesterone with a testosterone-like androgen added. Therefore, tibolone has beneficial effect on hot flashes, bone density, and libido (sex drive). The dose used for menopausal symptoms is 2.5 mg a day. Tibolone has no direct biological activity but it is metabolized in the body into active components. These components have different hormonal actions depending on the tissue type. It acts like estrogen in the bone and vaginal tissues, like progesterone in the lining of the womb (endometrium), and like testosterone in the brain.

Tibolone (Livial or Xyvion)
Category
Both antiresorptive and bone formation
Synthetic steroid
Manufacturer
Organon
Pivotal Fracture Trial
LIFT (using 1.25 mg daily)
stopped early because of strokes
Fracture Reduction
Spine
Nonspine

Indications
Not approved
Dose
2.5 mg pill once a day
Additional Information
Risk of breast cancer and colon cancer reduced by two-thirds

LIFT: Long-Term Intervention on Fractures with Tibolone

Despite widespread use of tibolone, its long-term safety and effects on fracture reduction were not known. The LIFT trial sought to fill the gaps of knowledge about this medicine. More than 4,500 women aged sixty to eighty with low bone density and a spine fracture or osteoporosis by bone density were randomly assigned to tibolone 1.25 mg or placebo pill each day.

The trial was stopped just short of three years because of safety concerns. Women in the tibolone group had an increased risk of stroke. Overall, they were twice as likely to have a stroke. Women over seventy had a fourfold increased risk. Although the numbers of strokes were small, the differences were significant between groups. Interestingly, there was no increased risk of clotting, as is seen with estrogens and SERMs.

Tibolone did reduce spine fractures identified on x-rays by 45 percent and nonspine fractures by 26 percent. Two unexpected findings were that tibolone reduced both breast cancer and colon cancer by two-thirds.

Almost one in ten women had vaginal bleeding. Women in the tibolone group were more likely to have a thickening of the lining of the womb, and four developed endometrial cancer. More women on tibolone stopped taking the study medicine because of vaginal discharge, vaginal bleeding, or breast discomfort.

For these reasons, the benefits of tibolone did not outweigh the risks. Tibolone in half the dose that is used for menopausal symptoms did pass the safety test. Therefore, where approved, tibolone is used in younger postmenopausal women who have a low risk of stroke to treat symptoms of menopause without increasing their risk of breast cancer

STRONTIUM RANELATE

Strontium is a naturally occurring mineral (element number 38 on the periodic table you studied in chemistry). Like calcium, strontium has two positive charges. Your body naturally contains about 320 mg of strontium, most of which is in bone. Strontium can replace calcium in some of its biochemical processes because of the similarity between the two elements. In the bone, strontium accumulates in the active remodeling sites. It is incorporated into the bone mineral and retained in your skeleton. Strontium in the form of various salts has medicinal uses. The compound strontium ranelate is used in other countries for treatment of osteoporosis.

As a medicine, it may have a dual effect on the bone. In animal models, strontium both prevents bone breakdown and stimulates bone formation. However, bone biopsies of women treated with strontium ranelate do not show this dual effect. The biopsies showed less bone breakdown but no evidence of increased bone formation. Bone markers showed only a modest effect on bone metabolism. Bone breakdown decreased by about 10 percent and bone formation decreased by 8 percent.

Using bone density, it is hard to tell if there is an actual increase in bone. Measurements by DXA overestimate the bone density because strontium is denser than calcium. Therefore, much of the bone density effect is a technical artifact due to the replacement of some calcium with strontium. The error in measurement is estimated at 10 percent above the "real" bone density. To get a better estimation of the correct reading, the use of mathematical formulas to adjust the DXA bone density measurements is recommended. However, these calculations are complex and based on multiple assumptions. In addition, because strontium stays in the bones, these adjustments will need to be applied to all future DXA results, even after treatment with strontium ranelate has ended.

Strontium ranelate
(Protelos or Osseor)
Category
Both antiresorptive and bone formation
Mineral
Manufacturer
Servier
Pivotal Fracture Trial
SOTI
TROPOS
Fracture Reduction
Spine
Nonspine
Indications
Not approved

Dose
2 grams in a sachet mixed into water once a day taken at least 2 hours after food, milk products, and calcium supplements
Additional Information
Rare allergic reaction

Two fracture studies have evaluated the effectiveness and safety of strontium ranelate. One was designed to look at spine fractures and the other looked at nonspine fractures. Before subjects were given strontium ranelate, calcium and vitamin D intakes were optimized. This phase was called FIRST (Fracture International Run-in Strontium Ranelate Trial).

After successful completion of FIRST, subjects were randomized to strontium ranelate 2 mg dose daily or placebo. Strontium ranelate comes in a sachet that is mixed in water to form a suspension. Subjects were instructed to drink this suspension as soon as it was prepared. The strontium ranelate suspension cannot be taken at the same time as food or calcium products, such as milk or supplements. The dose is taken at least two hours after eating or consuming these products, usually at bedtime.

SOTI: Spinal Osteoporosis Therapeutic Intervention

The SOTI trial included about 1,600 women with postmenopausal osteoporosis defined either by bone density at the spine or the presence of at least one spine fracture. Almost 90 percent of the participants, average age seventy, had spine fractures at entry. After three years, the reduction of spine fractures identified by x-ray was 38 percent. The study continued, and after four years, the decrease overall was 33 percent for spine fractures.

TROPOS: Treatment of Peripheral Osteoporosis

Only older at-risk women were targeted for this study. Entry criteria limited participation to women older than seventy-four years of age or women older than seventy who also had risk factors and low hip bone density. Over five thousand women participated in TROPOS. After three years, the reduction of nonspine fractures was 16 percent. The numbers of hip fractures were similar in the strontium ranelate and placebo groups.

A later analysis found that a subgroup of women over the age of seventy-four with low bone density (T-score of less than -2.4 at the neck region of the hip) had 36 percent lower risk of hip fracture. Consistent with the SOTI study, spine fractures identified by x-ray decreased 39 percent. However, x-rays were not available for about one-third of the participants. At the end of five years of treatment with strontium ranelate, the nonspine fracture reduction was 15 percent.

The most common side effects were digestive complaints—nausea, loose stools, and diarrhea. These symptoms tend to decrease after three months of use. Mild increases were seen in blood levels of an enzyme found in muscle, but there were no associated symptoms. A small increase in the number of clots in the deep veins was also observed.

After the medicine was approved in other countries, rare severe allergic reactions were reported, which caused several deaths. Patients taking strontium ranelate are advised to discontinue it immediately if any skin reactions appear.

According to my colleagues in other countries who prescribe strontium ranelate, it is reserved for those who could not tolerate bisphosphonates, and for whom tibolone or SERMs are not indicated. Also, it can be challenging to take, since individuals must wait two hours after dinner before they can take it as a drink. Patients often dislike it. Digestive side effects are common; many have to get up during the night to go to the toilet. Some doctors are hesitant to prescribe it both because the mechanism by which it works is still not clear and because it is difficult to measure response by analyzing bone density changes.

The use of other strontium salts is in development. Servier, the French manufacturer of strontium ranelate, has acquired the rights to an investigational drug, strontium malonate, which is also known as NB S101. Unlike the powder form, strontium malonate is in pill form for once-daily use. However, the new formulation does not change the effect strontium has on bone when it replaces calcium.

The Bare Bones

- Tibolone and strontium ranelate are medicines used in other parts of the world, but they are not approved for use in the US.
- In the pivotal fracture study of tibolone, the increased occurrence of strokes outweighed the benefits of reducing fractures.
- Strontium is a natural element that can take the place of calcium in bone.
- Strontium ranelate has a modest effect on bone turnover and fracture reduction and is used, where available, by patients unable to tolerate other medicines.

Complementary and Alternative Medicine

Introduction

Complementary and alternative medicine is a fascinating area for me. My first educational experience occurred in the 1980s while on a trip to China with a group of health professionals. Witnessing the effectiveness of acupuncture needles in providing complete anesthesia to a patient whose abdomen was wide open instantly made me a believer! Seeing acupuncture and a variety of other alternative techniques in action taught me to think about options outside of conventional medicine. In Chinese university-based hospitals, the doctors used a hybrid of Western and traditional Chinese medicine to treat their patients.

My personal experience with chronic back pain has led me to use many alternative medicines and complementary techniques. I had an open mind, which made me more receptive to alternative solutions. The pursuit of pain relief is always a strong motivating factor. With pain, you receive immediate feedback, and you will know whether the remedy is working. However, dealing with your bones, the problem is that you do not have the benefit of knowing the result for a long time.

We use complementary and alternative medicine therapies quite often, maybe even more often in my state—California. The problem is that evidence is scant or nonexistent for so many of the treatments. It is difficult to know what are the real benefits and risks of these alternative treatments.

The good news is that, just as I observed in China some twenty-five years ago, the increasing integration of the "two worlds" is happening here and now. The National Institutes of Health (NIH) established the National Center for Complementary and Alternative Medicine to foster research and provide information about this area. Many major hospitals and universities have set up integrative medicine centers. In the future, as conventional medicine broadens its view to encompass a more integrated approach, nothing will be "outside the mainstream." Meanwhile, more research is needed to provide answers on safety and effectiveness of alternative medicine.

Fosteum: A Food Product by Prescription

Fosteum® is a unique product that is categorized as a "medical food" and requires a prescription from your doctor. Fosteum's main ingredient is genistein, which is an isoflavone (one of the estrogen-like compounds in soy products). Each capsule contains 27 mg of genistein, a bioavailable form of zinc, which provides approximately 4 mg of elemental zinc and 200 IU of vitamin D (cholecalciferol). The prescribed dose is one capsule twice a day, approximately every twelve hours.

WHAT IS A MEDICAL FOOD?

Prior to learning about Fosteum, I thought medical foods were only nutrition products given to ill patients who could not take in regular foods, for example, special nutrient-rich liquids given through a tube directly into the stomach when someone is unable to swallow or eat solid food.

As defined by the Food and Drug Administration (FDA) under the Orphan Drug Act, "the term 'medical food' refers to a food that is formulated to be consumed or administered internally under the supervision of a physician and is intended for the specific dietary management of a disease or condition for which distinctive nutritional requirements, based on recognized scientific principles, are established by medical evaluation."

Originally, medical foods were designed for patients with rare, inherited metabolic diseases who needed special diets. These foods were considered drugs because they are used for medicinal purposes and were referred to as "orphan drugs" because so few individuals are affected.

To promote development of these types of products, the FDA reclassified them from drugs to foods. The FDA *does not* approve medical foods, but they are intended for use by patients under a doctor's supervision.

SOURCE: www.fda.gov

Effectiveness

Fosteum has only been studied in Italy, in two small, randomized trials of post-menopausal women. No study subjects had osteoporosis.

One study enrolled ninety women who were on average six to seven years past menopause. Subjects were randomly divided into one of three groups that received either Fosteum, continuous estrogen therapy pill, or a dummy placebo pill. At the end of one year, bone density increases of three to four percent were observed in both the Fosteum and estrogen groups. Therefore, in this small study, Fosteum appeared to protect against bone loss to a similar degree as estrogens. Hot flashes were reported by 40 percent of subjects in the placebo group, by 20 percent of those in the Fosteum group, and by only one woman taking estrogen. Information is not given about the percent of women reporting hot flashes at the start of the study. Therefore, the actual decrease in occurrence of hot flashes is not known.

The largest study started with 389 postmenopausal women, age fifty-four on average, with low bone density at the hip. They were randomized to groups that took either Fosteum or a dummy placebo pill. The study was planned to last for two years and about one-third continued in a one-year extension for a total of three years. At the end of two years, bone density for those in the Fosteum group increased 5 percent at the neck region of the hip and 6 percent at the spine. The placebo group had the same magnitude of loss at both sites. In the smaller extension group, at the end of three years bone density increased in the Fosteum group while the placebo group had a mirrored loss of 7 percent at the hip and 10 percent at the spine.

Since it is unlikely that women who were more than five years past menopause would have had such rapid bone loss, it raises questions about the results of this small study. In addition, the modest effect of Fosteum on bone turnover does not explain the observed robust increase of bone density.

Digestive complaints were more common with Fosteum. By the end of two years, one in five participants in the Fosteum group discontinued the study due to adverse events. The lining of the womb (endometrium) did not change with two years of use. The report of this study did not include any mention of hot flashes.

It is nice to see randomized clinical trials with Fosteum. However, the two studies combined have a total of just fewer than five hundred subjects. Since the main ingredient is genistein, other soy studies can be looked at to put the results of these two studies into perspective. Fosteum clearly has an estrogenic effect, which may be why the number and intensity of hot flashes are lower. Even so, one of the small Italian studies showed that Fosteum was less effective than estrogen in decreasing the frequency and intensity of hot flashes. Do not use Fosteum if you have a history of breast cancer or have other reasons you cannot take estrogen products.

Fosteum
(genistein)

Category
Antiresorptive
Phytoestrogen

Manufacturer
Primus Pharmaceuticals

Pivotal Fracture Trial
none

Fracture Reduction
none

Indications for Osteopenia and Osteoporosis
Prescription medical food product

Dose
1 capsule twice a day
Each capsule contains
27 mg genistein aglycone
20 mg citrated zinc bisglycinate
200 IU cholecalciferol

Additional Information
May increase bone density
May decrease hot flashes
Not for use in women with history of breast cancer

If you have hot flashes and good bone density to begin with, soy products may be helpful in reducing the number and intensity of those power surges. It may be the total daily dose amount of isoflavones in soy that is important rather than just the genistein. If that is indeed the case, you can get all you need in other less expensive soy products.

If you have established osteoporosis or have a history of broken bones and are looking for something else, you cannot rely on Fosteum to reduce your risk of fractures. I recommend that you look at FDA-approved medicines that show reduction in the risk of fractures in studies of thousands of people.

The Bare Bones

- Fosteum is a medical food prescribed by your doctor.
- It is a concentrated product of soy, called genistein, and contains zinc and vitamin D as well.
- Fosteum should not to be taken if you have a history of breast cancer.
- Fosteum is not proven to reduce fractures, but it may increase bone density and help in reducing hot flashes, although the data are scant.

Soy: Pass the Tofu?

I did not pay attention to soy until I reached menopause. I switched to a soy latte in the morning and increased the soy in my diet with the hope that my hot flashes and sweats would diminish. Plenty of other women are doing the same thing. Soy is everywhere. It's a common dairy substitute in the form of soy milk, soy cheese, or soy yogurt. Soy protein is in all types of products on the grocery shelves. Tofu has increased in popularity beyond use in Asian dishes. The whole soybean in its young, green stage is called edamame, its Japanese name, and is served as a healthy appetizer.

Soy is commonly used by postmenopausal women for health benefits, whether as a supplement or as a regular part of their diets. There is tremendous interest in the use of soy foods for protecting the bone.

A Natural SERM?

Soybeans are high in protein that is rich in isoflavones. Isoflavones belong to a class of plant compounds called phytoestrogens. Depending on the target tissue, these compounds have the ability to mimic or block the actions of estrogen. Their action is similar to the designer estrogens or SERMs, like Evista, which has both estrogen-like and anti-estrogen effects.

The soy isoflavones are genistein, daidzein, and glycitein. Like Evista, soy isoflavones bind to estrogen receptors. Therefore, you might expect similar effects: Benefit to the bone without causing stimulation of breast tissue or the lining of the uterus (endometrium). Research has focused on whether you actually get these effects with soy.

Effectiveness

Looking at women in Japan and China, where soy foods are consumed in large amounts, suggests that a diet high in soy is beneficial for bone health, since rates of fracture are lower there than in Western countries. Trying to pinpoint the key factor is the difficulty. Most likely a combination of factors that make up the Asian lifestyle contributes to the lower risk of fracture, not just a single factor. For those of us on Western diets, it is difficult to change our diets to match those of Asian women. In the research setting, the approach has been to try tablets or supplements to see if they result in bone density changes.

Several analyses of multiple small studies (meta-analyses) have shown mixed results regarding bone-protective effects of soy. Regardless of the findings, the results cannot be applied to US women because the majority of the studies included in the meta-analyses were based on Asian women. However, recent results from larger, well-designed, randomized clinical trials show little, if any, effect. The following are recent randomized placebo-controlled trials conducted for a year or longer in European or American women.

PHYTOS

The PHYTOS study used isoflavone-enriched biscuits and cereal bars in more than two hundred healthy, early postmenopausal Caucasian women for one year. The foods were enriched with a total daily dose of 110 mg of isoflavones from soy concentrate, which consisted of 60 to 75 percent genistein. Consumption of enriched foods containing 110 mg per day of soy isoflavone did not prevent bone loss and did not affect bone turnover in early postmenopausal women.

Soy and Bone Mineral Density in Older Women

This study looked at the addition of dietary soy protein and isoflavone in tablet form separately and in combination versus placebo. A total of 131 women with an average age of seventy-three began the clinical trial and three-quarters of the women successfully completed the study. In a group of late postmenopausal women, the addition of soy for one year did not affect bone density or bone turnover markers.

OPUS: Osteoporosis Prevention Using Soy

OPUS was a two-year study with daily supplementation of 80 or 120 mg of soy isoflavones in the form of a tablet versus an inactive placebo tablet. A total of four hundred healthy early postmenopausal women, average age fifty-five, participated. At the end of two years, bone density decreased in the 3 percent range at the spine and the 2 percent range at the total hip in all groups. Bone density declined regardless of soy treatment.

SIRBL: Soy Isoflavones for Reducing Bone Loss

SIRBL was a three-year study of daily 80 or 120 mg doses of soy isoflavones in 224 postmenopausal women, average age fifty-four. The soy isoflavones were extracted from soy protein and compressed into tablets. Approximately 2 percent loss in bone density was observed at the hip and spine with the 80 mg dose. However, the 120 mg daily dose showed a slowing of bone loss at the neck region of the hip only. No treatment effect was seen on bone turnover markers. These doses had no effect on the lining of the womb (endometrial thickness) and there were no reports of any adverse events.

The study interventions included the use of isolates of soy protein, isoflavone supplements, extracts from soy foods, and soy integrated into foods. Even though the studies used different types and dosages of supplements, the results are underwhelming. Although the active component of soy is considered to be the isoflavone component and not its protein, no significant differences were found. Older studies with the synthetic ipriflavone up to doses of 200 mg three times a day also failed to show bone benefits.

The effects of soy on bone may depend on the dose. A daily dose higher than 80 to 90 mg appeared to be required for any effect, and that was only minimal. This is considerably higher than the average soy dietary intake of 50 to 60 mg in Asia and the estimated 25 to 30 mg needed for heart benefits. Overall, the intervention trials examining the effect of soy isoflavones on bone density and bone turnover markers in Western population groups do not confirm the findings of the population studies and clinical trials involving Asian women.

The wide variability in response may relate to the ability to produce equol, which is a byproduct of the isoflavone daidzein. Only an estimated 30 to 50 percent of those in Western populations are able to produce equol. In contrast, Asians, who consume soy products with greater regularity, are more likely to be equol producers. The presence of equol may be a key factor in the positive effects of a diet rich in soy. Since this is not fully proven and has been contradicted, the verdict is still out on the production-of-equol theory.

Because soy protein and isoflavones (either alone or together) did not affect bone mass, they should not be considered an effective therapy for preserving skeletal health in postmenopausal women.

Is there a downside to use of soy supplements? Because they deliver levels of isoflavones that exceed the usual dietary intakes from soy, the safety of soy isoflavone supplements may be a concern. Soy products were well tolerated in short-term studies. The overall long-term effects on the breast and uterine lining are not known. However, if soy works like a SERM, you would not expect stimulation of breast tissue or the uterine lining. Also, Asian women have low rates of breast and endometrial cancer.

Right now there are two opposing lines of research on breast cancer and soy: Soy or its isoflavones may either protect against breast cancer or promote breast cancer. For heart disease, the benefits and risks are also being debated.

Remember, the research studies are based on soy protein or isoflavones, not the whole food. Just like any other nutrient, dietary soy is preferable to supplements. However, the few studies on dietary intervention did not show prevention of bone loss. Soy isoflavones in higher doses appear to suppress bone loss rather than induce bone gain.

The Bare Bones

- Intervention studies using soy supplements do not show treatment effects.
- The ability to produce equol may be needed to gain some health benefits, but the evidence is inconclusive.
- Increasing your dietary soy intake may be helpful for your overall health, but do not count on a boost for your bones.

Strontium Citrate:
Is It the Same as Ranelate?

Because strontium ranelate is not available in the US, many women have turned to the other strontium sources on the pharmacy shelves. The over-the-counter supplement strontium citrate is the most common. Strontium may be available in other salt forms. You may also find strontium carbonate, strontium chloride, or strontium gluconate. A totally different form, a radioactive isotope of strontium, is used as a treatment for bone pain caused by cancer in the bone. I mention that in case you hear of someone being treated with strontium in the hospital.

You cannot take strontium citrate at the same time as anything else. You must be very fastidious about taking it on an empty stomach. That means having no food, drink, or any other medicines or supplements for at least two hours before. The most convenient time is usually at bedtime. The doses of strontium citrate vary from a few micrograms to 1,000 milligrams in a multivitamin and mineral packet. The most widely available formulations of strontium citrate only contain 226 mg or 340 mg per pill, and the supplement dose is two a day for a total of 452 or 680 mg daily.

The above doses equate to about a quarter to a third of the amount of strontium in the strontium ranelate sachet. At those fractions of the prescription medicine dose, the strontium citrate is probably not going to work. The 2 gram or 2,000 milligrams daily dose of strontium ranelate only decreases bone turnover a small amount. Therefore, you are unlikely to see any changes with over-the-counter strontium citrate. Although a systematic study has not been done, colleagues who have followed patients taking strontium citrate have not seen any changes in bone turnover or bone density.

Effectiveness

What are the data for strontium citrate? At the present time, almost nothing. One small study at the University of California, Davis, will answer a few questions, but it will not be definitive. Researchers there are conducting a study titled "Effects of Strontium Citrate on Bone Health in Women." They are evaluating the 680 mg formulation taken daily for three months. A total of two hundred early postmenopausal women are being recruited and randomized to strontium citrate or placebo pills. Measures of bone markers and bone density will be done at baseline. However, because of the brief duration of the study, only bone markers will be followed.

The many curious patients who want to know if strontium citrate works will find that the UC Davis study will provide only limited results. The study's three-month duration will be too short to allow researchers adequate time to evaluate strontium citrate's effects on bone density. What we really want to know is whether strontium citrate decreases fractures. But that would require a huge study of thousands of people for at least three years. Such a study is unlikely.

The UC Davis study will only provide results for bone turnover markers collected in a controlled environment. If this study verifies what has been seen in the clinic, you should leave the strontium citrate on the pharmacy shelf and not waste your money.

Cannot Live without Strontium?

If you decide you cannot live without strontium and have absolutely *no* other option, take the medicine that has been used in clinical trials. Read the section titled "Other Medicines: Available Elsewhere But Not in the United States" (page 263) to get more information about strontium ranelate. If you are still interested after reading that summary, talk to your doctor about this medicine.

If you have a valid prescription, canadadrugs.com will fill your prescription and send it to a US address. If you and your doctor agree that strontium ranelate is a reasonable next step, ask him to write the prescription. The brand Protelos, which contains a dose of 2 grams of strontium ranelate, is stocked in boxes of twenty-eight sachets. Be sure to understand that you will need to find a DXA center that knows how to measure your bone density and adjust the measurement for the presence of strontium.

The Bare Bones

- Strontium citrate is a supplement containing a quarter to a third of the strontium in the medicine strontium ranelate, which is not available in the US.
- The supplement must be taken on an empty stomach at least two hours after food, drink, or other supplements or medicines, usually at bedtime.
- Based on limited information from individual patients rather than from trials, strontium citrate does not appear effective for increasing bone density and lowering risk of fractures.

Natural Products:
Still More Questions to Be Answered

In this section, you will find a list of supplements that is by no means complete, though it does cover the names of the majority of supplement components you may encounter. One problem with listing them separately is that many are used in combination with other supplements. Trying to isolate which one or two ingredients may be responsible for the main effect hampers studies of the natural health products. For instance, traditional Chinese herbal medicines tend to rely on the joint actions of many herbs mixed together.

The natural health products listed below include most products that are promoted as "effective" for bone health. However, there is little scientific evidence on the effectiveness of these various products for boosting bone health. Many of the natural medicines advocated for bone protection are used for reducing menopausal symptoms. You get immediate feedback when trying to quell hot flashes. In contrast, you just do not know if the treatment is effective for bone, since there is no relief of symptoms and you need to wait a longer time interval to see results.

Selected Natural Health Products Used for Bone Health
Alfalfa (*Medicago sativa*)
Black cohosh (*Cimicifuga racemosa*)
Black currant seed oil
Boron
Copper
Deer velvet
Dehydroepiandrosterone (DHEA)
Dong quai (*Angelica sinensis*)
Evening primrose oil
Fish oils
Flaxseed (*Linum usitatissimum*)
Fluoride
Ginseng
Hops (*Humulus lupulus*)
Horsetail (*Equisetum arvense*)

Licorice root (*Glycyrrhiza glabra*)
Manganese
Red clover (*rifolium pratense*)
Silicon
Stinging nettle (*Urtica dioica*)
Wild yam (*Dioscorea species*)
Zinc

This laundry list of natural health products is organized for discussion into the following groups: products with estrogen-like effects, oils, trace elements, and Chinese herbal remedies.

Estrogen-like Effects

These products may have effects like estrogen and theoretically, if strong enough, they may protect bone. Some may act like a "natural SERM." They are estrogen-like at the bone, inhibit estrogen at the breast, and may have other anticancer properties. Others may work by increasing circulating levels of estrogens. The products with the most scientific evidence are covered first.

Dehydroepiandrosterone, or DHEA, is a hormone made naturally by the adrenal glands, which sit atop each kidney. Levels of DHEA fall progressively after about thirty years of age. Since these hormone levels decrease with aging and diseases of aging, including osteoporosis, DHEA is touted as an effective "anti-aging" hormone supplement.

Does increasing DHEA to youthful concentrations improve or preserve bone health? Estrogen levels increase as a result of taking DHEA. Small positive changes in bone density were observed with use for one or two years at a daily dose of 50 mg for older women and 75 mg for men. However, these small changes were not consistently seen in the hip, spine, or forearm or in both men and women.

Since DHEA is converted into testosterone and estrogen, the long-term effects, especially risks of breast cancer or prostate cancer, are not known. In addition, DHEA has also been shown to decrease levels of "good" (HDL) cholesterol in women, and this could potentially increase the risk of heart disease. In the absence of long-term studies and with a potential for harmful effects, DHEA is not recommended until further information in known.

Red clover is a legume like soybeans. It contains large amounts of plant estrogens, or phytoestrogens, with the active isoflavone compounds genistein and daidzein, which are similar to soy, as well. Based on dry weight, red clover is said to contain ten times the phytoestrogens found in soy. Supplements made from extracts of red clover are increasingly popular as alternative therapies for hot flashes. One brand, Promensil®, contains 40 mg of red clover isoflavones in the standard tablet preparation.

The bone-preserving effects of red clover have also been examined, but the evidence is very limited. In a one-year clinical trial using a red clover-derived supplement, bone density was better than placebo at the spine. No difference was observed at the hip.

Flaxseed in a dose of 40 grams daily was given in a small clinical trial for three months. Flaxseed improved cholesterol but did not change bone turnover markers in postmenopausal women. In a longer one-year study in two hundred postmenopausal women, bone density was similar between the treatment and placebo groups.

Other plants, including alfalfa, horsetail, hops, and licorice root, have similar isoflavone properties, which may be responsible for their reported estrogen-like effects.

Black cohosh and wild yam are used as a "natural alternative" for estrogen therapy. The mechanism of action for black cohosh is not clear, and there is no information on its effect on bone. In a small study of Taiwanese women, wild yams increased levels of estrone, which is an estrogen produced in fat cells. No direct study has been done on its effect on bone. However, estrone positively correlates with bone mass in postmenopausal women in other studies.

Ginseng is used for a myriad of health reasons. The estrogen-like effects of ginseng are controversial. Estrogen activity is suggested by the fact that with large doses in postmenopausal women, vaginal bleeding may occur.

OILS

Plant-based and fish oils are essential fatty acids. These fatty acids are necessary for health, but your body does not make them so you must get them through food. The two types are called omega-3 fatty acids and omega-6 fatty acids. Some studies suggest that people who do not get enough of some essential fatty acids are more likely to have bone loss. The ratio of the fatty acids is also implicated. A higher ratio of omega-6 to omega-3 fatty acids is associated with lower hip bone density in both men and women.

Evening primrose oil and **black currant seed oil**, taken as supplements, contain an omega-6 fatty acid called gamma-linolenic acid. In a small pilot study using evening primrose oil in combination with fish oils and calcium, subjects showed less bone loss over three years than those who took placebo. In this study, after the first eighteen months, the placebo group switched to active therapy and all subjects had small increases in bone density.

Fish oils have a long list of benefits. I take fish oil for its purported heart effects. Dietary studies suggest that the omega-3 fatty acids are important for bone density. In five small supplemental fish oil studies, the effect of omega-3 fatty acids on bone density was variable. Small or no effects were observed.

TRACE MINERALS

In addition to calcium and vitamin D, certain minerals are required for the maintenance of healthy bone. Trace amounts, as the name implies, are all that is needed. Unless you are malnourished, your diet should be supplying what you need.

Copper, **manganese**, and **zinc** work with enzymes that manufacture the collagen fiber of bone as well as many other essential reactions in the body. In epidemiology studies pinpointing one element, zinc showed a correlation with higher bone mass. But if more is given in supplements, will that make a difference? No clinical trials have looked at this.

In the early 1990s, a colleague at the University California, San Diego, Dr. Paul Saltman, looked at a "cocktail" of trace minerals with and without calcium in a small group of women for two years. Since this study is widely cited as "proof," I am providing more detail. Each active supplement contained 15 mg of zinc, 2.5 mg of copper, and 5 mg of manganese. The calcium was 1,000 mg in the form of calcium citrate malate. A total of fifty-nine older women with an average age of sixty-six were divided into four groups. Bone density at the spine was evaluated at the end of two years:

Trace mineral only: slowed bone loss
Calcium only: slowed bone loss
Combination trace minerals and calcium: maintained stable bone density
Placebo: bone loss

Only the combination versus placebo comparison showed statistical difference.

Do you need more than a trace for "good measure"? There is no evidence to suggest that supplementation is needed or beneficial for people eating a normal diet. If you think you need more of one of these minerals, eat food rich in that nutrient. The food will supply it in balance with other essential nutrients.

Boron and its usefulness became a topic of discussion following my very first public lecture on the topic of bone health. The first question asked was, "Do I need boron in my calcium tablets?" There was no guiding data then, and more than twenty years later, there is still no evidence from clinical trials. In fact, its biological function has not been clearly established. Again, it is a "trace" element, and a trace is all you should need.

Silicon may confer bone benefits. In one observational study, higher dietary intake of silicon was associated with higher bone density. Beer was recently found to be high in silicon content. This finding led to many headlines, like "Beer, A New Treatment for Your Bones?" Just don't make a steady diet of it.

Horsetail also contains significant amounts of silicon. Horsetail contains an enzyme (thiaminase) that can cause deficiency of the B vitamin, thiamine. Some horsetail products may specify that they are "thiaminase-free," but there is not enough information to know if thiaminase-free products are safe. You may want to stay clear of this product.

Stinging nettle is a root that contains both silicon and boron. It is better known for its use as a diuretic.

Fluoride has a high affinity for calcium, so it can easily become part of the bone mineral structure. Years of research and development have investigated fluoride as a potential prescription medicine. There were high hopes for its success because it stimulates the bone-forming cells, osteoblasts. In 1993, three preparations were in final stages of clinical trials. Large increases in bone density, particularly at the spine, were achieved. The problem turned out to be that the denser bone was more prone to fracture. Fluoride did not prevent fractures. The mineral structure it created was more brittle.

Dr. David Baylink, at Loma Linda University in California, believes that there may be a small window of opportunity for fluoride. He uses it with a very special patient who needs a bone formation boost but cannot take Forteo. He must fastidiously follow blood levels of fluoride to get "just the right amount." He cautions people not to try this on their own.

TRADITIONAL CHINESE MEDICINES

Even though I am fascinated by Chinese medicine, I cannot begin to interpret the dozens of Chinese herbs that go into different concoctions. These prescriptions were produced by trial and error literally over centuries.

In general, the kidney is viewed as the controlling system for the bone. Therefore, stimulating the kidney with traditional medicines is thought to provide beneficial bone effects. However, it is unclear how the herbs actually influence the bone tissue. Many "tonics" are a combination of multiple botanicals.

Dong quai or *Angelica sinensis* is a common ingredient in prescriptions for bone fractures and osteoporosis. Clinical data has shown that these prescriptions reduce fracture healing time. This observation suggests that Dong quai speeds up bone formation. Researchers in the laboratory have shown that Dong quai increased production of proteins in cell culture, which may, in turn, increase bone formation.

Deer velvet from deer antlers is another product in common use. It contains ferulic acid, which seems to have estrogenic activity. In cell cultures, ferulic acid stimulates breast cancer cells. You should avoid using deer velvet if, for example, you are restricted from using estrogen because of a history of breast cancer.

Researchers are working to demonstrate the effectiveness of traditional remedies beyond the cell cultures. Usually, traditional prescriptions combine many herbal and mineral medicines. Although only one or two are responsible for the central effect, the supplemental ingredients may also be important in achieving the goal of a remedy.

WORDS OF CAUTION

These products do not require evaluation for safety and effectiveness by the FDA. The FDA has no requirements for the composition of supplements. As a result, some products may contain different amounts than stated on the label. For example, in a study of commercially available DHEA preparations, only half of products tested matched the stated ingredient amount on the package. The other half ranged from none to 150 percent of the claimed amount.

Under the Dietary Supplement Health and Education Act of 1994, the dietary supplement manufacturer is responsible for ensuring that a dietary supplement is safe before it is marketed. Good Manufacturing Practices (GMPs) for dietary supplements are modeled after those for food. They are designed to help prevent super-potent or sub-potent products, wrong ingredients, contaminants, or foreign materials in the supplements.

Natural products are not always innocuous. There is a false perception that these remedies are safer than manufactured medicines. An analysis of 251 Asian herbal products bought in the United States identified arsenic in 36 of them, mercury in 35, and lead in 24 of the products. Yikes!

Taking a blood thinner? Don't take these. If you are taking Coumadin, Plavix, Effient®, or anything else to thin your blood, do not take any of these products. It is playing Russian roulette with your body; some increase bleeding, others decrease blood-thinning effectiveness. Dong quai has blood-thinning properties like Coumadin. Other herbs including ginseng and red clover, may also increase bleeding. Others can reduce the effects of your blood thinning medicine, such as alfalfa, which contains a large amount of vitamin K. The American Society of Anesthesiologists recommends stopping all herbal medicines at least two weeks before surgery because of the risks of herbal and drug interaction as well as an increased chance of bleeding.

If you use these supplements, be aware that the data, if any, do not show support for bone health. Some supplements, like fish oil, may have other benefits for your general health, which may make them good choices to include in your daily regimen. However, your diet is the best way to get the nutrients you need and in the right proportion. Although many of these products may help diminish menopausal symptoms, longer-term effects on bone health have not been seen. Overall, clinical evidence is presently lacking to support their use as effective supplements for bone health.

The Bare Bones

- The research on these products for beneficial bone effects is scant or inconclusive.
- Although some of these products may help your hot flashes, don't count on getting bone benefits, too. Effects on bone overall are not seen.
- Choose wisely and stay clear of claims that sound too good to be true.
- Share with your doctor which supplements you are using.
- Recognize that the products you are taking are not necessarily harmless and be aware of potential side effects or interactions with medicines.

Vibration Therapy:
Good, Good, Good, Good Vibrations

Like the Beach Boys, Dr. Clinton Rubin has been delivering good vibrations for years in his laboratory experiments. Dr. Rubin's research at the State University of New York (SUNY) at Stony Brook focuses on how vibration affects bone. He and his team have been responsible for the lion's share of research in this area. Prior to his research, vibration was most often viewed as harmful to bone and muscle, particularly for generating low back problems among those who were regularly exposed to vibration in the workplace. As a result of those concerns, international safety standards were established to define thresholds for human tolerance of vibration.

Dr. Rubin's laboratory experiments started with "buzzing" turkeys with low levels of vibration. A true buzz was created at an international bone meeting when he showed the effect of low-intensity, high-frequency vibration on bone. Adult female sheep were treated for twenty minutes a day with low-level mechanical vibration at high-frequency, 30 cycles per second, for one year. The treated sheep showed a marked increase of 30 percent in the density and volume of the leg bone (femur) in comparison to the untreated. That is a tremendous amount of bone formation.

Vibration therapy is being explored as a drug-free intervention for preventing bone loss and building bone. Similar to drug development, a low-intensity version of whole body vibration has been tested in animals and small groups of subjects with promising results. Now, larger studies in high-risk individuals are being done, and the exact mechanism of action of how vibration is causing these changes is being worked out.

A SUBSTITUTE FOR EXERCISE?

This low intensity mechanical vibration at high frequency of 30 cycles per second may offer the benefits of exercise (without having to exercise) plus other positive effects. It would be a welcome addition to the "medicine chest" for treatment of osteoporosis, particularly in older individuals with fragile skeletons. The additional benefits of building muscle mass and improving balance in this high-risk group, who are prone to muscle loss and falls with aging, are particularly attractive. The recent findings that these low magnitude signals direct the bone marrow stem cell population to make more osteoblasts, or bone-forming cells, instead of becoming fat cells, is equally exciting.

Mechanical signals are critical to achieving and retaining bone health. The benefit of exercise is achieved through this mechanism. The bone's adaptation to mechanical signals can be influenced by a very few higher magnitude strain events or by many thousands of low magnitude strain events. Low-magnitude vibration signals basically mimic muscle contraction similar to maintaining a standing posture. The low-intensity mechanical signals produced by the vibration platform can change the fate of stem cells to become bone-forming cells instead of fat cells. This process is similar to what happens with higher impact signals from weight-bearing exercises.

Dr. Rubin and his team elegantly showed the ability of low-intensity signals to increase bone formation and at the same time decrease fat formation in several animal experiments. In one experiment, the overall number of stem cells was increased by almost 50 percent and more became bone-forming cells than fat cells. The end result was better bones, less fat, and more stem cells.

In another theory of how vibration may increase bone formation, experiments in the absence of weight bearing suggest that shaking back and forth causes fluid changes that can be sensed by bone cells. Dr. Janet Rubin, a professor of medicine at the University of North Carolina at Chapel Hill, is helping to work out the precise mechanism of action. (It is a family affair for the Rubins—they are brother and sister.)

EFFECTIVENESS

Several small pilot studies evaluated whether the observations seen in animal studies would also occur in humans. In the first clinical trial, seventy postmenopausal women were randomly assigned to either a treatment group that used a vibration platform delivering low-level mechanical vibration at high frequency, 30 cycles per second, or a control group that used an inactive platform. Subjects in each group stood on their platform for ten minutes twice a day for twelve months. At the end of one year, the treatment group maintained bone mass while the control group lost bone. The greatest benefit was seen in women weighing 143 pounds or less. In contrast to those in the vibration-active group, who had essentially stable bone density, those in the control group experienced bone density losses that averaged about 3 percent at the spine and 2 percent at the neck region of the hip.

One study looked at vibration therapy as an intervention for twenty children with conditions that limit exercise, such as cerebral palsy. The children stood on platforms five days a week for ten minutes each day; half of them received the active vibration. After six months, the treatment group gained 6.3 percent on measurements of the shinbone and the placebo group lost 12 percent. An 18 percent difference in just a half a year is *huge*. Keep in mind that this study looked at only a handful of subjects.

A one-year trial of fifty young women, ages fifteen to twenty, with a history of a fracture and bone density lower than the average for their peers was also done. Subjects were randomized to an active or an inactive vibration platform. At the end of one year, spine bone density in the active group, measured by CT scan, increased almost 4 percent. The muscle next to the spine showed a 10 percent increase; and a small increase in abdominal fat was noted. In contrast, women in the control group failed to increase their bone density or muscle area and had an almost 6 percent increase in abdominal fat formation.

Although this may all sound too good to be true, we are anxiously awaiting the outcomes of the current randomized clinical trials that use these low intensity vibration platforms for treatment of frail older patients with osteoporosis. Because falls, muscle strength, and balance problems raise the fracture risk in seniors, this intervention would be a boon for this population. Anyone who is unable to exercise may benefit; the applications may be boundless. Based on the animal research, you may be able to jump-start stem cells to make osteoblasts instead of fat cells.

Positive results would open a whole new approach, especially for the high-risk older patient. The mantra "no pain, no gain" may be trumped by this approach. How vibration therapy might interface with individuals on medicines for osteoporosis is another area for further research. Be on the lookout for the results of the clinical trials and the FDA approval of this low intensity vibration platform, which looks like an oversized laptop computer and weighs seventeen pounds. Availability of this device is anticipated in late 2011.

Not All Vibration Platforms Are the Same

A word of caution about those whole-body vibration platforms in your fitness center; they are different from the ones used in Dr. Rubin's experiments. Do you need to hang on for dear life while you are on the vibration machine? All that shaking is probably too much force. The high intensity whole body machines were developed to give elite athletes an extra edge. For us mere mortals, more is not necessarily better.

Just like there is a "therapeutic window" for many medicines and nutritional supplements, research indicates that a "mechanical window" also exists. Too little or too much may cause harm rather than good. Those platforms developed for use by elite athletes should not be used by anyone with a fragile skeleton. If you have good bone density and do decide to use one, make sure to *bend your knees*.

The potential to use low-intensity vibration in place of strenuous exercise to improve bone quality and quantity is an exciting new horizon. In addition, the stimulation of signals to the bone marrow to produce more of the bone-forming cells that tend to decline with aging may truly be the "Fountain of Youth" for bone and muscles. We will know soon from results of well-designed clinical trials whether Dr. Rubin has found the sweet spot with his device that delivers low-intensity vibrations at high frequency. If so, this portable low-intensity vibration platform will be a surefire blockbuster.

If more research demonstrates that low-intensity vibration results in a remarkable decrease in production of abdominal fat in preference for making bone, we will all be making a beeline to get this device. And we will look forward to idly standing around for fifteen to twenty minutes a day while good vibrations do their thing.

The Bare Bones
- Low-intensity vibration may be a substitute for high-impact physical activity.
- Mechanical signals do not need to be large to produce positive effects on bone.
- Low-level, high-frequency mechanical signals produced by a vibrating platform appear to promote bone formation.
- If proven effective in clinical trials, this simple device may be a drug-free therapy for osteoporosis.

Physical Measures: Integrating Movement

Picture daybreak in a city. Hundreds of people are moving yet it is eerily quiet. That was my experience on a trip to China in 1988, where millions and millions of people practice tai chi. Just after dawn, parks and street corners filled with men and women moving slowly and fluidly through a complete range of motion over their natural center of gravity. When I looked closer, I discovered that most of the participants were older and some were quite elderly. They all moved gracefully, floating from side to side. It was an amazing sight—I was transfixed—and I witnessed the same scenes, again and again, in the early morning light, in every city I visited.

Tai chi is just one of the meditative mind-body exercises growing in popularity in the US. Yoga, Pilates®, and Feldenkrais® are other common low impact forms of exercise that focus on the mind-body link. You will find that most fitness clubs provide classes or individual instruction in yoga or Pilates. However, you may need to search for a Feldenkrais practitioner in your area if you wish to learn that method, as there are currently only eight to ten thousand in the United States. Health departments often sponsor free tai chi classes, and local tai chi societies also offer introductory sessions.

TAI CHI

Tai chi has been practiced in China for more than a thousand years. Tai chi has its roots in martial arts, but it has developed into a practice of flowing meditative movements. Some styles of tai chi retain more of a martial arts focus with the sharp release of power. Slow and smooth movements that involve all the major muscle groups characterize this low-impact weight-bearing exercise. The sway of movement is centered with constant shifting of body weight, which improves leg and core strength as well as balance. The body's weight is transferred back and forth between the legs with both knees slightly bent at all times. I like to visualize the expressive names of the movements, like "white crane spreads wings" or "carry tiger to the mountain."

Tai chi has been touted to have health benefits for just about every ailment. Tai chi is based on the same principles as acupuncture and herbal therapies—to balance the yin and yang and the flow of life force called qi or chi. For bone health, tai chi is helpful for balance, posture, muscle strength, and flexibility.

Studies of tai chi's effects on bone density have been mixed. From the bone perspective, tai chi's real value is in fall prevention, which plays an important role in decreasing fracture risk.

Tai chi practiced in the controlled environment of trials has shown a positive impact on older people, including frail adults. The observed benefits included directly reducing the risk of falls and fear of falling and improving muscle strength, balance, and flexibility, as well as performance of usual activities of day-to-day life. The benefit lasts only so long as tai chi is being regularly performed.

YOGA

"Yoga" means something different to each of us, probably because the variations seem innumerable. Yoga is a systemic exercise that combines posture, breathing, and stretching to promote physical and mental well-being. Some types are very strenuous and difficult while others are gentler, with more of a focus on alignment and stretching. According to yoga master B. K. S. Iyengar, "Words cannot convey the value of yoga—it has to be experienced." In his book, *Light on Life*, Iyengar writes, "Physical health is not a commodity to be bargained for. Nor can it be swallowed in the form of drugs and pills. It has to be earned through sweat. It is something that we must build up."

As with any exercises or movement, if you have already had a spine fracture or are at high risk for one, you will need to adapt some of the exercises that involve flexion or bending forward, since that would increase forces on your spine. Therefore, the emphasis should be on maintaining a neutral spine position that is neither bent forward nor extended back.

PILATES

Pilates studios and classes at fitness centers have sprouted up like mushrooms everywhere. Joseph Pilates was a German rehabilitation specialist who developed the exercise in the 1920s. The Pilates regimen offers neuromuscular reeducation via exercises integrated with a yoga-like conscious breathing pattern. Pilates may be done as a series of floor-mat exercises or by working with specialized machines. There are many adapted regimens, as well. The emphasis on centering and breathing is akin to the concepts in yoga and tai chi.

The focus in Pilates is on contracting muscle for power and developing a strong core. Pilates is also valuable for improving balance. Maneuvers on the Pilates machines are designed to lengthen and stretch the spine. Initially, focus is on posture of the spine and learning to use core muscles during controlled breathing. After one learns to maintain control of the spine, exercises gradually progress to incorporate arm and leg movements while maintaining control of the spine. Mat classes are similar but are done without the resistance of the machines. There are certain positions in Pilates that should be avoided if you have osteoporosis of the spine or history of spine fractures. The best approach would be to work first with an individual instructor before joining any group class. Ask your instructor to help you modify exercises so that they are appropriate and can be done safely.

Pilates is a whole body exercise that emphasizes core strength and correct body mechanics via specific exercises. These may help with balance, muscle strength, and reducing fall risk. Pilates has not been studied systematically in formal research studies on bone health. Modified programs have been adapted for use in older women at risk for fracture.

FELDENKRAIS

Feldenkrais focuses more on the brain to orchestrate movement. You are taught to think about any movement before you make the actual physical motion. By practicing Feldenkrais you learn to visualize your movement and to make the changes necessary for improving action and alignment. You create a new pattern of movement.

The best way to explain this method is by telling the story of its inventor, Moshe Feldenkrais. He applied his knowledge as a physicist and Judo master to "fix" his own knee injury by reteaching himself how to walk. He focused on the links between his brain and the rest of his nervous system in an effort to "rewire" his muscle responses. Based on this work, which he extended to therapy on others, he formulated the method known by his name in the 1950s. Now practitioners are taught and certified by the Feldenkrais Guild.

The technique has two major forms, group classes or individual sessions. A series of guided exercises in a class with a Feldenkrais instructor is called "awareness through movement." If you observe a class, you will see participants rolling from hip to hip with fluid movements. These and other simple movements that involve standing or sitting rewire the brain to direct correct movement.

The other approach, called "functional integration," involves the Feldenkrais practitioner making a series of gentle manipulations with movement. The practitioner's role is to look at how you move and to teach your brain to make the muscles move in the right directions. I call this "bodywork." You lie fully clothed on a massage-like table for about an hour while the practitioner moves you. This works on breaking habitual patterns of movement that may be the cause of problems like neck or back pain.

Anyone who has limitations as a result of fractures, illness, or just plain bad habits may benefit. Several small studies with guided exercises over short periods of time showed improvement in balance and mobility and decreased fear of falling. Keeping your body more finely tuned will help with muscle strength, balance, vitality, and decreasing risk of falling.

WANT TO BEGIN ONE OF THESE PROGRAMS BUT YOU'RE NOT SURE HOW?

Most of the people who practice one form or another of these techniques usually become strong advocates for their method of choice. However, at present there is not much science available on these mind-body physical measures in the area of bone health. Any activity that helps you improve strength, balance and coordination, posture, mental outlook, and overall vitality makes sense. It will complement and enhance your other efforts.

Participating in any form of these physical measures or exercises is always a good idea; doing so may be your road to longevity. If you are interested, check out the opportunities available in your community and take an introductory class.

I have tried all four of these methods. As a geriatrician, I was so fascinated with the vitality of the older Chinese who practice tai chi that I took up the practice of tai chi myself and continued for a couple of years after I returned from my trip to China. Now that I have reminded myself of its benefits, it is time to restart! The other techniques were recommended to me for relief of back pain. I am most familiar with Feldenkrais. A wonderful and insightful Feldenkrais practitioner treated me for years, but unfortunately she moved away. I was unable to replace her experience and expert eye with another practitioner.

Finding the right person with the right touch is a challenge, just like finding an expert in anything. The fit many times depends on the individual instructor, so it might take a bit of trial and error. Whatever your fitness level and interest, you will be able to find a class or instructor to fit your level and needs. If you have osteoporosis or previous spine fractures, some programs will need to be modified. There are positions in Pilates and yoga, particularly forward bending with a rounded back, which should be avoided.

The Bare Bones
Physical measure that utilize the mind-body link complement other therapies and are beneficial for:
- Improving balance and coordination
- Improving posture and muscle strength
- Building confidence
- Reducing pain

After a Major Fracture

New Spine Fractures:
Ways to Cement a Recovery

The majority of spine fractures are silent. You are not even aware that a fracture has happened. One clue may be loss of height. However, other common causes of height loss with aging include changes in your posture and decreases in the disc spaces, which are the cushions between your vertebrae. Silent fractures are discovered with some types of imaging like an x-ray or a DXA scan of the entire spine.

On the other hand, a fracture may be painful. However, back pain can have many other causes and it may be hard to sort out whether the pain is the result of a fracture or some other cause. Do not ignore back pain and think it will just go away. See your doctor. Get an evaluation ASAP.

LOCATION OF SPINE FRACTURES

There is a tendency for fractures to occur in the midback (T7–T9) and at the junction between your mid and lower (T11–L1) regions of the spine. As you can see on the diagram, these levels correspond to the areas between the shoulder blades and at the waistline in the small of the back. Do not ignore pain in those regions of your back; that is how some fractures may get missed. Talk with your doctor about getting an x-ray (or he may use the DXA machine in his office for a vertebral fracture assessment) as part of your evaluation of the pain.

Tim Gunther, gunthergraphics.biz

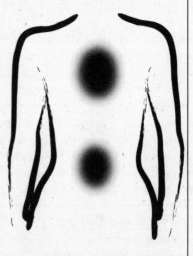

Common areas of back pain caused by spine fractures

Back pain caused by a fracture usually starts suddenly. The fracture may occur following a fall or after lifting a heavy object. Many times it just happens spontaneously and no precipitating cause is identified. The pain is localized to a spot over the area of the back where the fracture occurred. Then the area of pain tends to expand, as the muscles next to the spine become tight and go into spasm. The intensity of pain varies from person to person. It may start as "take your breath away" pain and then ease with time. Typically, the pain is made worse when standing up and when trying to work with your arms in front of your body, as in lifting a heavy pot or doing dishes.

MANAGING ACUTE PAIN

The priority first and foremost is to feel better. Pain relief can be a challenge. Multiple approaches may be needed to achieve the goal of eliminating pain.

Conservative measures. Your doctor may prescribe pain medicines and muscle relaxants. Be careful while taking these medicines. The risk of falling is increased while taking prescription pain medicines and muscle relaxants. You do not need another fracture. Lessen your risk of falling by taking your time when changing positions. Sit down if you feel lightheaded and ask for assistance if you need it. You may not tolerate the combination of pain and muscle relaxant medicines as well as when you were younger. Lower the dose if needed to keep your wits about you and your balance steady. Pain medicines also tend to cause constipation. Take a stool softener or fiber product along with plenty of water to prevent constipation. A trial of calcitonin by shot or nasal spray may be worthwhile. If it works, pain usually diminishes within five to seven days.

Additional therapies your doctor may recommend include physical therapy, acupuncture, electrotherapy with a "TENS" unit, and local anesthetic administered at a pain clinic. Sometimes the pain does not respond to these measures and a short hospital stay is needed to control the pain.

Cement Reinforcement. If the pain is too severe for control by conservative measures, another option may be cement reinforcement. The injection of special bone cement into the fractured bone stabilizes it like an internal splint and may even reinflate the bone. The majority of patients get pain relief that can be immediate because the cement prevents movement of the bone while it heals.

There are two types of these procedures: vertebroplasty and kyphoplasty. Many times they are lumped together, but they are distinct. Both techniques are controversial, as there is some uncertainty as to whether they help alleviate or actually create problems.

The procedures can be done on an outpatient basis in the radiology department or operating room. Under x-ray or CT guidance, cement is injected into the center of the broken bone in the back. Local or general anesthesia is used. You are allowed to go home as soon as two hours after the procedure.

Does cementing make a difference? Orthopedic studies tend to be short-term not long-term. My own back pain sojourn taught me that it is necessary to look at a longer time frame in evaluating any procedure. The initial reports of good pain relief are tempered by reports of fractures after the procedures. Several randomized trials using placebo comparison showed no effect. This additional information paints a not-so-rosy picture.

What is the difference between kyphoplasty and vertebroplasty?

Characteristics	Vertebroplasty	Kyphoplasty
Who typically performs the procedure?	Radiologist	Orthopedic or spine surgeon
Balloon expands the bone before cement	No	Yes
Height of vertebra	Not usually restored	May be restored
Cement leakage	Common	Uncommon

Vertebroplasty. The bone cement is injected under pressure, and it basically "freezes" the bone. Usually, it is not possible to increase the height of the broken vertebral bone. A common problem is the leaking of cement from the bone into surrounding tissue during the procedure. Cement leakage typically does not cause any symptoms, but has the potential for side effects.

Kyphoplasty. The company Kyphon developed this newer technique, hence the name. Kyphon is now part of Medtronics. The aim is to restore some height to the collapsed bone before putting in the cement. A balloon is inflated inside the bone (vertebral body) to create a space for the cement to be injected. Therefore, less pressure is needed to push the cement in. The lower pressure plus the creation of a space makes the cement more likely to stay in the confines of the bone and not leak out. The drawing depicts the vertebral body before and after a kyphoplasty. The height of the bone is increased. The angle of forward flexion is lessened, which helps restore the spine's center of gravity.

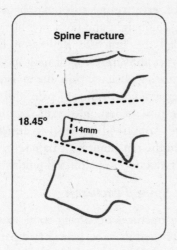

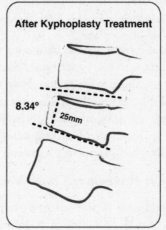

SOURCE: Adapted with kind permission from Springer Science and Business Media: Gaitanis IN et al. *European Spine Journal* 14 (2005): 250–60, figures 6a–b.

In studies comparing those who had cement with those who received conservative therapy, both types of procedures reported good pain-relief results in the short term. Compared with patients treated conservatively, those treated with either vertebroplasty or kyphoplasty experienced prompt reductions in pain and improvements in physical functioning within a day after either procedure. Many of the cement-treated patients were able to stop their pain medicines within twenty-four hours of the procedure. However, when a longer horizon was examined, no differences in pain were seen between groups at one year.

The real proof comes from a comparison of treated and placebo groups. To do this type of study, one group has to actually have the same procedure but with no injection of cement. Two small randomized trials done in that manner with vertebroplasty found no difference in pain relief or quality of life benefit. In both studies, patients with painful osteoporotic spine fractures underwent either vertebroplasty or a simulated procedure without cement. No difference in overall pain improvement was observed between the groups at the one-month mark in one study and at the three-month mark in the other. A larger European study that is planned to last at least one year is currently recruiting subjects with acute pain due to fracture.

As you can imagine, recruitment of participants for a study of this sort, which uses a sham procedure, is difficult. In addition, it raises ethical issues. Selecting the right individuals who may benefit is another challenge. Fortunately, most people improve spontaneously with no intervention. However, those with acute severe pain that is not relieved from conservative measures may benefit from a cementing procedure. The goal of retaining height and posture is also desirable.

A randomized two-year trial called the Fracture Reduction Evaluation (FREE) study compared kyphoplasty with nonsurgical treatment in three hundred subjects who had experienced fractures with acute pain due to osteoporosis. As expected, those with kyphoplasty experienced relief of pain and improved quality of life earlier than the nonsurgical group. However, by the end of twenty-four months, no differences were observed between treatment groups except for a small statistical difference in the ten-point back pain score, with the kyphoplasty group reporting a greater reduction in pain (-0.8 points).

Do Cement Procedures Cause New Spine Fractures?

After several case reports of new spine fractures occurring soon after a vertebroplasty, the Mayo Clinic in 2006 published its experience of all patients who had the procedure. Twenty percent of the 432 patients had new fractures. Subsequent studies reported the same rate. Are new fractures a result of underlying fragile bone or are they the result of the recent cementing procedure?

Fractures in the level above or below the cemented fracture, which happened about two months after the vertebroplasty procedure, were thought to be a result of the cementing. In contrast, fractures in other levels of the spine not next to the cemented level occurred later and were not thought to be due to the procedure.

However, later studies of biomechanics suggest that the cementing procedure may have more than just a local effect. The newly cemented vertebral body is harder than the adjacent ones. Not only are the local mechanical properties changed but the loading of the spine may be different. So it may take less force to cause a fracture anywhere in the spine.

In addition, once one level in the spine has fractured, one is at high risk for subsequent fractures. In the FREE study, almost half of those in both the kyphoplasty and nonsurgical treatment groups had new fractures identified by spine x-ray in the twenty-four-month-follow-up. The majority of the new fractures occurred in other levels of the spine not adjacent to the original fracture.

Factors Associated with New Fractures after a Cement Procedure

- On steroids
- More than one level cemented
- Two or more previous spine fractures
- Previous spine fractures next to the repaired fracture
- Fracture at the junction of the thoracic and lumbar spine (more motion back and forth)

Research into improved cement materials may help to solve the problem of adjacent-level fractures. New cements are being formulated with the main mineral components of bone. The goal is to find cement that more naturally mimics the composition of bone. The combination of cement and a titanium implant device, called OsseoFix®, has been approved for sale in Europe and is under investigation in the US.

An evaluation of Mayo Clinic patients after vertebroplasty showed fewer refractures in those who participated in a rehabilitation exercise program. The instruction incorporated isometric muscle strengthening of the back extensors that support the spine, as well as postural retraining. A structured therapy program after any fracture with or without cementing is a good idea.

YOUR STORIES . . .

Laurie, age sixty-two, and her husband were making a move to a smaller place a few miles away. They were downsizing because their youngest child had graduated from college and had taken a job out of state. Laurie's husband quipped that the move was to ensure "no room at the inn" for boomerang children. In the middle of packing, Laurie picked up a box and had stabbing pain in between her shoulder blades. The pain immediately took her breath away.

Over the course of the next several days, the pain became unbearable. She had her husband take her to the emergency room. A fracture of the eighth thoracic vertebra (T8) was found. Her pain was decreased in the emergency room to a tolerable level. She was sent home with pain medicines and a muscle relaxant.

However, the next day the pain returned with a vengeance. She went to see her primary doctor, who suggested another regimen for pain and put in a referral for physical therapy. In addition, he reviewed the DXA scan report that had been done about a year and half earlier. At that time, her bone density was reported as "osteopenia," with a lumbar spine T-score of -2.

Unfortunately, pain medicine and therapy was not helping to break the pain cycle. One night, when she couldn't even get comfortable lying down, she had her husband take her back to the emergency room. She was admitted to the hospital for pain control. A spine surgeon saw her in consultation and ordered an MRI and doctors from the pain clinic were helping manage her pain. The spine surgeon recommended proceeding with a kyphoplasty. At that point, she wanted to do anything to get rid of the pain. The kyphoplasty was performed and she had immediate relief of pain. She was discharged from the hospital later the same day.

She and her husband finally finished the move into their new home. Her physical therapy continued for two weeks, where she learned exercises and proper body mechanics. In the meantime, she read up on the options her doctor offered her to prevent a future fracture. She had another DXA scan, which showed that the lower two lumbar vertebrae actually had arthritis changes that falsely elevated her bone density scores. When only the first and second lumbar vertebra (L1 and L2) were used for analysis, her spine T-score was in the osteoporosis range, at -3.2.

Two years later . . .

Laurie's big incentive was to avoid pain ever happening again. She had had no more fractures at the two-year mark. She went all out to improve her bones and overall health. She and her husband joined the local YMCA and now go most days of the week. They do a combination of aerobics and weight exercises. Calcium and vitamin D are regular supplements. She cooks healthier foods and no longer stops at the fast-food places. She took Forteo for two years without problems and is now on generic alendronate. Her bone density after completing Forteo therapy showed an 11 percent increase using the total of L1 and L2, while her hip remained stable.

IF A SPINE FRACTURES HAPPENS, BE AGGRESSIVE TO PREVENT ANOTHER

The initial enthusiasm for the use of cement procedures after spine fractures has waned. Although the initial pain course may be shortened, over the long term it does not appear to make a difference. Afterward, the problem is that the strongly cemented vertebral body may overpower the rest of the other fragile vertebral bodies and cause new fractures. Different, more natural cements are being studied, as are other devices. In the meantime, the jury is still out. However, a small subgroup of patients with debilitating pain from a recent fracture may benefit from the procedures.

You still have a high risk for fracturing again in the natural course, even without cementing. Make sure there is no other cause of your fracture. Reassess every relevant detail of your life to look for ways you can make improvements; small changes can make a big difference. Consider a two-year course of Forteo. It is the only option that builds bone and reestablishes broken connections. Of note in the pivotal fracture trial, back pain was lower in the Forteo-treated group. Be aware of your body movements. Build up your back muscles and improve your posture in physical therapy. Learn to keep your back neutral and not bent forward as you go through your everyday activities.

The Bare Bones

If a painful fracture occurs...

- The first priority is pain control.
- Initial treatment includes pain medicines and physical therapy. A trial of calcitonin may be beneficial.
- Injection of cement may be considered in select individuals who have severe pain.
- Cement injection may increase the risk of more fractures.
- Be aggressive to prevent future spine fractures.

Hip Fracture: What to Expect

The risk of hip fracture is a clear and present danger for an eighty-year-old person. On average, a hip fracture occurs within five or six years after reaching that age milestone. An estimated one-third of Caucasian women who reach age ninety will suffer a hip fracture. That is a large number! However, the overall lifetime risk of hip fracture for Caucasian women is lower—14 percent—because many women will die earlier of other causes. About 17 percent of Caucasian men surviving to age ninety will sustain a hip fracture. If you are long-lived, you are at high risk. By educating yourself and your family, and by taking the appropriate measures now, you can make a difference: Hip fractures are not inevitable.

I hope neither you nor your loved ones ever suffer a hip fracture. But if you or they do, things happen quickly, so you must be prepared. In this section, I write from the perspective that the person who has sustained a hip fracture is one of your parents. Because the typical hip fracture occurs in an eighty-something woman, who is living at home, "your mother" will be the patient.

Your mother falls at home and can't get up. She activates her medical alert necklace that dials 911. An ambulance responds to the call and takes her to the nearest emergency room.

EMERGENCY ROOM

In the emergency room, the diagnosis of the fracture is confirmed by x-ray. Making your mother as comfortable as possible is the immediate goal. She will be given pain medicine, fluids by vein (IV fluids), and oxygen. The admitting physician will be contacted to come to the emergency room to evaluate your mother and admit her to the hospital. Depending on the hospital setup, the admitting doctor may be the orthopedic surgeon, a hospitalist (doctor based in the hospital), or her regular doctor. Some hospitals have a designated team organized to handle patients with hip fractures. Others may have set protocols that help deliver a consistent quality of care.

More often than not, the admitting physician is someone who does not know your mother. Giving an accurate picture of your mother's normal functioning status and medical history is critical to her management. With pain medicines on board, she may not be the best historian. You may need to help provide her medical history, or at least direct hospital doctors to her regular internist, family doctor, or specialist, who will be able to fill in the gaps.

Medicines. The medicines that your mother takes will matter greatly to the medical staff caring for her. I cannot stress this enough! Unfortunately, it is often the case that not all medicines are accounted for or specified correctly. Incomplete information can have disastrous (and I emphasize *disastrous*) outcomes.

I do not want you to just bring a list. You need to gather up all of her medicines and supplements from home. Check the bathroom, the kitchen, and her bedside table to be sure you have them all. On average, women in their eighties take ten to twelve different medicines and supplements. Put all the medicines and supplements in a bag and take them to the hospital. Doctors call review of the medicines "the brown bag assessment." They will thank you for taking this extra step to ensure complete information.

Do not take the medicines home until each of the treating physicians has physically seen what is inside the bag. A common medical error is not continuing your mother's regular medications. The medicines she takes at home tend to get lost in the shuffle between the emergency room and the hospital floor, and eventually the rehabilitation center or nursing home.

Even if you tell the emergency room staff, the information may not be correctly transmitted to the admitting physician, anesthesiologists, or anyone else responsible for her care. The ball can be dropped in a big way. Think of the childhood game "Telephone," and you will understand. The first person whispers a sentence or phrase to the next. Each player thereafter whispers the message as he or she heard it. The last player announces the statement, which usually differs significantly from the original. This is amusing if you are playing the game. In real life, such errors can be dangerous.

Critical decisions will be based on her regular medication regimen. If the doctors do not have the whole picture, that may contribute to a poor outcome.

Okay, you have gotten the message about the bag of medicines. Now, it is time to get her admitted to the hospital and up to a room. (If your mother is relatively healthy and has not eaten recently, sometimes she will go directly to surgery from the emergency room.)

PREPARING FOR SURGERY (PRE-OP)

In the hospital room, the bed may be set up with traction (a small amount of weight) to temporarily stabilize the fracture. Pain control is a balance between too much and too little. In order to reduce the chances of blood clots, special stockings will be placed on each of your mother's legs. These stockings will intermittently inflate and deflate to keep the blood flowing. She will continue with oxygen, IV fluids, and get nothing to eat or drink.

The ideal timing for surgery to repair the hip fracture is within twenty-four hours of admission. This does not provide much time to get "tuned up" for the operation. The medical doctors (hospitalists, internists, and cardiologist) may be involved in optimizing your mother's medical status prior to the surgery. Her underlying chronic medical problems will be taken into consideration for planning the type of surgery and anesthesia that will be used. Juggling a complex combination of medical conditions can be very challenging. The last time your mother ate or drank, as well as the medicines she is taking, will also be part of the decision-making.

Some situations may delay surgery beyond twenty-four hours. For example, if your mother was taking Coumadin to thin her blood, it may take several extra days before it is safe to operate because of the risk of bleeding. Once her blood's ability to clot is closer to normal, then the surgery can proceed.

Meeting with the anesthesiologist. The sage chair of surgery during my medical school training, Dr. Hiram C. Polk, taught us that the most important factor in a successful surgery is the anesthesiologist, not the surgeon. The anesthesiologist assigned to your mother's case will also see her before surgery. He will take a history, perform a physical examination, and review laboratory tests, electrocardiogram (EKG), and other records. Based on that information, the doctor will discuss the options for anesthesia.

What Are the Options for Anesthesia?

Plan A: Spinal Anesthesia. The first choice for anesthesia is a spinal, but it is not appropriate for everyone. Many people just want to be "put out." However, your mother should be assured that she will be kept comfortable and that she will be drowsy but most likely won't remember anything. This approach decreases the risk of complications involving the brain and heart. In addition, less blood loss will occur because blood pressure will be more stable during the operation.

Plan B: General Anesthesia. General anesthesia is necessary in certain situations. The most common reason spinal anesthesia cannot be used is blood thinners like Coumadin (warfarin), Plavix (clopidogrel), and Effient (prasugrel). Your mother may be on blood thinner if she has stents in her heart or legs, irregular heart rhythm called atrial fibrillation, a history of a clotting problem, peripheral vascular disease, or has had a stroke or temporary stroke (TIA). Use of Coumadin may delay the surgery for several days, since her blood's normal clotting function will have to be restored in the absence of Coumadin. If she has taken Plavix or Effient within the last seven days, she must have general anesthesia because of concerns about bleeding.

Another common problem is a heart valve problem called aortic stenosis. The narrowing of the aortic valve requires higher blood pressure and precise fluid management during surgery, which is better managed under general anesthesia. Previous back surgery in the low back area may also prevent the use of spinal anesthesia.

Meeting with the surgeon. By the time you have a chance to sit down with the surgeon, you will probably feel as if you are a character in the movie *Groundhog Day*. You will think: But I have already told this story to ten people, and I have already given the bag of medicines to at least half that many! Take a deep breath and rewind again. This will not be the last time you recount the information. After going through the same scenario with the surgeon, you will get a different response. He will explain where the fracture is and how he intends to repair it. The options are based on the location of the fracture and whether or not it is displaced (no longer lined up correctly). The surgeon may use nails, plates, or screws to hold the pieces of the broken bone together and allow it to heal. If that is not possible, more involved surgery, which includes replacing the hip, may have to be performed. If there are arthritic changes in the hip joint, a total hip replacement, including the socket may be necessary. The location of the fracture and what has to be done surgically determine the recovery process. Procedures requiring less surgery, such as inserting screws to secure the neck region of the hip, allow for a faster recovery; a total hip replacement involves a longer, tougher recovery.

What the Surgeon Is Talking About: Parts of the Hip and Types of Fractures

The "femoral neck" is the narrowest section of the hip. It lies between the ball and bony projections called trochanters. The major hip muscles attach to the trochanters. The greater trochanter can be felt on the lateral side of your hip. If you have little padding, that area is particularly vulnerable when a fall to the side occurs. The lesser trochanter is internal to your inner thigh. The area between the two trochanters is called the "intertrochanteric" region. Below that is the "subtrochanteric" area—meaning "below" the trochanters.

In addition to the parts of the bone, the blood supply is also shown. Many people are surprised to see these blood vessels because they do not think about the blood flow to and from the bone. The old saying

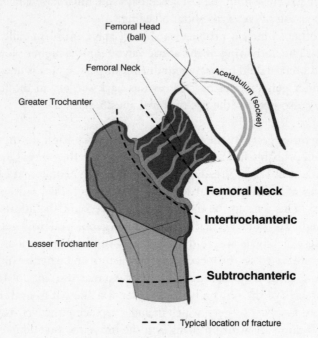

3 Major Types of Hip Fractures

Femoral Head (ball)

Femoral Neck

Acetabulum (socket)

Greater Trochanter

Femoral Neck

Intertrochanteric

Lesser Trochanter

Subtrochanteric

– – – – Typical location of fracture

Tim Gunther, gunthergraphics.biz

"dry as a bone" is a misnomer. Though it would make the orthopedist's job a lot easier if bone were, in fact, "dry," the truth is that it's not.

If the blood supply is interrupted, the hip will need replacement. This happens when the broken parts of the bone are "displaced"; that is, when they are not lined up anymore. Also, the location of the fracture may be associated with a greater risk of blood loss. This is particularly true for breaks across the subtrochanteric area.

Fortunately, subtrochanteric fractures are uncommon. Of the three major types of hip fractures in older persons, subtrochanteric fractures account for less than 10 percent. The majority of hip fractures are split about equally between femoral neck and intertrochanteric fractures.

The best-case scenario is a femoral neck fracture that is not displaced. In such cases, a small incision of less than two inches will be made so that the surgeon can insert about three screws to stabilize the fracture. The surgery will take only thirty to forty-five minutes.

SURGERY

Less than a day has gone by and your mother has most likely already been to the operating room. The duration of the surgery was dependent upon which type of surgical repair was performed. The risk of blood loss was related to the location of the fracture, the repair, and the anesthesia.

With spinal anesthesia, the anesthesia slowly wears off and small amounts of pain medicine are gradually increased. In contrast, after general anesthesia a patient will wake up and immediately experience pain, so pain management will require larger doses of medicine right away. Unfortunately, pain medicine and older age are not a good combination. Quite often, patients wake up confused or entirely disoriented.

After the surgery is completed, the surgeon will come out to the waiting area. He will give you a brief description of what was done and how your mother did during surgery. Once she has awakened in the recovery room and the activity has quieted down, the recovery room nurses may invite you to go to her bedside. Otherwise, you will meet her back in the hospital room.

AFTER SURGERY CARE (POST-OP)

Control of chronic medical problems and prevention of postoperative complications are both key to a smooth recovery. A respiratory therapist or a member of the nursing staff will provide breathing treatments every two to four hours to prevent pneumonia. Control of your mother's pain and her reaction to pain medicine tends to be "a wild card." Also, factor in sleep deprivation, the trauma of surgery, waking up in a strange place, and constant poking and prodding.

All of these may contribute to confusion and disorientation. If there were pre-existing memory loss issues, they may be heightened during this time. Unfortunately, sometimes the confusion never clears. Patients who have had general anesthesia are at even higher risk of permanent memory problems. It is imperative for you or a designated person to stay with your mother in her hospital room, if at all possible.

Which brings me to an important point: You need to take care of yourself and get some rest. You cannot be there twenty-four hours a day. Inquire about using "sitters" during the night, particularly if confusion and disorientation are a problem. Sitters are usually trained health aides, who will sit by your mother's bedside with a watchful eye and tend to her needs. They will also ensure her safety.

Management after surgery focuses on mobility as soon as possible. This is a good predictor of long-term success. The day after surgery, the physical therapist will start to work on getting your mother moving. If she had screws or nailing of the fracture, she will not be able to put weight on her repaired leg for four to six weeks. If she had a hip replacement, a physical therapist will get her standing right away.

The energy expended in physical therapy is sometimes much more than the energy expended during one's physical activity prior to surgery. Heart problems may be unmasked, such as angina (chest pain) or even a heart attack or congestive heart failure.

Common Problems after Surgery

- Infections
  —pneumonia
  —bladder infections
  —infection of the surgery site
- Confusion
- Constipation
- Fluid overload and heart failure
- Heart attack
- Blood clots in the leg or to the lung

Later problems
- Pressure sores
- Poor nutrition
- Depression

Discharge planning. Preparing for the next step, rehabilitation, starts almost as soon as your mother is admitted to the hospital. Length of stay depends on the extent of the surgery and how smoothly the recovery goes. A person who specializes in discharge planning will meet with you and will explain your mother's options. You will usually have more than one choice of rehabilitation facilities. Some are located in skilled nursing facilities (SNFs) and others are dedicated rehabilitation facilities, which are typically staffed by physiatrists, who are physicians that specialize in rehabilitation medicine. Be sure to visit each facility during the day to see the staff in action. You can schedule appointments with the admissions coordinators at each rehabilitation site. Talk to whomever you can during your visit: patients, their family members, the therapists, etc.

It is natural to feel overwhelmed by all of this. You may feel as though you need to be in more than two places at once, so schedule some help—family, friends, or professionals—to cover for you at the hospital.

REHABILITATION

In rehabilitation, the focus is not only on therapy for the hip but also on optimizing care for chronic problems. Medicines may need to be modified and adequate vitamin and mineral supplements need to be put in place. Often times, nutrition falls by the wayside. Supplementation of the diet with protein may be helpful to boost healing and recovery of strength.

Fall Prevention. Risk of falls is high following hip surgery and preventing them will require vigilant attention. Vitamin D plays an important role in fall prevention, not only for the bone but also for muscle function. The vitamin D blood level needs to be above 30 ng/ml. Improved muscle function will decrease the risk of falls. Fear of falling is also a common problem. The physical therapist and staff will help ensure safe mobility by teaching your mother to use a walker or cane and by building her confidence. Hip protectors that cushion the hip to decrease the blow of a fall are a great concept. However, in clinical trials so far, the materials used do not prevent hip fractures. In addition, they are bulky and difficult to put on, so people do not like using them.

Consider Reclast. The risk of another fracture within a short period of time is quite high. Increasing bone density in a short period of time can make a difference in lowering risk. Only one medicine, Reclast, has been tested in a clinical trial of patients after a hip fracture. Not only did the patients receiving Reclast have fewer fractures, their death rate over three years was 28 percent lower. This is more than an added bonus of its use, considering the high rate of death after hip surgery. Reclast is given by vein once a year.

When should the first annual dose of Reclast be given? Giving the first dose of Reclast any time from two to twelve weeks after hip fracture shows effectiveness in decreasing risk of fracture and death. Because of the cost, the nursing home may not want to administer it during the rehabilitation phase. You can make arrangements after that time period, if necessary. You may consider other medicines, but this is the only one tested in this situation. However, reduced kidney function may prohibit its use.

Medicare Part A. Medicare covers the cost of rehabilitation up to a total of one hundred days, as long as progress is being made in therapy (the clock starts with the day of admission to the hospital). Many frail patients simply cannot meet the therapy requirements, so therapy is stopped and they are forced to transition to another facility before they have reached their full rehabilitation potential. Unfortunately, this is a common scenario.

THE NEXT STEPS

Recovery will be dependent both on your mother's level of function prior to the fracture and on the progress she made in the hospital and during rehabilitation. Be prepared to plan for a change in her living situation. Most likely, your mother will not be able to live independently. In less than two months, both your mother's life and your life will have drastically changed. A seemingly never-ending series of decisions will have been made in a short period of time. These changes are stressful. Be on alert for depression in your mother and for your own sheer exhaustion. It will be a difficult and challenging time. Keep your wits and stamina by getting plenty of help and support from your family and friends. By talking about it, you will discover others who have been down the same road with one of their parents, which will provide important information, as well as comfort and support. You will find *that you are not alone*.

The Bare Bones

Hip fracture is an all-too-common event for women and men in their eighties. Here is some essential information for getting your parent through the ordeal:

- Take all her medicine and supplement bottles to the hospital.
- A thorough medical and heart evaluation prior to surgery should be followed by close monitoring.
- Pain medicines should be prescribed in the lowest amounts needed to achieve pain control.
- Spinal anesthesia is preferred during surgery, unless contraindicated (for example, if Plavix had been used prior to the fracture).
- Adequate nutrition should be maintained; protein supplements may be helpful.
- Blood levels of vitamin D should be boosted above 30 ng/ml; supplements may be required.
- Intensive physical therapy and fall prevention measures should be put in place.
- Prevent another fracture; look for other illnesses or medicines that may contribute to the risk.
- Consider Reclast or another treatment to increase bone density and decrease the risk of another fracture.

Other Concerns

How Do You Monitor Your Progress?

Once a year, review bone-specific topics as part of your annual health check-up with your primary care physician. Discuss what you have been doing and decide whether anything needs to tweaked. General lifestyle factors are a good topic for discussion, too, not only for your bones but for the rest of your overall health.

Just as with measuring blood pressure and cholesterol to see if diet, lifestyle changes, and/or medicines, are improving your health, you can also measure prevention and treatment steps for osteoporosis. Measurement of height, bone density, and bone markers may be helpful. None of these tell the "whole story," since other factors such as nutritional status, muscle strength, and balance also contribute to fracture risk. These factors should also be included in your routine evaluation.

HEIGHT

Having your height measured once a year should be part of your annual physical with your primary care physician. Height loss may be a clue that a silent spine fracture has occurred over the past year. If you have lost an inch of height, your doctor should search for an underlying cause. If a DXA is planned, a scan of your entire spine (vertebral fracture assessment) can be performed to look for silent fractures. Another option is a lateral spine x-ray (thoracic and lumbar) to further investigate height loss.

DXA SCANS

The most precise way to measure response to therapy is repeating a bone density scan of your spine and hip. The repeat bone scan is usually done no sooner than one year after an initial scan. The recommended interval is two years because of expected changes in bone density with therapy. Also, insurance reimbursement is set at this time frame.

There is some controversy about length of time for follow-up scans and also whether they are needed at all when you are on therapy. Just as with any medicine, one size does not fit all. You may have had a similar experience with blood pressure or cholesterol. Some medicines may work well, others not as well. The medicines for osteoporosis were shown to be effective for the majority of subjects in clinical trials. However, those participants are typically not as diverse as the general population, since study participants are thoroughly screened to eliminate other problems that may have an impact on bone. In addition, study participants are monitored closely to ensure that they take their medicine as directed. As with treatment using any other medicine, you want to monitor its effect to make sure it is working. DXA is currently the best method available. Bone density is the best surrogate measure for bone strength. It is not perfect by any means but no surrogate measure is.

If you start on a bone-specific medicine, expect the greatest improvement in the first two years, with a smaller improvement in the subsequent three to four years. In general, you will have a larger increase in bone density at the lumbar spine than at regions of the hip. It may take longer than the first two years to see a significant change at the hip.

The definition of treatment success or "response to therapy" is bone density that remains stable or increases. A gain or loss of bone density must be "statistically significant" to be clinically meaningful. All scientific measurements have a degree of variability between repeat readings. The machine, the patient, and/or the technician performing the test can influence a DXA measurement. Each DXA center should have a calculation for its variability in doing follow-up tests. The interpretation of the test results should take this variability into account to determine if the change seen on your bone density exceeds the range of variability for that DXA center and is therefore considered to be a clinically important difference.

If bone loss that is statistically significant occurs while you are on therapy, reasons for the loss need to be investigated. A new problem may have developed since the initial evaluation was conducted. With aging, some illnesses that affect bone become more common. A previous evaluation may not have uncovered a hidden problem. Other problems can masquerade as postmenopausal osteoporosis. Low bone density itself does not equal osteoporosis.

Tests Your Doctor May Order

- Twenty-four-hour urine for calcium, sodium, and creatinine
- Complete blood count (CBC)
- Erythrocyte sedimentation rate

- Liver enzymes and albumin
- Calcium and phosphorus
- Kidney tests: creatinine, blood urea nitrogen
- Thyroid hormone and TSH
- Vitamin D
- Parathyroid hormone (PTH)
- Antiendomysial antibodies or equivalent for celiac disease
- Multiple myeloma screen
- PSA and testosterone for men
- Bone turnover marker

Your clinical situation will determine which tests are ordered in looking for other causes of bone loss. These are some of the tests that may be ordered. A twenty-four-hour urine collection should be done for everyone with osteoporosis. Yes, it is cumbersome to collect but it is also necessary.

BONE TURNOVER MARKERS

Bone turnover markers are complementary to DXA scans. As a dynamic measure, markers provide another tool to quantify response to therapy. Instead of waiting two years for results from a repeat DXA, bone markers can be used to see the effect on bone metabolism in a matter of days or months, depending on the medicine. However, bone markers have not been widely used because of their variability. In general, a change of 30 percent or more is considered significant.

Bone turnover markers are helpful as part of your evaluation if you have lost bone density while on bone-specific medicines. For example, the results of markers may suggest that the medicine is not being absorbed.

YOUR STORIES...

Rosemary, age seventy-three, started Fosamax after a screening bone density showed that she had osteoporosis. She is taking generic alendronate now and has been on therapy for a total of eight years. She had two follow-up DXAs that showed good response to therapy and she had no fractures. Her last DXA was four years ago. This year, she asked about going off of her medicine for a "holiday." Her doctor ordered a bone density. This time, it showed a significant loss at both the spine and hip.

Her doctor ordered additional tests, which revealed a slightly high calcium blood level and a high parathyroid hormone level. Everything else was normal, including a vitamin D level of 46. The blood test suggested a problem called "hyperparathyroidism," which is when the parathyroid produces too much of its hormone. High levels of parathyroid hormone cause bone loss.

A special scan of her parathyroid glands (four of them sit adjacent to your thyroid, which is located in the neck) showed that one was larger in size and quite active. She was referred to a surgeon who successfully removed the culprit, called an adenoma. This resolved the cause of her bone loss. She continued on a regimen that included good nutrition, vitamin D, calcium, exercise, and alendronate.

WHAT IF YOU FRACTURE?

The goal is to reduce your risk of fracture. Medicines, with even small changes in bone density, may decrease fracture risk by about half. Medicines reduce risk but do not eliminate fractures.

Should you change your medicine after a fracture? The temptation is to make a switch. Reassess. Look for other factors that could contribute. Did you start a new medicine or develop another problem? Go back to square one. The same evaluation used for assessing bone loss applies. Do you need to work on balance and build up core muscle strength to prevent falls? Talk with your doctor about lifestyle, nutrition, exercise, calcium, and vitamin D.

Although the measurement of height, bone density, and bone markers is useful, these measures don't account for all factors, such as bone microstructure, or those factors not associated with the skeleton, like fall risk. Studies suggest that taking your medicine as prescribed is itself a good predictor of success in reducing fracture risk.

> ## The Bare Bones
> "Success" is measured by...
> * No height loss
> * An increase or no change on DXA scan
> * A bone marker decrease of 30 percent or more
> * Taking your medicines as prescribed

Living and Coping with "Osteopenia" and Osteoporosis

"Osteopenia" is not a disease. Strike this word from your vocabulary. That is what the experts in the bone field are doing. "Low bone density" is the term replacing osteopenia. Why is that? The attempt is to try and disassociate the finding of low bone mass with disease. A T-score on DXA between -1.0 and -2.5 is "low bone density."

Thin bones do not necessarily mean weak bones. Your fracture risk is what is important. In fact, the majority of fractures occur in women with low bone mass. Age is a huge factor. Measurement of bone density does not account for the microstructure or the fragility of bone that occurs with aging. That is where fracture risk assessment comes in to play. The use of tools like FRAX will help determine if you are at high risk. The younger you are, the less likely you are to fracture. Age and previous fracture are major risk determinants.

In addition, you cannot go by only one bone density test. One snapshot in time will not tell if your bone density is stable or if you are at risk for fast loss of bone in the next year.

Assess your risk with your doctor. By having a bone density measurement, your awareness of your bone health is increased. In addition, knowing those numbers forces you to re-examine your lifestyle and hopefully make positive changes to improve your bone health and overall health.

DIAGNOSIS OF OSTEOPOROSIS BY BONE DENSITY ALONE

Discovering you have any "silent disease" is always a shock. You most likely had the test just because your doctor recommended it but you did not expect to find anything wrong. Emotions run high after learning a test is "abnormal." A new diagnosis creates an instant sinking feeling. I, myself, have had that reaction. I know how traumatic it is.

Dealing with a new diagnosis of low bone mass or osteoporosis is challenging. All of a sudden, there is a major imbalance between how you look (healthy) and how you feel (fragile, vulnerable). You are in disbelief. You feel frustrated. Typically, the first question is, "How can I have osteoporosis when I am healthy and I have done everything correctly?"

As an eternal optimist, I ask you to see the glass as half full. It is better to know than to not know. Once a silent problem is uncovered you have the advantage of being able to do something positive about it. Just as when you discover that you have high blood pressure or high cholesterol you can take steps to improve those conditions to decrease your risk of heart attack or stroke, you are going to do the same with osteoporosis and take steps to lessen your chances of fracture.

Do not panic. Although there is no cure, you have plenty of options to help you strengthen your bones and decrease your risk of fractures. Learn all you can. Share the information with your family members so that their awareness is heightened and they can offer you support.

After your discussion with your doctor, do not feel "rushed" into anything, especially when you may be skeptical about taking medicines. It is natural to be terrified of medicine and possible side effects. By getting the facts and carefully weighing the risks and benefits, hopefully you will be able to make better-informed decisions.

You have *time* to decide about what do. In the clinical trials, women diagnosed by bone density who had not experienced fractures continued to have low risk of fractures over three years regardless of treatment assignment. Those in the placebo group, who took calcium and vitamin D, having become conscious of their diagnosis, also improved their lifestyles. As a result, they, too, had low numbers of fractures.

In most cases, bone loss is a very slow process, so take your time, do your research, change your diet, and increase or augment your exercise. But if you are eighty-plus or are experiencing rapid bone loss from taking medicines like steroids or aromatase inhibitors for breast cancer, you do not have the luxury of time. You need to make a treatment decision.

Start by taking small steps. Do not try to change everything at once, although that is what you may feel you should be doing. Make an intelligent plan.

Attention to detail and lifestyle is essential. Daily exercise, a well-balanced diet, adequate calcium intake, and vitamin D supplementation are keys to bone health. Be sure that any other problems are well controlled. Even if you are already doing all of these things, there will still be room for improvement. You will have to make some adjustments in your physical activity, such as learning to lift objects by bending your knees and activating your core muscles—instead of bending forward. However, do not think that you should stop physical activities altogether.

Beware of information overload! Support groups are a wonderful way to meet others who have similar concerns and interests. Members of support groups share stories and knowledge and can help you sort out all of the new information you will have to confront. They still do happen in various communities on a regular basis but in the new media era, support groups are more readily available via the Internet. You will have twenty-four-hours-a-day, seven-days-a-week backup.

If you want to talk with someone locally and a support group is not available in your community, ask your doctor if there are other patients who might be willing to talk with you. Also, a support group does not have to be disease specific.

DIAGNOSIS WITH FRACTURES

Falls should not result in broken bones. One study even suggests that fractures with trauma may be related to underlying structure problems. Under normal circumstances, a fall from standing height, even if you "hit hard," should not cause a fracture. Many times, you or even your doctor may not connect the dots that you have a bone health problem that needs attention. Even if your bone density shows that you are above the "osteoporosis" range, the fact that you have fractured means that your bones are fragile. If an evaluation to look for other causes finds none, you will be diagnosed with osteoporosis based on the fracture.

Many people are shocked to find out they have osteoporosis after they have sustained a fracture. It is discouraging to learn that the odds of another fracture occurring right away are high and that this high risk persists for about ten years. Once again, the cup is half full. There is always a positive solution to every problem. Armed with your new knowledge, you can make a difference to lower your risk. It will take some energy and persistence to get there but you can achieve it.

When fractures negatively impact your physical quality of life it is difficult to maintain your mental quality of life. Unfortunately, little attention is paid to the emotional ramifications and burden of fractures. Medical professionals tend to focus on the physical aftermath of problems associated with fracture without including psychological impact. In addition, if fractures have changed your physical appearance, redrawing your body image is scary.

It is healthy to express fears. Keep talking. Keep connecting. You will find help where you least expect it. You may complain that others do not realize or cannot understand the emotional turmoil caused by fractures. The feeling of being alone, in any situation, is difficult to cope with. Emotional support is paramount. Connect with others; this is how communities and support groups work.

The Bare Bones
- "Osteopenia" is not a disease. The preferred term is "low bone density."
- Think in terms of risk if you have "low bone density."
- If you have osteoporosis, be aware of the possibility of fracture and take steps to decrease your risk.
- Connect with others through support communities that may be available locally and online.

Expert Medical Advice:
Asking the Right Questions

Your primary care doctor—internist, family physician, or obstetrician/gynecologist—is the person who takes care of your general health needs and bone health. This doctor is a fundamental part of your overall health. As part of your annual check-up, talk with your doctor about bone health. If you are over fifty, you should see your doctor at least once a year, even if you do not think it is necessary.

An informed patient gets the best care. You have to be your own advocate. If your doctor does not mention bone health, you will need to raise the topic and initiate the discussion. You will have a lot to cover with him, and the subjects may run the gamut from your mother's health to your marital problems.

YOUR ANNUAL CHECK-UP

The challenge for your annual primary care doctor's visit is covering everything in a short amount of time. Your doctor will have an agenda and a scheduled time allotment. He will want to talk with you, perform a physical exam, make health-care plans, and counsel you. In addition, you have topics that you will want to cover. It may be difficult to thoroughly cover both of your agendas.

Therefore, prior to your visit, make a list to help you better organize your medicines, your questions, and your concerns. Place all of your medicines *and* supplements in a bag and take them with you to your appointment. Do not take only a list of your medicines and supplements. Hand your questions to your doctor or his staff when you are taken to the exam room. However, time may not allow absolutely everything to be addressed. In addition, information from more blood work or other tests may be needed in order to answer your questions. Schedule a follow-up appointment to continue the dialogue and the process.

For bone health, questions you may ask depend upon your age or your stage of life. Everyone, no matter what age, should discuss daily calcium and vitamin D requirements, exercise, and nutrition. For women in the transition to menopause or postmenopause, questions should include when to measure your bone density. Bone density serves as a basis for your assessment of fracture risk, along with other factors from your medical history.

Questions You Should Ask Your Doctor

1. How much calcium do I need each day?
2. How much extra calcium should I supplement to my diet?
3. How much vitamin D supplement do I need?
4. Should my vitamin D level be checked as part of my annual lab tests?
5. Do you have exercise and diet tips to recommend?

If your bone density is in the osteoporosis range, it does not automatically mean you have postmenopausal osteoporosis. Further testing may be indicated to look for other causes. Postmenopausal osteoporosis is the most common reason for low bone density; even so, make sure everything else is "normal." Vitamin D is the most common abnormal test. If no other problems are found, discuss your options for therapy. You may want to work on optimizing "everything else" in your lifestyle before beginning a medicine. Unless you are losing bone quickly due to a medicine such as steroids or you have had a previous fracture, time is on your side. Take it one step at a time. You need to work on reducing the risk of falls. This is paramount at any age.

Questions to Ask When You Are Perimenopausal or Postmenopausal (Men Should Ask, Too)

1. When should I get a bone density DXA scan?
2. If you have already had a DXA scan: When should I get another one?
3. If your bone density is low: What is my risk of fracture?
4. If your bone density is in the osteoporosis range: What other tests will I need to undergo to look for other causes?
5. If I am at high risk for fracture or have osteoporosis: What are my options?

When should you ask about seeing a specialist or getting a second opinion?

Most of you will be well taken care of by your primary care physician. A primary care physician can manage the majority of people with osteoporosis. At times, the evaluation or treatment may be beyond either the level of expertise of your primary care doctor or his comfort zone. In some situations, a second opinion or consultation with a specialist is helpful. For instance, if you do not have a "typical" presentation, are not responding to therapy, or have other problems complicating the picture, referral to an osteoporosis specialist should be considered. Your comfort zone is important, too. If you feel a second opinion would be beneficial, raise the issue with your doctor.

Second Opinion

When a referral may be appropriate:
- Young individual with fracture not due to trauma
- Normal bone density, but fractures anyway
- Unusual laboratory findings on the evaluation
- Declining bone mineral density while on therapy
- Fracture while on therapy
- Unable to tolerate therapy
- No desirable therapy choices
- Multiple other illnesses
- You and/or your primary care physician want another opinion

---

There are no board qualifications for doctors specializing in osteoporosis. In your community, the specialists who have a focus on osteoporosis may be endocrinologists, rheumatologists, or sometimes a nephrologist or geriatrician. Your doctor will know which specialist is best for you. Many university medical centers have an osteoporosis center or metabolic bone unit. Finding a specific *type* of doctor is less important than finding a doctor with knowledge.

In addition, your choices may be limited to what is available through your insurance or healthcare plan. If you want to go to, or your doctor wants to send you to, a doctor whose services are not covered, you may need to pay out of pocket for the consultation. Most specialists' consultation costs are in the $200 to $300 range. If you are paying on your own, a discount may be available. Also, any additional testing recommended by the consulting doctor may be directed to your primary care physician who can order the tests.

YOUR STORIES...

Tara, age fifty-four, started on Fosamax after her baseline DXA showed osteoporosis. Her lowest T-score was -2.9 at the lumbar spine. Her two-year follow-up DXA revealed a significant loss of six percent at her lumbar spine. She had some additional testing done. A low vitamin D blood level of 18 ng/ml was discovered. Her physician recommended that she take an additional 1,000 IU a day of vitamin D on top of her calcium supplement of 1,200 mg a day, which also contained 400 IU of vitamin D.

She was scheduled for a repeat bone density in one year because of her physician's concern over the bone loss even in light of her vitamin D deficiency. In the interim, her vitamin D level was rechecked during the summer and was 42 ng/ml. On the new one-year follow-up DXA, her spine showed loss again and the hip density was not significantly different. She and her doctor decided that a further investigation was needed and an endocrinology consultation was requested.

The endocrinologist reviewed her medical history and laboratory records and performed a brief physical examination. He ordered several tests not previously done to look for possible hidden causes. Her vitamin D level drawn in March was lower at 27 ng/ml. Her twenty-four-hour urine showed too much calcium. The rest of the tests were normal.

In reviewing total calcium intake, the endocrinologist determined that she was taking more than she needed. Her diet and supplements averaged a total of 2,200 mg a day. Therefore, he advised her to decrease her calcium supplement use from 1,200 mg a day to 400 mg of calcium citrate. In addition, he increased her supplemental vitamin D to a total of 2,000 IU a day.

After six weeks of an average of 1,200 mg of calcium daily from diet and supplements, she repeated the urine collection. The follow-up twenty-four-hour urine was still high in calcium. The next step to decrease the calcium loss in her urine was the use of a water pill called a thiazide diuretic in low dose. Another urine collection after eight weeks of taking the diuretic resulted in the normal range for calcium. The new diuretic therapy was effective in preventing excessive calcium loss in her urine. Her endocrinologist expects to see a bone density increase the next time it is checked, in one to two years.

Sometimes it is challenging to find doctors who will listen to you and take the time to answer your questions and concerns. They definitely exist, and I believe that they are in the majority. If you are not happy with your current arrangement, let your doctor know which of your needs are not being met. If you cannot accommodate one another, it is time to find someone else. Having a doctor with whom you can communicate is crucial to your health.

The Bare Bones
- You have to be your own advocate for all healthcare matters.
- Bone health tends to be low priority or is not addressed at all.
- Ask your primary care doctor questions about bone health.
- Your primary care doctor should be able to manage most people with osteoporosis.
- A second opinion with a specialist may be appropriate in some situations.

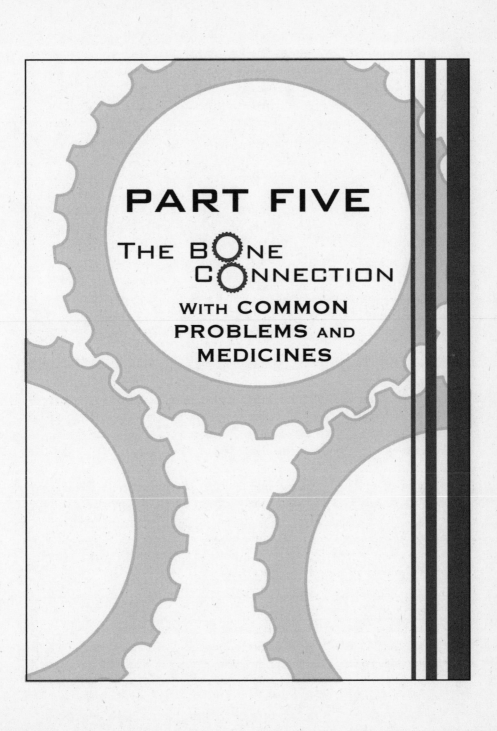

PART FIVE

THE BONE CONNECTION WITH COMMON PROBLEMS AND MEDICINES

Pregnancy and Breastfeeding

A frantic e-mail message arrived in my inbox from a friend who was about to become a grandmother. "HELP!" was written in the subject line. The body of her e-mail expressed her fears: "My daughter, Brittany, is seven months pregnant, and she broke her foot. Does she have a problem with her bones? I know you lose bone during pregnancy, do you think she's losing too much?"

I talked directly with Brittany. As it turned out, she had gotten her little toe caught on the leg of her desk and had fallen. She was not worried about anything except the pain. She said her "worrywart" mother had all of the concerns.

The good news is that fractures of toes are not considered to be osteoporotic fractures at any age. Just as Brittany was entering the "waddling stage" of pregnancy, she might have become very uncomfortable and wondered when the pain would go away. However, she did not have to worry about the possibility that her broken toe was a sign of osteoporosis.

Substantial changes do take place in bone metabolism during pregnancy and breastfeeding. Combined, these may result in a loss of 3 to 10 percent of bone. The next question is whether these changes lead to lower bone density and the long-term consequences of fracture. In general, bone loss during and immediately after pregnancy is short-term. Bone density is regained after weaning and resuming menstrual periods.

PREGNANCY

As you would expect, pregnancy increases the body's calcium needs to meet the demands of the growing baby. For women age nineteen and older, the calcium recommendation during pregnancy and breastfeeding is 1,000 mg daily. During pregnancy, it is estimated that 2 to 3 percent of the mother's total body calcium content is transferred to the growing baby. The greatest transfer takes place during the third trimester, when the growing baby's bone development peaks.

By the end of nine months, the baby's skeleton has amassed about 30 grams of calcium. About 80 percent of the calcium is deposited rapidly during the third trimester. This corresponds to a daily calcium demand of about 250 to 300 mg during the third trimester.

How is this demand met? Fortunately, the body has built-in compensation measures. To counteract the calcium loss, the main adaptation in pregnant women is that more calcium is absorbed from the intestine. In this way, a higher percentage of the calcium that is eaten or supplemented is taken up into the blood to meet the demand of the growing baby. A smaller contribution comes from lower levels of calcium loss in the urine. Some calcium may also come from the breakdown of bone. This is minor, so long as expectant mothers are taking enough calcium each day. However, if enough calcium is not provided through dietary and supplemental sources, the mother's skeleton provides the calcium to make up the deficit. The body is a finely tuned machine, as long as you supply what it needs.

In numerous observational studies of postmenopausal women with normal or low bone density, no association was found between their number of pregnancies and bone density or fracture risk. What is actually happening in real time during pregnancy is difficult to study. Since the current best test for measurement of bone density uses low-dose radiation, you cannot use that measurement during pregnancy. The dynamic bone turnover markers have also been evaluated. Interpretation of the data is difficult because the growing baby and the womb contribute to higher levels of bone metabolism.

Women after delivery were found to have 2 to 9 percent lower bone density in comparison with a control group of women of the same age. To get a better idea of what is happening, several clever studies recruited women who were planning a pregnancy. A baseline prepregnancy bone density was compared to a follow-up bone density after delivery. The results were variable based on when the postdelivery bone density was obtained. If the follow-up bone density was done within one to two weeks after delivery, bone density was not different from the prepregnancy measurement. However, when the follow-up bone density was done four to six weeks after delivery, bone density was at the lumbar spine was found to be 3.5 to 4.5 percent lower. These later results might have been influenced by breastfeeding rather than pregnancy.

Although these studies yielded conflicting results that do not entirely answer the question, you can cautiously conclude that there is no net loss of bone density during pregnancy. If there are changes during pregnancy, they do not result in long-term changes in bone density or risk of fracture in postmenopausal women.

Fractures during Pregnancy

In contrast to Brittany's toe fracture, occasionally an apparent fragility fracture (one without significant trauma) may occur during pregnancy or in the first few weeks after delivery. In most instances, the possibility of low bone density before pregnancy cannot be excluded. One's history may reveal an underlying problem that may be a contributing cause, such as the use of steroids. Other considerations include excessive bone breakdown that released calcium from the skeleton because of low dietary calcium intake and vitamin D deficiency during pregnancy. An increased rate of bone turnover is an independent risk factor for fracture. A thorough investigation should be done to look for underlying causes.

POSTPARTUM—AFTER DELIVERY

Effects of Lactation

Calcium demands during breastfeeding are huge. The mechanism for supplying the calcium differs from the mechanism during pregnancy. Hormonal changes ensure a sufficient supply of calcium to the breast milk in most new mothers and, therefore, to the nursing infant. The main source appears to be the mother's skeleton. However, the control of calcium loss from the bone during breastfeeding is not fully understood. Lactation results in the loss of bone. Changes associated with breastfeeding are temporary. The good news is that bone is regained after weaning.

Breastfeeding is associated with a loss of 300 to 400 mg of calcium daily in breast milk. The duration of breastfeeding and the time until the return of regular menstrual periods are both associated with the amount of measurable bone loss. Breastfeeding for six months is associated with a 5 percent bone loss on average, despite the body's attempt to maintain calcium. The calcium drain, in part, explains bone loss during breastfeeding. Nutrition, as well as physical activity, may also play a role in the regulation of bone mass.

The pattern of bone density changes during lactation has been systematically studied by comparing breastfeeding women with women using formula only. Among those in the formula-feeding group, no loss of bone density or a small decrease occurred in the first three months. After that, there was a general increase of 1 to 3 percent over twelve months postpartum. For breastfeeding women, the skeletal site and amount of bone loss varied.

One study showed a redistribution of the bone density in the hip. The neck region lost bone density while another area, the trochanter, gained bone density. Despite the changes that occur during breastfeeding, in the end, no differences were seen between those who breastfed and those who did not. There is no evidence that the duration of lactation has a major effect on bone density. Bone density appears to be restored by approximately six months after stopping breastfeeding. The research data supports the observation that lactation is not associated with increased fractures in later life.

Resumption of Periods

In general, formula-feeding women resume menstruation within three months. For breastfeeding women, the duration of lactation is associated with restarting menstrual periods. When one breast-feeds for less than six months, periods occur close to or slightly after stopping lactation. If one breast feeds for longer than six months, menstruation tends to return before the end of lactation. The resumption of normal hormonal status is thought to contribute to bone density gains.

Timing between Successive Pregnancies

In the case of "Irish Twins"—that is, two babies born in one year—the recovery of bone density is a question. It is not known whether the gain in bone density observed after weaning or resuming menstrual periods can occur if one becomes pregnant before or shortly after weaning. Closely spaced pregnancies might have the potential for long-term effects.

HOW MUCH VITAMIN D?

A physician colleague shared her good news with me. Finally, after multiple attempts, she was pregnant at the tender age of forty-two. She had been in tune with calcium and vitamin D requirements, but later was surprised by her lab results. She told me, "My OB (obstetrician) checked my vitamin D level, and it was only 21. I had been taking 1,000 international units a day and thought that was enough." Her vitamin D level needed to be a minimum of 30 ng/ml.

Another friend told me that her OB instructed her to stop taking her extra vitamin D supplement of 1,000 IU and to take only the recommended prenatal vitamins. "Was a vitamin D level measured?" I inquired. "No," she said. "How much D is in your prenatal vitamins?" I asked. She replied, "400 IU."

Since prenatal nutrition is definitely not within the scope of a geriatrician's expertise, our conversation spurred me on to further investigation. I headed to a local drugstore to inspect the prenatal vitamins. The standard vitamin D content was 400 IU of cholecalciferol, which is vitamin D_3. But is that enough? One condition OB/GYNs fastidiously monitor for is pre-eclampsia, which is associated with low levels of vitamin D.

I was curious about what OB/GYNs did as part of their routine practice. So I conducted my own survey, asking twelve physicians from various parts of the country, "What laboratory tests do you order for your pregnant patients?" Granted, it was not a "scientific survey," but in my small sample, only once did an OB/GYN mention checking vitamin D levels of patients.

My colleague's experience points out that you cannot know how much vitamin D to take without actually having your level measured. You may think you are getting "enough," but so many variables come into play. Vitamin D is essential for calcium absorption from the intestine. Older studies that looked at pregnancy focused primarily on calcium supplementation and did not take into account vitamin D.

At the Medical University of South Carolina, researcher Dr. Bruce Hollis and neonatologist Dr. Carol Wagner are changing that. In almost five hundred newly pregnant women of three ethnicities (African American, Hispanic, and Caucasian), they found that 82 percent had vitamin D levels less than 32 ng/ml. African American women had the lowest vitamin D levels, with an average of 15.5 ng/ml. In general, women in their first pregnancy were most likely to have low vitamin D levels, pointing out the need for education of new mothers-to-be.

In addition, Doctors Hollis and Wagner are conducting intervention studies of pregnant and breastfeeding women. In one completed study, the women were assigned randomly to three different daily doses of vitamin D supplementation: 400 or 2,000 or 4,000 IU. The 4,000 IU dose, which is about seven times the recommended daily dose of 600 IU, yielded an average vitamin D level of 50 ng/ml. Those taking the 2,000 IU dose had a vitamin D level of 40 ng/ml on average and those taking 400 IU reached an average level of 29 ng/ml. Clearly, ten times the 400 IU dose did not result in ten times the vitamin D level. This points out that larger doses of vitamin D may be required to bring up the vitamin D level to over 30 ng/ml, which is considered the target level.

Higher vitamin D levels were associated with lower numbers of infections and preterm births. I inquired whether their study showed a reduction in pre-eclampsia, as suggested by cross-sectional studies. Dr. Hollis said, "We saw it trend down but it was not significant. However, when we lumped the complications of pregnancy (pre-eclampsia, gestational diabetes, and blood pressure) together, then it was significantly reduced."

How much vitamin D is enough? Again, for bone health and nourishing the growing baby, mothers' vitamin D levels need to be at a minimum of 30 ng/ml. Even higher levels may provide more protection and further reduce the likelihood of potential problems in pregnancy. To help more fully answer the question, additional clinical trials are underway using different amounts of vitamin D supplements during pregnancy and breastfeeding.

INFANTS

The American Academy of Pediatrics' latest recommendation from 2008 is to give all breastfed infants 400 IU of supplemental vitamin D daily. The updated

2010 *Dietary Reference Intakes for Vitamin D* by the Institute of Medicine concurred with the daily intake of 400 IU for infants up to twelve months of age. Infant formulas contain vitamin D in the amount of 400 IU per liter. Supplementation for exclusively formula-fed babies is not needed. However, it is still a need if the baby is fed a combination of formula and breast milk.

One small, six-month study done at the Medical University of South Carolina showed that infants could achieve high enough vitamin D levels exclusively through breastfeeding; but it took supplementation of 6,400 IU of vitamin D each day by the mothers. Their vitamin D levels ranged around the 50 ng/ml level and the vitamin D content of their breast milk increased eightfold from the start of the study.

Vitamin D is a basic requirement for the growing skeleton. Researchers in England looked at bone density in a huge study of almost seven thousand ten-year-old children. Local weather information was used to estimate the mothers' ultraviolet light exposure during the last trimester of pregnancy. Children of mothers whose last trimester occurred during sunny months tended to have larger bones than mothers with less sun exposure. Their research suggests that expectant mothers' vitamin D levels during the time of greatest prenatal bone growth may have lasting effects on children's later bone development. If the benefits persist into adulthood, the researchers concluded, mothers' vitamin D levels during pregnancy might affect their children's bone health into old age.

It is not clear what role vitamin D may play in the long-term prevention of other diseases beyond bone health and in establishing lifelong health. This is an area of hot debate and active research. Just ensure that you and your children or grandchildren have adequate vitamin D intakes. At least be vigilant during the part of the year when there is not enough sunshine for the body to produce its own vitamin D.

Back to the frantic query regarding Brittany's broken toe: Her mother was worried that she had osteoporosis. Major fractures during pregnancy have been reported but they are rare. Brittany was just starting her third trimester, the period of greatest calcium demand. Since her toe fracture was quite painful, she had a built-in reminder about bone health.

If you, a family member, or a friend are planning to become pregnant, the best advice is to start with good nutrition, an adequate vitamin D blood level above 30 ng/ml, 1,000 mg of calcium daily between diet and supplements, and regular exercise. Even better: All of these measures may help conception, too!

The Bare Bones

- During pregnancy and breastfeeding, extra demands require special attention to your calcium and vitamin D intakes.
- Calcium 1,000 mg is *essential* each day.
- Supplements are needed to ensure you are getting enough vitamin D—you cannot just count on the sun.
- Bone lost during breastfeeding is usually recovered after weaning.

Premenopausal Women

Osteoporosis in a premenopausal woman is a rare diagnosis. Nevertheless, I am constantly surprised by the number of younger women labeled with this diagnosis. The rate is higher than expected because the diagnosis is being applied incorrectly. A low bone density alone does not establish a diagnosis of osteoporosis. In premenopausal women, the association of bone mass and fracture risk is not the same as for postmenopausal women. The number of fractures that occur in premenopausal women is very low compared with the frequency of fractures in older postmenopausal women. At any given level of bone density, the risk of fracture increases with age because of progressive loss of bone microstructure.

LOW BONE DENSITY ON DXA SCAN

Screening bone density scans are not recommended for premenopausal women. When bone density machines were new and first installed in many doctors' offices or clinics, staff members acted as volunteers to test the machines. Commonly, the staff members were young women who happened to have low bone density. If the criteria for postmenopausal women were applied using their T-score results, their diagnosis would be "osteopenia" or osteoporosis. Understandably, these staff members went into panic mode when they were given one of these diagnoses. However, T-scores *are not* used in premenopausal women, men under the age of fifty, or children, according to guidelines established by the International Society of Clinical Densitometry.

Z-scores that compare the bone density results to individuals of the same age, ethnicity, and sex are used instead. For example, if you were a thirty-two-year-old Asian woman, your results would be compared with other thirty-two-year-old Asian women in the database. If the Z-scores were higher than -2.0, the results would be considered "within the expected range for age." If the lowest Z-score were -2.0 or lower, the results would be considered "below the expected range for age." Approximately 2.5 percent of premenopausal women will fall into this category.

Since bone density measured by DXA scan is two-dimensional, it does not take into account bone size. A petite woman with small bones will have a result lower than a woman with larger bones, although they may have the same actual bone mineral content. This is a limitation of the measurement device.

One low bone density measurement does not mean you are actually losing bone. Serial measurements are needed to determine loss. Bone density for the US female population is distributed from low to high in a bell-shaped curve. This means that not everyone can be average or above normal. A low bone density may mean that you are on the low end of the bell-shaped curve.

Measurement of bone density is recommended only in situations such as disease or medicine exposure that may cause bone loss or low-trauma fracture of the hip or spine.

UNDERLYING CAUSES

A thorough history and physical examination may provide the majority of clues that explain low bone density. Additional investigation with appropriate laboratory evaluation is also indicated in searching for an explanation for major fracture or low bone density below the expected range for age.

Research has shown that the most common cause of fracture or unexpectedly low bone density in younger women is steroid use. Other underlying causes were found in at least half of women, including other medicines (cancer chemotherapy or older seizure medicines), low estrogen status, and malabsorption. Low estrogen status can be the result of medicines (such as low-dose birth control pills, Depo-Provera®, and treatment of endometriosis) or the lack of menstrual periods. Diseases affecting the intestine (celiac disease or inflammatory bowel disease) may prevent adequate nutrition and absorption of vital nutrients, including vitamin D and calcium.

Recent research has raised concern about other medicines, including antidepressants, called SSRIs, and acid reflux medicines, called proton pump inhibitors (PPIs). The bone connection with common problems and medicines are explored in more detail in subsequent sections.

The majority of premenopausal women with low bone density and no fractures have stable bone density and no underlying causes. This means that repeat DXA scans do not show significant bone loss. Most likely, these women have low peak bone mass and their short-term risk of fracture is low.

MANAGEMENT

The usual general measures of good nutrition to maintain a healthy weight, exercise, and adequate calcium and vitamin D are indicated for everyone. Decreasing risk factors, such as avoiding smoking and limiting alcoholic beverages, will also help.

If an underlying cause is found, lessening the effect of the medicine or disease is the goal. Osteoporosis prescription medicines are approved for use only in premenopausal women who are taking steroids. Although data is limited, treatment studies show that premenopausal women taking steroids, such as prednisone, do not appear to be at high risk for fracture. The bisphosphonates, Fosamax and Actonel, are FDA-approved for premenopausal women taking steroids. These medicines should not be given to women who are actively trying to become pregnant or are breastfeeding.

Sometimes the cause of low bone density is decreased bone formation. Therefore, bisphosphonates would not be expected to improve bone density. Treatment with Forteo, which increases bone formation, is being evaluated in research studies. Therapy with Forteo may be an option in the future for select premenopausal women.

The perimenopause-to-menopause transition period is an appropriate time to readdress bone density and fracture risk. With the loss of estrogen, bone loss accelerates unless measures are taken to prevent bone loss.

The Bare Bones

- Osteoporosis in premenopausal women is uncommon.
- Low bone density in premenopausal women is not associated with the same increased risk of fracture that occurs in older women.
- An underlying cause of low bone density (below expected range for age) or low-trauma fracture should be investigated.
- If a cause is found, the goal is to remove the cause or lessen the effect of medicines and illnesses.
- Prescription osteoporosis medicines are not regularly used in premenopausal women because the short-term risk of fracture is low.

Birth Control: Pills and Shots

Birth control pills are the most common means of preventing pregnancy in the US. The Pill is also prescribed for other reasons, including painful periods, irregular or heavy periods, premenstrual syndrome (PMS), migraine headaches, and acne. Birth control pills are a synthetic form of the hormones estrogen and progesterone. Over the past thirty years, the strength of hormones contained in the Pill has gradually decreased to lessen the risk of side effects such as blood clots.

The current lowest dose birth control pills contain 20 micrograms (mcg) of an estrogen called ethinyl estradiol in combination with another hormone called progesterone, which may vary according to different manufacturers and brands. It is common practice for doctors to prescribe these low-dose pills for women of all ages. Though low-dose pills may be good for thirty-something women through those making the menopausal transition, they are *not* good for teenagers and young adults.

Until recently, very little attention has been directed toward the effect of different doses of the Pill on bone growth during the teen years. In fact, many doctors who prescribe the low-dose 20 mcg pill are not aware of its potential harmful effects on bone mass. The Pill works by maintaining consistent estrogen and progesterone levels. Without the mid-cycle estrogen surge, the average monthly estrogen levels for pill users are significantly lower than those of women with regular cycles. These lower-than-average estrogen levels associated with low-dose birth control pills may not support normal bone growth. Sufficient estrogen is critical for optimal bone growth in the teen years and for attainment of peak bone mass.

LOW-DOSE PILL EFFECTS ON BONE DEPEND ON YOUR AGE

More than 40 percent of your bone mass accumulates during the teen years. In contrast, when you reach your thirties, you have reached your peak bone mass and have a slow steady loss of bone mass until the menopausal transition. For those reasons, growing teenagers need more estrogen support than older premenopausal women who have already reached their peak bone mass.

Teenagers and Young Women

Recent studies have scrutinized the pill dose of estrogen necessary for optimal bone growth in teenagers and young women. Researchers observed that young pill users had less increase in bone density compared with young women not using the Pill. Studies of the low-dose pill with 20 mcg of ethinyl estradiol cast doubt on its ability to support bone growth and the achievement of optimal peak bone mass.

Use of higher-dose birth control pills that contain 30 to 40 mcg of ethinyl estradiol has no demonstrated detrimental effects on bone density in teens and young women. There is consistent evidence that birth control pills containing 30 mcg of ethinyl estradiol are adequate to ensure sufficient bone accrual during adolescence and normal bone health into adulthood.

The research findings make sense if you think about how birth control pills work. The suppression of hormones with low-dose pills does not allow sufficient estrogen support for the growing skeleton, and this results in less bone mass. The impact of birth control pills is largest during the time of highest bone mass growth. Unfortunately, we do not have information about what happens after teenagers discontinue their use of low-dose pills. Questions remain about the use of low-dose birth control pills by teenagers and young adults. Are the negative effects on bone reversible after stopping the Pill? Is there a long-term risk for osteoporosis and fractures later in life?

It is important to ensure that teenagers and young women achieve the strongest bones possible. For this reason, it is best to limit the use of birth control pills or to use higher-dose pills instead of low-dose preparations. A gynecologist friend told me that a common request for the Pill comes from teens and their mothers for use in control of acne. Instead, she advises them to use local measures and, if needed, consider antibiotics. She says that when these same girls return later for an office visit, she often finds out that they are taking birth control pills that their dermatologists have prescribed, since acne is an indication for its use.

Please understand the implications of using low-dose birth control pills during the teen years. You do not want to jeopardize bone health. If the use of birth control pills is warranted, it is preferable to use preparations containing at least 30 mcg of ethinyl estradiol to ensure proper bone development.

Thirties and Forties (After Attaining Peak Bone Mass)

Premenopausal bone loss starts soon after attaining peak bone mass in the late twenties to early thirties. The rate of bone loss at the spine is estimated to be up to 1 percent each year. The dense bone sites, such as the hip and forearm, have much lower rates of loss. The low-dose birth control pills contain enough estrogen to prevent or slow bone loss, particularly at the spine.

Older studies show that bone density was protected using higher dose pills (30 to 40 mcg of estradiol) for five to ten years. Spine bone density may increase one percent for each year of use. The greatest protection of bone is seen with ten or more years of use of the higher dose pill.

Perimenopause

During the menopausal transition, or so-called perimenopause, women with irregular periods are more likely to lose bone than women who continue to have regular periods. No evidence of bone loss is seen in perimenopausal women who continue normal menstruation. Once menstrual periods become irregular due to low estrogen production during the transition to menopause, bone loss starts to accelerate; bone loss will typically be about 2 percent a year.

Perimenopausal women who use low-dose pills (20 mcg of ethinyl estradiol) can preserve and even increase their bone mass. The biggest effect is seen at the spine, which has the fastest bone metabolism. Without protection against bone loss, a long menopausal transition may signify an additional risk factor for low bone mass and osteoporosis. Low-dose pills make sense for the perimenopausal women, both for protecting the bone and preventing the "oops" baby.

The changes that occur in the bone at different ages should be an important consideration when determining which birth control pill to prescribe. Of specific importance is the estrogen content of the pills. Low-dose pills may be good for women over thirty through the menopausal transition, but they are not good for teenagers and young adults. Teens are not "little adults." Pills with a higher dose of estrogen are needed for support of bone growth. However, low-dose pills may prevent bone loss in women who have attained peak bone mass, and they may even boost bone mass in perimenopausal women.

DEPO-PROVERA

Depo-Provera (depot medroxyprogesterone acetate) is another effective birth control method that contains only a type of progesterone. Depo-Provera is sometimes an appealing choice for women because it is a shot given every three months, so you don't have to worry about taking a pill everyday.

Depo-Provera prevents pregnancy by a different mechanism than the Pill. A slow release from the injection site provides the prolonged action. It stops the master gland of the body, the pituitary, from producing the messenger hormones that signal the ovary to release an egg during the middle of the normal menstrual cycle. As a result, a woman has no menstrual periods and has decreased production of estrogen.

Unfortunately, the effectiveness of Depo-Provera comes with a downside for the bone, particularly for teenagers and young adults. Use of Depo-Provera for two years is associated with an average bone loss of 6 percent at the spine and 5 percent at the hip in all ages of users. The longer the drug is used, the greater the bone loss. In teens, this loss may be due to lack of bone mass accrual rather than actual loss.

As a result of these research findings, in 2004 the FDA issued a prominent boxed warning in the product label, referred to as a "black box" or "boxed" warning, which can be found in the package insert for Depo-Provera. Because of the bone loss associated with Depo-Provera and the concern that it may not be completely reversible, the FDA recommended that use of Depo-Provera be limited to two years or fewer.

More recent studies indicate that the bone loss observed may be fully or at least partially reversible, with significant increases in bone density occurring after discontinuation. However, bone density improvements after stopping Depo-Provera may be blunted if Depo-Provera is followed by taking low-dose birth control pills. Limiting use of Depo-Provera to two years or fewer appears to be the best option for limiting bone loss.

Nevertheless, the American College of Obstetricians and Gynecologists in a 2008 Committee Opinion concluded that the need for effective birth control to prevent teenage pregnancies outweighs the risk of bone effects. They stated that when Depo-Provera is the best option to prevent pregnancy concerns regarding its effect on bone density "should neither prevent practitioners from prescribing Depo-Provera nor limit its use to two consecutive years." Long-term use for reasons other than prevention of pregnancy should be avoided.

The Bare Bones

- Your choice of birth control may affect your bone health.
- Birth control pills act differently on bone depending on your age.
- Prolonged use of low-dose birth control pills in teens and young adult women may result in lower bone density.
- In teens and young adults, higher-dose pills should be considered for support of their growing bones.
- Low-dose birth control pills in the menopausal transition are protective against bone loss.
- Use of Depo-Provera shots should be limited to two years because of bone loss.

Menstrual Problems: No Periods and Endometriosis

Regular monthly menstrual cycles are a part of every woman's life for more than thirty years. Sometimes menstrual periods make an unexpected visit, sometimes they are very heavy, and sometimes they do not show up at all. Bone loss occurs much more rapidly when women reach the age where periods skip, then stop for good. The end of periods with transition to menopause may be a welcome relief for many women who view menstrual periods as "the curse."

I liked the practice portrayed in Anita Diamant's novel *The Red Tent*. Women gathered in one place, "the red tent," with other women who were all cycling together for the duration of their periods. They were off the hook for all of their duties during that time—wishful thinking for modern times!

Problems may arise when teens and younger women have only irregular, unpredictable periods. Some teens may fail to start their first period, others may have periods that come regularly for a while but then stop. Adult women with a history of menstrual disorders during their teenage years have decreased bone density when compared to their same-age peers. Women typically in their thirties who experience pelvic pain or infertility may have a problem called "endometriosis." Medicines that treat this condition have profound effects on bone. This section highlights the connections between bone health and women who have menstrual disturbances.

NO PERIODS

Loss of menstrual periods, called amenorrhea, may be a sign that something is wrong. The associated lack of estrogen and other hormones can cause bone loss. As few as three months without a period may cause bone loss. The longer you go without having a period, the lower your bone density. This may be caused by increased bone loss and, in adolescents and young adults, by failure to accrue new bone, as well. The pattern of bone loss is dependent on the type of bone. Bone loss occurs first in the higher turnover bone of the spine. A longer duration of five to six years of amenorrhea is associated with changes in the dense cortical bone of the hip.

The teenager with amenorrhea gains bone throughout adolescence. However, the amount of bone mass is lower compared with regularly menstruating teenagers. The absence of periods for an extended time makes it unlikely that optimal peak bone mass will be achieved.

What Is Amenorrhea?

The word "amenorrhea" is a compound word constructed from three Greek roots: *a* = no; *men* = month; *rhoia* = flow. No monthly flow. In this section, the term refers to no menstrual period during the expected time between puberty and menopause. This is abnormal in a woman who is neither pregnant nor in the months immediately following delivery.

Amenorrhea is categorized into two types:

Primary amenorrhea is a delay in the start of menstruation (no menstrual period by the age of sixteen-and-a-half years).

Secondary amenorrhea is the absence of a menstrual cycle for at least three to six consecutive months in a woman who has previously menstruated.

Some causes include decreased body weight or weight loss, endocrine and other medical disorders, certain medicines, strenuous exercise, and even stress.

SPORTS, WEIGHT, AND MENSTRUAL PERIODS

Menstrual problems are expected in young, very lean athletes. We think of these young women as healthy but they are the most likely group to have menstrual problems. Athletic girls tend to experience their first period later than nonathletic girls. The average age of first menstrual period in healthy American girls is twelve years. Athletes who participate in a wide variety of sports typically have their first periods one to two years later.

The delay may be due to insufficient nutrition, the stress of training, or low levels of body fat. Alternatively, it may just reflect the athletes' physique, which tends to be slender with low levels of fat. However, athletes who begin training before age twelve may experience a later start of periods compared with girls who begin training after their first period occurs.

Prolonged amenorrhea may lead to diminished bone mass from the associated decrease in estrogen secretion. A decrease in frequency or intensity of training may allow resumption of regular periods. However, most athletes view the loss of periods as a blessing—no worries about cramps or bleeding, which might negatively impact their performance.

Participation in sports where a thin appearance is required can also put girls at risk. Women who participate in lightweight rowing at the international level cannot individually exceed 130 pounds, and the average weight for the entire crew of the boat is 126 pounds. They need to "make weight." At rowing events, all participants are weighed at check-in to make sure the weight requirement is met. Women's wrestling, which was added to the Olympics in 2004, is gaining popularity in the US; participants have weight-class requirements they must meet. Other sports, such as gymnastics, figure skating, diving, synchronized swimming, ballet, and ballroom dancing, though they do not have weight requirements, do encourage maintenance of a thin, lean body shape.

Athletes participating in these sports and activities may have a tendency to decrease their dietary intake as a way to lose weight. Sometimes the weight loss is too much and they end up "underweight." Most girls do not realize that their eating habits have repercussions that will ultimately reduce their physical performance. Exercising intensely and not eating enough calories is harmful. Periods may become irregular or just stop. The subsequent bone loss puts them at risk for immediate problems such as stress fractures. When disordered eating, amenorrhea, and "osteoporosis" occur together, it is called the "female athlete triad." The common manifestations of this triad are weight loss, irregular periods or no periods, and stress fractures.

Even girls who begin their periods at a later age and have a lower weight during their teen years have lower bone density when compared with their peers. Practically every teenage girl is trying to lose weight, even if they are normal weight or underweight. Weight loss is also associated with amenorrhea. It may be a function of how much body fat is present. Weight loss may be from excessive dietary restrictions as well as malnutrition. Weight gain usually restores regular menstrual cycles and hormone levels that result in increased bone density.

Teens should be counseled about how nutrition is a necessary fuel for their physical activities and health. Adolescence is a delicately balanced and hormonally supercharged time. Get help if you need it.

ENDOMETRIOSIS

Any woman who has menstrual periods can develop endometriosis, but it is most common among women in their thirties and forties. The name comes from the word for the lining of the uterus or womb, "endometrium." Endometriosis occurs when this tissue grows outside of the uterus on other structures, typically in the pelvis or abdomen. These endometrial cell "implants" cycle as if they are still contained in the uterus. Therefore, this condition typically causes pain with menstrual periods, but pelvic pain may be constant as well. Some women may have no symptoms at all. It is commonly found during an infertility evaluation, and it may be present in almost half of women with infertility.

There is no cure for endometriosis. Treatments are focused on pain relief and promoting fertility. Since estrogen appears to promote the growth of endometriosis, medical therapy is directed at reducing estrogen by causing amenorrhea. These hormonal treatments include birth control pills, Depo-Provera, or other progesterone preparations, and medicines that chemically cause "temporary menopause."

Medicines of this type include a daily nasal spray (Synarel®), an implant put under the skin once a month (Zoladex®), and a shot once a quarter (Lupron®). Lupron is the most commonly used. Called gonadotrophin-releasing hormone agonists or GnRH agonists, these treatments target the master gland, the pituitary, to decrease production of the messenger hormone that stimulates the ovary. As a result, estrogen levels drop dramatically. Similar to menopause, regular periods stop and symptoms such as hot flashes, poor sleep, and vaginal dryness occur.

In addition, bone loss from the spine occurs rapidly, just as though your ovaries had been surgically removed. These agents are used for an average of six months. Even though it is a short time, bone loss of 2 to 7 percent is common during a six-month course of GnRH agonist therapy. Once these are stopped, estrogen levels rapidly return to normal. However, bone density may take up to twelve to twenty-four months to return to normal. Once the medicines are stopped, monthly periods return, along with the potential to get pregnant. However, if pain with endometriosis had been a problem, it may recur. Careful monitoring of bone density is needed if consecutive six-month courses of therapy are used. Sometimes a small amount of estrogen is "added back" along with these drugs to counter the side effects and bone loss. However, it is difficult to find a dose that protects the body from substantial bone loss but does not interfere with the treatment of endometriosis.

The Bare Bones

- Delayed start of regular menstrual periods or stopping after starting during teen years may prevent the development of optimal peak bone.
- Those at high risk for menstrual problems and lower bone density are young athletes in high-intensity training.
- Young women participating in sports that require attention to weight may be at higher risk for weight loss, irregular periods or no periods, and stress fractures.
- Short-term treatments for endometriosis may cause rapid bone loss but bone density is usually regained in the one to two years following cessation of therapy.

Eating Disorders:
Anorexia and Bulimia

Somewhere along the line our idea of beauty was transformed from the shapely, buxom Hollywood actress Marilyn Monroe to the androgynous British supermodel Twiggy. Monroe, the woman idolized as a sex symbol, wore a size twelve dress. By today's standards, that would be considered chunky or even "fat." Although Twiggy turned sixty-two in 2011, her super skinny look, which was popularized in the mid to late 1960s, continues to be idealized. Today's ultrathin models depict the "ideal beauty" in our advertisements and create a skewed definition of what is considered "normal." Practically every woman thinks she needs to lose weight. Weight loss products and programs abound.

We come in all different colors, shapes, and sizes, and few fit these idealized pictures. Our young women are barraged with media messages that may be harmful to their body images. Preteen and underweight models portray this unrealistic image of "physical perfection." Teenagers and young adults are especially vulnerable to feeling dissatisfied with their own bodies.

Victoria Beckham, who rose to fame in the late 1990s with the all-girl pop group the Spice Girls, was dubbed Posh Spice. She revealed in her autobiography *Learning to Fly* that magazine and newspaper articles labeling her "Podgy Spice" or "Fat Spice" led to her eating disorder. She wrote that those articles affected her perception of herself. She would think, "Yes, you're disgusting. Society says you've got to be thin." Doctors and other concerned groups are calling for a stop to the promotion of unhealthy, ultrathin bodies that make eating disorders appear glamorous.

Other well-known women have let the public know about their struggles with eating disorders. The late Diana, Princess of Wales, revealed that she suffered from bulimia. Outwardly, she looked gorgeous and composed, but inside she was at war with herself. Princess Diana's decision to publicize her harrowing battle with an eating disorder resulted in a more than doubling of the number of sufferers coming forward for treatment. Doctors dubbed it the "Diana Effect."

Pressures out of the limelight are just as great. Today, more kids are overweight than ever before. First Lady Michelle Obama chose the fight against childhood obesity as her mission. We have to be smart about how we approach the subject of weight with kids. Too many have the tendency to go to extremes, and others lose weight even if they do not need to. Advice on dieting should balance warnings about overeating with discussion of the dangers of extreme dieting.

Eating disorders cause problems with bone health that may not be reversible. A woman who was a patient advocate for osteoporosis vividly brought the long-term consequences to my attention. In front of a congressional committee, I heard this woman in her early forties give emotional testimony about the pain and suffering from four spine fractures. She had a visible hump in her upper back and looked older than her years.

She wove her story around her fractures. First one, then a second, and a third fracture drastically altered her life. She had the "million dollar" work-up to look for uncommon problems or obscure diseases. Finding none, her physicians were dumbfounded. Finally, one day she came "clean." She confessed to her doctors that she had had anorexia since her early teens, and it had lasted over a decade. She was testifying that day and revealing her medical story in hopes of helping others avoid the pain and misery that she was experiencing.

WHO IS AT RISK?

Teenage years are the most common time for eating disorders to start. Approximately one in every two hundred adolescent girls develops anorexia nervosa. An estimated 1 to 4 percent of college-aged women have the disorder. Even larger numbers of adolescents have disordered eating without meeting the full criteria for anorexia nervosa. Teens who are underweight may escape detection because the focus of healthcare is on overweight and obese kids. Although we think of this illness as predominantly affecting girls and young women, 5 to 10 percent of all cases occur in males.

ANOREXIA IS DOUBLE TROUBLE FOR THE BONES: NUTRITION AND HORMONES

More than 90 percent of adolescents and young women with anorexia have low bone mass. Bone density may be lower not because they are actually losing bone but rather because they are missing the accrual of bone that occurs rapidly during the adolescent growth period. In as little as six months, permanent effects on bone density can develop.

Chronic caloric restrictions may occur either from failure to take in calories or from purging. Sometimes it is a combination of both. Even too much exercise may contribute. The end result is low body weight. The loss of body fat takes away the necessary building blocks for sex hormones, and menstrual periods stop (amenorrhea). Anorexics have *even lower* bone mass than young women with amenorrhea who are of normal weight. Poor nutrition coupled with lack of sex hormones means double trouble for bone.

Approximately 90 to 95 percent of the skeleton's foundation, called peak bone mass, is built by age eighteen. Approximately 40 to 60 percent of this peak bone mass is acquired during the adolescent years. By missing the important building blocks during this time, it is unlikely peak bone mass will be achievable. Bone mass may not be recovered at a later time even after weight is regained. An unexpectedly high rate of persistent low bone mass is reported following recovery from anorexia. Age of onset and duration of illness are the best predictors of decreased bone density.

Lower bone density leads to an increase in fracture risk in later years. Adult women with a history of anorexia lasting an average of six years have an annual fracture rate seven times greater than the fracture rate of healthy women of the same age. During the active phase of anorexia, a higher rate of fracture is also reported. Recent research shows evidence of lower bone strength in young adult women with anorexia. Therefore, less load or force on the bone, such as with a fall, is needed to cause a fracture.

Bone loss in anorexia nervosa is a result of *both* increased bone breakdown and reduced bone formation. Bone remodeling continues but bone formation associated with growth and bone mass accumulation is reduced. This pattern is in contrast to bone loss in postmenopausal women, which is characterized by increased bone breakdown without interference in bone formation. The amount of bone "loss" in anorexia is more than that observed in early postmenopausal women, who may lose bone rapidly with loss of estrogen.

Researchers at Children's Hospital Boston found marked increases of fat content in the bone marrow of young women with anorexia. Paradoxically, anorectic young women with no body fat have fat in their bone marrow. The bone-forming cells, osteoblasts, are made from the bone marrow's stem cells. However, these same mesenchymal stem cells can also become fat cells. Hormonal changes associated with malnutrition trigger the stem cells to become fat cells instead of osteoblasts. As a result, more fat in the bone marrow means less bone formation.

The rate of bone formation increases with increased nutrition. Therefore, bone formation may be reduced by malnutrition while lower levels of estrogen cause increased breakdown. It is probably not that simple, with a whole host of factors contributing to the bone effects. Other hormonal abnormalities associated with amenorrhea and poor nutrition may affect the bone. Elevated levels of the hormone cortisol and lower production of growth hormone and other related growth factors have also been implicated. In addition, low body weight results in less muscle strain on bone; in the absence of mechanical strain, the activity of bone breakdown cells increases and bone formation decreases.

Treatment: Food First

Psychiatrists usually lead the treatment of patients with anorexia. Multiple approaches are used to control the disorder and restore health. From the bone perspective, bone density improves with weight gain. The challenge is to achieve this goal. Some researchers find that a bone density scan can serve as a strong motivating factor for recovery. Although outwardly the patients may not see a problem, the abnormal bone density is an indisputable measure of the problem.

A common approach to increasing bone density has been the use of birth control pills or estrogen therapy. However, low-dose birth control pills may cause lower bone mass and are not useful in increasing bone density. Estrogen therapy given by pill has not helped, as shown in numerous studies. Estrogen skin patches are being investigated. However, since multiple causes contribute to bone loss, this may not be enough.

Continued poor nutrition may sabotage the effectiveness of estrogen. Estrogen does help decrease bone breakdown. However, without sufficient weight gain, new bone-building cells will not be put in motion. Bone formation is still suppressed. The key to recovering bone density is restoring bone formation. This is done by nutritional support and weight gain.

Since Forteo is the only medicine that increases bone formation, it makes sense that Forteo may be useful for treating these patients. Clinical trials are evaluating the effect of Forteo in this setting. Other researchers are using a hormone that is decreased in anorexia, called IGF-1, which is short for insulin-like growth factor. In small pilot studies, IGF-1 in combination with estrogen showed some benefit. IGF-1 did not show increases when used alone without estrogen.

The bisphosphonates, Fosamax and Actonel, have been shown to improve bone density at the spine and hip in clinical trials. They may be considered for an older woman who is past childbearing.

Of course, adequate vitamin D and calcium are important to bone health in all circumstances. The role of exercise in bone recovery is not clear. Some studies show a benefit from weight-bearing activities. However, if excessive exercise is a factor, then exercise needs to be decreased.

Some of the medicines prescribed by the psychiatrists may also impact the bone. For example, the use of antidepressants, called SSRIs, contributes to bone loss in other patients treated for depression.

The bottom line is that only nutritional recovery works. Even after restoring and maintaining normal weight and regular menstrual periods, the majority of women with a history of anorexia have low bone density. This puts them at higher risk for fractures for the rest of their lives.

Anorexia often begins with normal dieting that gradually escalates to extremes. This pattern must be identified as a problem right away. With earlier intervention, it might be possible to limit bone loss and decrease the high risk of osteoporosis in later life.

BULIMIA

Bulimia nervosa is characterized by binge eating followed by purging behaviors that are used to avoid weight gain. These may take the form of self-induced vomiting, laxative abuse, or the use of diuretics, enemas, calorie restriction, or excessive exercise. As opposed to anorexia nervosa, typical patients diagnosed with bulimia nervosa are often of normal weight. However, some 30 to 40 percent have a past history of anorexia nervosa. This history, rather than the bulimia, puts them at risk for low bone density and fractures. This is a consistent finding in multiple studies that show appropriate bone density for age in normal-weight bulimic patients without a history of anorexia. Normal levels of bone turnover markers also support this finding.

The Bare Bones

- Anorexia nervosa causes a lasting effect on bone health.
- Since this occurs commonly in teenagers, they fail to attain optimal peak bone mass.
- No established treatment is available to improve bone density in young women with anorexia nervosa. Weight gain will partially restore bone density.
- In the eating disorder bulimia, sufferers binge and purge, but do not have lower bone density unless they also have a past history of anorexia nervosa.

Intestinal Problems: Celiac Disease and Inflammatory Bowel Disease

Celiac disease made the "What's In" list for the decade 2010 in the *Washington Post's* "Ranking What's Out, What's In." The number of people diagnosed with the disorder seems high enough to call it "epidemic." Everyone is talking about it. Celiac disease has had top billing on the popular daytime talk show *The View*. Co-host Elisabeth Hasselbeck is increasing awareness by talking about her struggles with the disease. More than two million people in the US have celiac disease. An estimated one in one hundred children has the disease, yet the majority of those afflicted are not diagnosed. The symptoms at any age can range from severe—diarrhea, vomiting, and weight loss—to vague, such as an upset tummy, bloating, being out of sorts, or even *none at all*.

That is the problem! Years may go by with celiac disease undiagnosed, which puts your health, including bone health, in jeopardy. Gluten, which is found in wheat, rye, and barley, is toxic to the bowel. In the small intestine, little mini fronds called "villi" provide increased surface area for absorption of nutrients. Villi means "shaggy hair" in Latin. Basically, the shaggy hair gets a bad buzz haircut with celiac disease. The villi become damaged and inflamed nubs. This damage and inflammation in the small intestine leads to poor absorption of vitamins and nutrients that are vital for your health.

The treatment for celiac disease (also referred to as gluten sensitivity or intolerance) is a strict gluten-free diet. I mean strict! Gluten is hidden in hundreds of common food products that you would not suspect. No soy sauce on your sushi! Just an eighth of a teaspoon of gluten is enough to harm your intestine. You have to be a true sleuth and become familiar with what you can and can't eat. This is a *huge* lifestyle and nutrition change that is socially challenging.

In the past, this diet was extremely difficult to manage. Now "gluten-free" has gone mainstream. My local supermarket has a gluten-free section; other supermarkets offer lists of gluten-free products available in their stores. Labels are explicit: "No gluten ingredients used" or, conversely, "Made on equipment that processes wheat." Even so, you still need to be savvy and informed about what to eat. That is the reason Hasselbeck put together her *New York Times* best-selling book *The G-Free Diet*.

First, celiac disease needs to be diagnosed.

CELIAC DISEASE: HIDDEN CAUSE OF LOW BONE MASS AND FRACTURES

A number of studies have identified the presence of celiac disease without obvious symptoms in middle-aged women with low bone density. These findings have led to the use of screening blood tests for celiac disease in the evaluation of people with low bone density. The tests look for proteins, called autoantibodies, that react against the body's own tissues. The common markers have long technical names: antiendomysial antibodies, antigliadin antibodies, and tissue transglutaminase. Your doctor may include one or more of these tests to detect celiac disease.

Osteoporosis is more common in people with celiac disease than in the general population. At the time of diagnosis, low bone density is common in both children and adults. Before starting a gluten-free diet, osteoporosis may be present in up to one-third of adults with celiac disease. Typically, bone density increases about five percent during the first year of adhering to a gluten-free diet. However, bone density tends to remain lower than the average range. Early reports showed that the association of celiac disease with osteoporosis was found in up to 20 percent of postmenopausal women evaluated for osteoporosis. These reports tended to be from specialty clinics. Later reports from more general populations found much lower rates. Approximately 2 to 3 percent of women were reported to have the combination of previously undetected celiac disease and osteoporosis.

The fracture risk in patients with celiac disease varies across different study populations. Overall, fractures are more common among patients with celiac disease than in the general population. Specific risk factors for fracture include: young age at the onset of celiac disease, failure to follow a gluten-free diet, undernourishment, and low vitamin D and calcium intake.

Low vitamin D is common in celiac disease. Low bone mass and high fracture risk may be due to the intestinal inflammation itself, which is triggered by gluten, and the reduced absorption of calcium and vitamin D. The exact mechanism of bone loss in celiac disease has not been fully worked out.

A blood test for celiac disease should be considered as part of your evaluation if you have been diagnosed with low bone mass or a recent fracture. Celiac disease should also be considered as a possible cause if you have a low calcium level measured in a twenty-four-hour urine test or bone loss despite therapy with an osteoporosis medicine.

Based on screening guidelines, bone density evaluation (DXA scan) is recommended for adults with celiac disease.

INFLAMMATORY BOWEL DISEASE: CROHN'S DISEASE AND ULCERATIVE COLITIS

Despite the name, inflammatory bowel disease also causes health problems outside of the digestive system. Low bone mass is a common finding in inflammatory bowel disease (IBD)—Crohn's disease and ulcerative colitis. The frequency of low bone mass ranges from 11 percent to a high of 78 percent. This wide range is a result of the populations studied and the large variation of the diseases. The location, extent, and severity of the diseases all play a role in its effect on bone, as does drug treatment, especially steroids. Some studies indicate that Crohn's patients are at higher risk than those with ulcerative colitis, while other studies found no bone mass differences between the two groups.

Fracture risk is estimated to be 20 to 40 percent higher than for the general population. Fracture rates increase with age, and postmenopausal women are at the highest risk. Fractures do not necessarily correlate with bone density. In one study, over half of those with fractures had normal bone density. Bone density measurements need to be considered in association with risk factors.

Risk factors for low bone mass and fractures include the general risk factors for osteoporosis, in particular older age, being female, and being underweight. Other factors related to inflammatory bowel disease include steroid use, surgical removal of parts of the small intestine, vitamin D deficiency, and activity and duration of the inflammatory process. Onset of the disease before age eighteen, during the phase of large bone mass gains, may prevent attaining optimal peak bone mass and height.

The rate of bone loss is highest in postmenopausal women. Bone loss rates of 3 to 6 percent a year are reported for the spine during periods when the diseases are active. After remission for longer than three years, the rate of bone loss appears to follow average bone loss for age and gender. Bone loss is most closely related to steroid use. A high lifetime dose of steroids is associated with low bone mineral density at the hip and spine. Steroids, even in low doses of less than 7.5 mg of prednisone, may accelerate bone loss. Use of intermittent high-dose steroids may cause greater bone loss than long-term low doses.

However, the effect of steroids is difficult to separate from disease activity. Those with severe disease are more likely to receive steroid treatment. Even before the use of steroids, patients with inflammatory bowel disease have lower than normal bone density. Certain inflammatory factors, called cytokines, are overproduced. These are thought to contribute to bone loss as well.

Inadequate vitamin D along with poor absorption of calcium is a big problem in Crohn's disease. Since Crohn's disease commonly affects the part of the small intestine where vitamin D and calcium are absorbed from the gut, this is not surprising. Those with a history of surgery to remove part of the small intestine are at particularly high risk for vitamin D deficiency. Testing of vitamin D levels is essential in order to know how much supplementation is needed for maintenance of adequate vitamin D levels.

Poor nutrition as a result of chronic inflammation of the digestive system can have an additional impact. During flares, getting enough calories is a challenge and absorption of nutrients may be decreased. Frequently, patients lose weight, including muscle mass. Bone loss is associated with the weight loss, which may be rapid during an acute flare. The good news is that a return of bone is possible after successful treatment of the disease.

Increased awareness of the risk of low bone mass and fractures is essential in the management of inflammatory bowel disease regardless of the cause of bone loss. The American Gastroenterological Association's guidelines published in 2003 recommend assessment of risk factors and use of bone density (DXA) in select high-risk patients. I would add that there is a need to evaluate all inflammatory bowel patients to prevent fractures in the future. All will benefit from awareness about general bone health measures.

Recent advances in the management of inflammatory bowel disease have provided more treatment options. These include both steroid and nonsteroidal drugs. Entocort® (budesonide) is a steroid that acts locally in the intestine and has been in use for some time. Due to its inactivation in the liver, Entocort is less harmful to the bone and has limited general effects. Other combinations of biologic agents (monoclonal antibodies) and immunosuppressive drugs are being investigated, which may one day provide "steroid-free" treatment and remission.

The Bare Bones

- Low bone mass is common in celiac disease and inflammatory bowel disease.
- Celiac disease may be a hidden cause of bone loss and osteoporosis.
- Age at onset, steroid treatment, and disease activity correlate with bone health in inflammatory bowel disease.
- Nutrition, vitamin D, and maintaining body weight are crucial for maintaining bone health.

Thyroid Problems

My research career as an epidemiologist or "disease detective" began with an investigation of the effect of thyroid hormone on bone, working with Dr. Elizabeth Barrett-Connor in the early 1990s. Starting in 1972, she spearheaded a study designed to follow the residents of Rancho Bernardo, California, a community just northeast of San Diego. The original study focused on factors that might increase one's risk for heart disease. Dr. Barrett-Connor continued the study and expanded it to include other diseases and problems. The first osteoporosis-focused clinic visit started in 1989, when one of the first bone density machines, a central DXA, was made available for research purposes.

My first research project was to study the effect of thyroid hormone on bone density. My intellectual curiosity about this topic came from a group of patients that I referred to as "thyroid junkies." These were patients who had been on thyroid hormone for many years yet did not feel well unless they were taking higher than the needed replacement doses. Each time I lowered their doses in an effort to get their blood test results into the normal range, they would complain about how sluggish the lower doses made them feel. As a result, they would just resume a higher dose of thyroid hormone on their own. I kept telling them that this was not good for their health. They were putting themselves at risk for bad effects on their heart, such as irregular heart rhythms, and for damage to their bone.

Their response was, "Prove it to us!" When I looked into the literature on thyroid and bone, the information was primarily about the effects on bone from an overactive thyroid, or hyperthyroidism. Little information was available about replacement doses of thyroid hormone and bone. As a result, we did a systematic study of the women in the Rancho Bernardo Study. Our findings were novel. We hit the publication "jackpot"—the lead article in an issue of the *Journal of the American Medical Association* (*JAMA*) with an accompanying editorial. My research publication career started at the top!

THYROID DISEASE

When the thyroid goes awry, it either accelerates or puts on the brakes. A more sensitive blood test now helps doctors discover over or under activity of the thyroid earlier in the course of disease. Obvious presentations of overactive "hyper-

353

thyroidism" or underactive "hypothyroidism" are seen much less frequently in doctors' offices today. Thyroid disease is more common in women than in men.

Thyroid Hormones

The master gland, the pituitary, produces thyroid-stimulating hormone or TSH. As the name suggests, it stimulates the thyroid to produce thyroid hormones. Thyroxine, abbreviated T4 for its chemical structure, is the principal hormone. T3 or triiodothyronine is the other. A synthetic version of thyroxine T4 is the most common "replacement" for hypothyroidism. The thyroid hormones send feedback both to the hypothalamus (a region of the brain that produces hormones to control multiple functions, including thyroid-releasing hormone to activate the pituitary gland) and the pituitary.

If too large a quantity of thyroid hormone is produced, as in hyperthyroidism, or you are taking too much thyroid hormone medicine, the pituitary stops producing TSH. This is termed "suppression," and the TSH level will be low to undetectable.

If too small a quantity of thyroid hormones is circulating, the pituitary produces more and more TSH, trying to get the thyroid to make more thyroid hormones. The TSH level in this case will be high, indicating an underactive thyroid status or hypothyroidism.

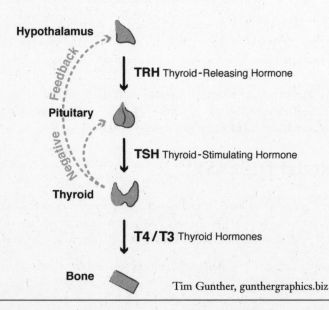

Hypothalamus

Negative Feedback

TRH Thyroid-Releasing Hormone

Pituitary

TSH Thyroid-Stimulating Hormone

Thyroid

T4/T3 Thyroid Hormones

Bone

Tim Gunther, gunthergraphics.biz

HYPERTHYROIDISM

Thyroid hormones play a major role in your body's metabolism and also influence bone metabolism. Hyperthyroidism revs up bone turnover, just as it revs up the whole body. Bone loss is a result of increased bone turnover. Too much thyroid hormone appears to be more detrimental to the dense cortical bone found in the hip and forearm than to the spongy trabecular bone found in the spine.

The main causes of hyperthyroidism are Graves' disease, toxic multinodular goiter, and toxic thyroid nodules. Hyperthyroidism is more common in women, and risk of hyperthyroidism increases with age.

The majority of studies of hyperthyroidism and bone have focused on postmenopausal women. Bone breakdown activity by the osteoclasts is increased out of proportion to bone formation by the osteoblasts. In addition, the normal duration of the bone remodeling cycle is shortened. These changes lead to a net loss of bone and increased fracture risk at the hip, spine, wrist, and foot.

An increased risk for hip fracture is reported in women with a history of hyperthyroidism. Other studies report that the risk of spine and forearm fractures is increased as well. The effect of this condition may worsen with age-related bone loss. After successful treatment of hyperthyroidism, small increases in bone density have been observed in postmenopausal women. However, complete reversibility is not usually possible.

In contrast, hyperthyroidism does not have an effect on the bone density of premenopausal women and men. Estrogen may provide bone protection to younger women who have not yet reached menopause. Few men have been systematically studied.

Fortunately, with the development of sensitive TSH assays and more frequent screening, hyperthyroidism is generally identified early.

HYPOTHYROIDISM

Bone metabolism slows down with hypothyroidism. In the early months of giving thyroxine (T4) replacement to normalize function, a transient increase in bone loss may be observed. This is "catch-up" loss of bone that would have been lost had the thyroid been functioning normally. Fortunately, this transient increase in bone loss is followed by resumption of a normal rate of bone loss. Today, an underactive thyroid condition is usually found by blood testing if hypothyroidism is mild, with few if any symptoms. However, those who never or rarely see doctors may be diagnosed from obvious signs of the disease.

THYROID HORMONE TREATMENT

The brand name Synthroid® (levothyroxine sodium) is the most common thyroid hormone prescribed for hypothyroidism. Synthroid is usually one of the top ten prescriptions dispensed in the US each year. The data from 2010 show that name or generic levothyroxine ranked fourth with a total of 70.5 million prescriptions dispensed. More than 10 percent of postmenopausal women take thyroid hormones.

The correct thyroid hormone replacement dose is the dose that maintains a normal TSH level. Up to 20 percent of postmenopausal women are estimated to be "over replaced." Younger adults usually require a higher dose of thyroid hormone replacement than older adults. This is related to the amount of lean body mass. With age, lean body mass, or muscle mass, decreases. Therefore, smaller doses may be required for replacement with aging.

However, it is all too common to be on the same dose without change over many years, even though the measured TSH may drop lower and lower. This is a sign that your thyroid hormone prescription probably needs an adjustment to a smaller dose. Advances in the measurement of TSH with more sensitive assays have contributed to lowering the doses of thyroid hormone over the last fifteen years.

The best way to monitor your dose of thyroid hormone replacement is to have your T4 and TSH levels checked each year as part of your annual laboratory evaluation. In that way, you will not run into the problem of "over replacement." Clinically, this is referred to as "subclinical hyperthyroidism." Subclinical hyperthyroidism is the term used for normal levels of thyroid hormone, T3 and T4, with a TSH below the normal reference range. With "over replacement," bone loss is greater at the hip than at the spine. Irregular heart rhythms are more common, particularly atrial fibrillation. The replacement dose of thyroxine should maintain normal thyroid hormone and TSH levels. Blood levels are followed to individualize and adjust your dose as needed.

What we found in the Rancho Bernardo Study on thyroid hormone and bone was interesting. In this population of older postmenopausal women, those who were taking more than "replacement doses" had lower bone density than those on appropriate doses of thyroid hormone. This finding confirmed other studies. The new observation was that those women who were "over replaced" *and* taking estrogen therapy had been spared the harmful bone effects. Their bone densities were higher at all sites, including the hip, spine, and forearm. Estrogen appeared to protect the bones when too much thyroid hormone was given.

Limited information is available on premenopausal women. Similar to what was observed in the Rancho Bernardo women, estrogen may provide premenopausal women with protection against acceleration of bone turnover and bone loss.

Thyroid disease is much less common in men than in women. Therefore, fewer studies have been conducted and less information is available. However, it appears that the influence of thyroid hormone on bone in men is less impressive than the influence of thyroid hormone on bone in women. In our evaluation of men in the Rancho Bernardo Study, we found that bone mineral density was not decreased in those taking thyroid hormone. This observation has been consistent in other studies as well.

As long as the levels of TSH remain in the normal range so that thyroid hormone is truly "replaced," bone density is not affected and, most importantly, fracture risk does not increase.

SUPPRESSIVE DOSES OF THYROID HORMONE

Thyroid hormone tablets are also prescribed to thyroid cancer patients to prevent recurrence of cancer. Larger amounts of thyroid hormone are given to "suppress" TSH to basically "undetectable" levels. Several other thyroid problems, such as a single benign thyroid nodule or an enlarged thyroid, called a "goiter," with multiple nodules, may require suppressive thyroid hormone therapy. These doses are not as high as those used for cancer.

In premenopausal women, thyroid hormone suppression does not cause any significant decrease in bone mineral density. On the other hand, bone loss is observed in postmenopausal women. The amount of bone loss is related to the number of years a person has been on suppressive thyroid hormone doses. This effect is not observed in women taking estrogen therapy. A few studies in men observed no effect of thyroid hormone on bone density.

PREVENTION AND TREATMENT OF THYROID HORMONE–ASSOCIATED BONE LOSS

The best approach is to prevent bone loss by identifying an overactive thyroid as early as possible and by taking the lowest possible thyroid hormone dose to maintain a normal range of TSH. Hyperthyroidism can adversely affect bone, and it is associated with higher risk of fracture in postmenopausal women. Therefore, assessment of bone mass is recommended for all hyperthyroid patients.

Thyroid hormone replacement that results in normal TSH levels has no effect on bone. Since maintaining normal TSH levels with this therapy does not have a significant negative effect on bone, recommendations for bone health and DXA screening follow those for the general population.

Thyroid hormone suppression of TSH for thyroid cancer, goiter, or nodules may have an adverse effect on bone that is greatest in postmenopausal women. Assessment of bone mass is recommended along with use of the lowest effective dose to minimize bone loss and fracture risk.

Adequate calcium intake and vitamin D supplementation are general measures for everyone. Estrogen therapy has fallen out of favor even though it can effectively protect postmenopausal women from thyroid hormone–associated bone loss. Bisphosphonates are the preferred choice if prescription treatment of low bone density is needed.

In summary, the harmful effects of excessive thyroid hormone on bone are observed only in postmenopausal women, not in premenopausal women or men even with suppressive doses. However, in postmenopausal women receiving both estrogen and thyroid hormone, bone appears to be protected. This does not mean that it is okay to take too much thyroid hormone as long as you are on estrogen therapy! Thyroid hormone has other possible harmful effects, especially on your heart. Also, keep in mind that these observations of estrogen therapy were done when estrogen was still "in vogue," prior to the Women's Health Initiative findings. This brings me back to my "thyroid junkies." The Rancho Bernardo research findings ultimately helped convince my patients to follow doctor's orders.

The Bare Bones

- Hyperthyroidism causes bone loss and is associated with increased risk of fracture.
- Bone density testing is recommended for all individuals with a history of hyperthyroidism.
- Thyroid hormone replacement with normal TSH levels appears to have no effect on bone. However, you may need lower doses with aging.
- Thyroid hormone suppression of TSH for thyroid cancer, goiter, or nodules may accelerate bone loss, particularly if you are post-menopausal.

Weight Loss, Including Surgery for Weight Loss (Gastric Bypass)

G iven our obsession with dieting and weight loss, this subject strikes a chord with just about everyone. Weight is associated with bone mass. In general, a heavier person has higher bone density than a lighter weight person. Unfortunately, the relationship is not as simple as it seems.

When screening women for clinical trials, I thought that I could pretty well predict who was going to have low bone density by looking at their weight. After screening thousands of postmenopausal women with DXA scans for eligibility, I was astonished to find overweight and even obese women with low bone mass and osteoporosis.

What is most important to bone density is weight change or the fluctuations in your weight. Weight loss is beneficial for protecting against most health problems but it seems to be detrimental to bone health. That is the bad news!

DIETING: INTENTIONAL WEIGHT LOSS

Dieting that results in weight loss is associated with bone loss. Regaining weight does not necessarily increase bone mass. Yo-yo dieting, as well as sustained weight loss, can cause significant bone loss. Losing as little as one percent of your body weight may accelerate bone turnover.

Fighting midlife weight gain is a common battle. During the menopausal transition, along with all the hormonal changes, weight gain averages one pound a year. The Women's Healthy Lifestyle Project looked at dieting and exercise during this time period. They followed bone density changes across menopause in women with normal weight. Nearly four hundred perimenopausal women were randomly assigned to either a lifestyle intervention group or the control group, which had no intervention. The intervention focused on weight control, healthy diet, and exercise.

After the first year and a half, women in the lifestyle intervention group lost an average of seven pounds compared with women in the control group, who gained an average of one pound. Women in the intervention group also lost twice as much bone density at the hip as the women in the control group. Weight change was not related to changes in bone density at the spine.

At the end of four and a half years, the intervention group maintained a lower average weight than the control group, with a six pound difference. Hip bone density remained lower in the intervention group. Of note, the women who started on estrogen therapy in the transition did not lose as much bone mass. Spine bone density was similar in both groups.

Physical activity was primarily walking, which may not have provided enough high impact resistance to make a difference. The Women's Healthy Lifestyle Project proves that cutting back on calories and exercising works to fight weight gain but does not spare the bone, at least with walking as the sole exercise. Similar results have also been observed in premenopausal women who exercised while engaging in dieting that resulted in weight loss.

There is little information about the type or amount of exercise needed to balance the negative effects of weight loss on bone health. The exercise program might require more intensity, such as weight lifting (see the discussion of the BEST program in the section titled "Exercise: On Your Mark, Get Set, GO!").

If you are dieting, be aware that you are at risk for bone loss. You will probably need a rigorous exercise program. Of course, you will also need adequate calcium and vitamin D supplements along with adequate dietary intake of protein to lose weight safely and, one hopes, to spare your bone.

If you are postmenopausal or in the menopause transition and have a history of weight loss due to sustained or yo-yo dieting, you should have an evaluation to measure your bone density with a DXA, along with a general risk assessment.

More clinical trials are needed in this area to determine exactly which exercises and other interventions will prevent bone loss during dieting. Further research on the mechanisms of dieting-induced bone loss may offer other strategies for prevention of bone loss.

UNINTENTIONAL WEIGHT LOSS ASSOCIATED WITH ILLNESS

In older adults, weight loss may be a marker for poor health. Bone loss associated with unintentional weight loss may parallel loss of muscle mass. With chronic or acute illnesses, there is a tendency toward unintentional weight loss, particularly among older adults. Physical limitations and immobility along with the underlying illness may contribute to bone loss and higher risk of falls and fractures. Bone loss and frailty due to weight loss with illness may compound the risk of hip fractures among individuals who are already at high risk.

WEIGHT LOSS SURGERY: GASTRIC BYPASS

Surgical therapy for obesity, termed "bariatric surgery," has rapidly grown with the advent of new surgical techniques. Surgery using small incisions and an instrument with a camera on it, called a laparoscope, can be performed on an outpatient basis.

The gastric bypass surgery basically creates a smaller stomach, which limits food intake and leads to weight loss. The most common procedures reduce the size of the stomach either by placing a band around the stomach, the popular LAP-BAND®, or by stomach stapling.

A more extensive surgery, called "Roux-en-Y," not only reduces the stomach size but also reroutes the intestine. The surgeon creates a small sac from the stomach that is connected to the middle portion of the small intestine. This results in the upper segment of the small intestine being bypassed. Some Roux-en-Y procedures may combine use of the stomach band with the intestinal bypass. As a result of the bypass of the upper portion of the small intestine, some essential nutrients are not absorbed, and some fat malabsorption also occurs.

This gastrointestinal "rearrangement" surgery creates a higher requirement for vitamin D and calcium because less area is available for absorption. "Restrictive" procedures that exclusively use banding or stapling are much less invasive because neither the stomach nor the intestine is cut. These procedures are less likely to create higher vitamin D and calcium requirements because the intestinal tract follows its normal course.

Multiple health benefits are derived from bariatric surgery. However, bone health may suffer. After gastric bypass surgery, there is a dramatic increase in bone turnover and bone loss. Studying a small group of patients who underwent the Roux-en-Y surgery, Mayo Clinic researchers found that 20 percent had fractured a bone within seven years of surgery. Their fracture rate was nearly double the expected fracture rate in a comparable group of people of similar age and sex.

Findings from another small series of patients treated at Columbia University with the Roux-en-Y procedure showed that bone density at the hip declined proportionally to weight loss. During the first year following surgery, the average weight loss was a hundred pounds. Bone density decreased by 8 percent at the total hip and was stable at the spine and forearm. The researchers found evidence of calcium and vitamin D malabsorption despite marked increases in calcium (100 percent) and vitamin D (260 percent) intake. Other studies have reported finding bone loss at both the hip and spine.

Awareness of bone health starts before gastric bypass surgery. Since vitamin

D is stored in the fat, the more fat you have, the more vitamin D you need. Many patients are vitamin D deficient before surgery. Therefore, it is important to optimize vitamin D well before the surgery.

After surgery, it can be a challenge to provide enough calcium and vitamin D, as observed in published reports of patient cases. The type of surgery makes a difference in determining vitamin D and calcium requirements. Calcium is absorbed all along the small intestine. Most absorption occurs in the first two parts of the small intestine, called the duodenum and jejunum. Since the Roux-en-Y procedure connects the stomach directly to part of the jejunum, the opportunity for vitamin D and calcium absorption is greatly diminished.

Supplemental calcium and vitamin D are required. Those who have undergone a Roux-en-Y procedure may have difficulty maintaining adequate calcium and vitamin D. Therapy with portable light boxes that produce vitamin D in the skin is currently under investigation with patients who are unable to maintain sufficient levels with oral supplementation. Measurement of vitamin D levels will help guide the amount of supplements required to maintain vitamin D levels above 30 ng/ml. Other laboratory tests may be needed to monitor bone health status; these may include parathyroid hormone, serum calcium, serum phosphorus, and twenty-four-hour urine for calcium.

A DXA scan is recommended with a follow-up study in about two years. Fortunately, since most men and women who have gastric bypass start with high bone density, they do not typically reach osteoporosis levels even after significant bone loss. However, this loss may translate into higher than normal fracture rates.

If osteoporosis is found, an evaluation should investigate additional causes. Consideration for osteoporosis therapy should include other routes of delivery besides pills. These will include medicines administered by vein or by shots under the skin.

If you or a loved one has had gastric bypass surgery, assessment of bone health should be followed closely as part of the overall management plan.

The Bare Bones
- Weight loss from any cause appears to have harmful effects on bone health.
- When dieting, be aware that you may be at risk for bone loss.
- Be vigilant about calcium, vitamin D, protein, and nutrients, along with the number of calories you take in while dieting.
- Weight loss associated with illness may place vulnerable individuals at even higher risk of falls and fractures.
- Gastric bypass surgery that causes a large amount of weight loss may put you at high risk for broken bones.

Steroid Use: Prednisone

Mention the word "steroids" and most people think of body builders trying to bulk up their muscles or professional athletes such as Major League Baseball players such as Alex Rodriguez, who confessed to using performance-enhancing drugs. "Great," you might think, "I'll take steroids to look buff." Unfortunately, instead of building muscle, the anti-inflammatory type of steroids, such as prednisone, can lead to muscle and bone loss.

These are called corticosteroids or glucocorticoids, in contrast to the "anabolic steroids" that athletes sometimes abuse. "Glucocorticoid-induced osteoporosis" is the most common type of osteoporosis after postmenopausal osteoporosis or age-related causes. You may also see the term "GIOP" used for short. For simplicity's sake, the less formal "steroids" will be used to refer to glucocorticoids in this chapter.

Steroids are given to millions of people to counteract allergic or inflammatory conditions. Common problems treated with steroids include lung problems (such as asthma or emphysema), rheumatoid arthritis, and severe psoriasis.

What Are the "Steroids"?

Steroids are usually referred to by their generic name. Selected brand names are also listed just in case your pill bottle or packet is labeled by brand. The most common glucocorticoid steroid is prednisone. Other common oral steroids are shown in the table below with the dose that corresponds to 5 mg of prednisone.

Generic Name	Brand Name	Dose Equal to Prednisone 5 mg
prednisone	Deltasone®, Orasone®	5 mg
prednisolone	Orapred®, Prelone®	5 mg
methylprednisolone	Medrol®	4 mg
hydrocortisone	Cortef®	20 mg
cortisone	Many brands	25 mg
dexamethasone	Decadron®	0.75 mg

STEROIDS: BONE LOSS AND
INCREASED FRACTURE RISK

Mechanism of Harmful Effects on Bone

Steroids affect bone through multiple pathways. Bone loss is primarily due to the effect of steroids on osteoblasts. Steroids decrease the birth rate of osteoblasts, suppress their activity, and cause earlier death of the osteoblasts. Initially, these bone-breakdown cells increase in number and activity.

Other effects of steroids include decreased production of estrogen and testosterone, decreased calcium absorption from the small intestine, and increased loss of calcium in urine. Muscle loss and weakness may occur with long-term use. As a consequence, there is increased risk of falls. Falls, in turn, increase the risk of fractures independent of bone loss.

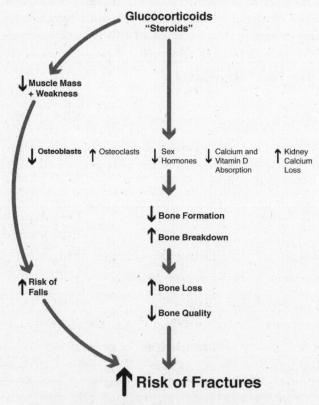

[Effect dependent on dose, length of use, age, disease being treated]
Tim Gunther, gunthergraphics.biz

Steroids are powerful medicines that are useful in many situations. The downside includes a multitude of side effects. Bone is one of the places where steroids are harmful. Individual responses to steroids are variable. One's sensitivity to steriods may be related to the dose of steroids, the duration of use, the disease or problem treated, age, and hormonal status. Postmenopausal women are at highest risk for steroid-induced osteoporosis.

Bone loss with steroids use is most marked in the spongy trabecular bone sites, like the lumbar spine, wrist, and ribs. Steroids also affect the hip and other sites of dense cortical bone. Steroid therapy is associated with early, rapid bone loss within the first few months up to six months, followed by a more gradual but constant decline. Bone density loss is dose-related and may be accentuated in the presence of other risk factors for osteoporosis.

The typical pattern of bone loss during the first year of therapy is 8 to 12 percent at the spine and 2 to 3 percent at the hip when the average dose is 7.5 mg per day of prednisone. In subsequent years, the annual decline is less. *Practically, no dose is without negative side effects.* However, the amount of bone loss is related to the daily dose of steroids. Bone loss increases markedly for doses over 20 mg of prednisone per day.

Initially, bone turnover may be increased due to an increase in the number and activity of osteoclasts. It is followed by a reduction in bone turnover after the first six to twelve months of steroid therapy, which is reflected in the pattern of bone loss. Bone formation is decreased due to the negative impact of steroids on osteoblasts. As a result, thinning of bone structure with steroids exceeds the thinning observed in those with postmenopausal osteoporosis, who have normal bone formation.

It is important to realize that among steroid-treated individuals fractures occur at a higher level of bone density than is seen in postmenopausal osteoporosis. This reflects changes in bone structure and quality as well as bone mass. Steroids affect osteocyte viability and induce the disruption of the osteocyte network. Since osteocytes play an important role in the maintenance of bone quality, this is thought to contribute to increased bone fragility and the risk of fractures at higher levels of bone mineral density. Therefore, the risk of fracture may be underestimated by using results of DXA alone.

Fracture risk may increase within three months of starting steroids. Spine fractures are the most common. However, the majority of these are silent with no symptoms. Even doses of prednisone less than 2.5 mg per day increase the risk of spine fractures by 50 percent. Doses of prednisone over 7.5 mg per day increase fracture risk by 500 percent. In general, the rate of spine fractures is increased four- to fivefold and the rate of hip fracture is increased twofold.

The FRAX calculator includes steroid use in its estimation of ten-year fracture risk. This is applicable only to men and women ages forty to ninety. The absolute risk of fracture in premenopausal women and younger men is generally low unless a fracture has already occurred. Since the FRAX calculation uses bone density of the hip rather than the spine measurement, and the spine is where dramatic bone loss may occur, it may underestimate your fracture risk. Your doctor must take into account your dose of steroids and be very aware of the bone risk involved.

After stopping steroid therapy, some but not all of the lost bone may be added back. However, the fracture risk does not return to pretreatment levels, though it will be lower than it was during steroid treatment.

When steroids are used at high doses or for long periods of time, loss of muscle mass may occur. As a result, the risk of falls increases and this leads to an increased risk of fractures independent of bone density.

INHALED STEROIDS: "MAYBE" BONE LOSS

The chronic use of inhaled steroids may cause bone loss. Inhaled steroids are less likely to have the effects of oral steroids. However, in higher doses and for long periods, enough may be absorbed to harm the bone. Lower bone density measurements at the spine, hip, and forearm have been observed in studies that compared users of inhaled steroids to nonusers. However, it may be hard to separate the effects of underlying disease and previous use of oral steroids from the effects of inhaled steroids.

Inhaled steroids are commonly used for asthma and emphysema or COPD (chronic obstructive pulmonary disease). The largest clinical trial to investigate inhaled steroids and bone was part of the Towards a Revolution in COPD Health (TORCH) study. No difference in bone density or fractures was observed between placebo sprays and inhaled therapies after three years of use. However, the researchers' main concern was that the majority of participants, both men and women, had low bone density.

If you have chronic lung disease and use steroid inhalers, a measurement of bone density along with an evaluation of your risk factors for fracture should be done. Even if the inhalers are not causing problems, your lung disease or previous use of steroids may be.

NASAL STEROIDS: NOT WITH USUAL DOSES

Limited data is available for nasal steroids. Only a few cases have been reported in the literature. Dr. Angelo Licata, an endocrinologist at the Cleveland Clinic in Cleveland, Ohio, reported on a forty-eight-year-old postmenopausal woman with nasal allergies who used her nasal steroid spray more frequently than pre-scribed. Over one year, she lost 10 percent of bone density at the spine and 5 percent at the hip despite being on estrogen therapy. In addition, she had other physical findings that raised suspicion about excess use of steroid spray. Whether these effects were from increased nasal absorption or from swallowing the excess liquid spray was unclear.

Using nasal steroids as prescribed does not appear to produce harmful effects on bone.

BONE PROTECTIVE THERAPY

The lowest possible dose is always desirable when it may not be an option to completely stop steroids. Decrease or eliminate all other risk factors, such as excessive alcohol use and smoking. General measures should include adequate calcium and vitamin D intake, a regular exercise program, and taking steps to reduce the risk of falling. However, for many patients taking steroids, these measures are not enough. Because many variables come into play, you must be attentive to your bone health while on steroids.

As seen in several clinical trials, subjects in the placebo groups who took cal-cium plus vitamin D had less bone loss than expected. Vitamin D blood levels need to be monitored, since steroids may decrease absorption. Higher doses of vitamin D supplements may be required to maintain levels above 30 ng/ml.

Four of the osteoporosis medicines have been tested in steroid users and approved by the FDA for this indication. The diverse group of individuals taking steroids complicates treatment studies. Studies combine adult men and women of all ages with different diseases who are taking different medicines in a variety of doses. Most of the clinical trials studied postmenopausal women with smaller numbers of premenopausal women and men included.

Use of osteoporosis medicines for steroid users is classified into two types:

1. *Prevention*: For individuals who are at risk for loss of bone as a result of beginning treatment with steroids.
2. *Treatment*: For individuals who have lost bone due to long-term steroid therapy.

In general, the steroid studies enroll smaller numbers of subjects and bone den-sity changes are the main outcome, not fractures. Prevention studies are usually twelve months in duration and focus on prevention of bone loss. Treatment studies may be up to three years in length. Due to the smaller number subjects, few fractures are observed.

BISPHOSPHONATES AND FORTEO

The two most common medicines used are generic alendronate (Fosamax) and Actonel. In steroid-treated patients, these agents increase bone density at the spine by 3 to 4 percent compared with placebo over one year. These agents also decrease the risk of spine fractures.

Reclast is gaining in popularity because it does not interfere with oral medicines and is given by vein only once a year. This is helpful for steroid users because, on average, people on steroids take a total of six to eight different medicines.

Forteo is also an appealing choice because it counters the effects of steroids on bone formation. Forteo directly stimulates the osteoblasts *and* inhibits their breakdown, which may reverse the key effects of steroids on bone formation. Forteo improves both bone density and bone quality, which results in rebuilding microstructure.

One three-year study compared Forteo and Fosamax at 10 mg a day in over four hundred high-risk patients who were taking long-term steroids. Bone density increased in patients receiving either Forteo or Fosamax. However, patients receiving Forteo had larger increases in BMD and fewer new spine fractures. Therefore, Forteo should be considered as a first-line therapy in high-risk patients.

FDA-Approved Medicines to Prevent Bone Loss from Steroids

The addition of an osteoporosis drug may be necessary for preventing bone loss while you are taking steroids. Clinical trials evaluated these drugs in men and both premenopausal and postmenopausal women using oral steroids. The FDA has approved the following drugs for the indication of "glucocorticoid-induced osteoporosis." You may also see the term "GIOP" used for short.

Brand Name	Generic Name	Indication
Actonel	risedronate	Prevention and Treatment
Forteo	teriparatide	Treatment
Fosamax	alendronate	Treatment
Reclast	zoledronic acid	Prevention and Treatment

As long as you are taking steroids, therapy with osteoporosis medicines will prevent bone loss. If you are on long-term steroids but discontinue bone-protective therapy, you may experience significant bone loss, particularly at the hip. In one study of Fosamax, patients who were taking a dose of 6 mg or more of prednisone a day and stopped taking Fosamax lost bone density rapidly. In a three- to four-year follow-up after stopping Fosamax, spine density decreased 5 percent. In contrast, bone density remained stable for those who continued Fosamax. At the neck region of the hip (femoral neck), bone density decreased 9 percent for those who discontinued Fosamax. Those who continued Fosamax had a small loss of less than 1 percent.

HORMONE THERAPY

Since steroids can lead to a decrease in estrogen and testosterone, replacing these hormones has been shown to be beneficial. A few small studies have evaluated hormone therapy in both men and postmenopausal women receiving steroid therapy. Estrogen use in women increases bone density at the spine over 3 percent with no significant change at the hip over one year. Testosterone replacement in men showed similar increases in bone density.

However, because of the increased risk for breast cancer and cardiovascular disease, hormone therapy is no longer recommended as treatment for steroid users. Hormone therapies are usually reserved for improvement in symptoms such as vasomotor symptoms, loss of libido, and loss of potency. Hormone therapy may enhance quality of life and may be given for reasons other than bone protection. Replacing these hormones must be balanced with consideration of the risks of use.

TREATMENT GUIDELINES

In 2010, the American College of Rheumatology updated its guidelines for patients starting or on steroid therapy. For all individuals, basic measures of calcium, vitamin D, and fall prevention are part of the overall treatment. They recommend that management decisions for prescription osteoporosis medicine use be based on assessment of fracture risk and consideration of your age and sex.

This is a synopsis of the recommendations for anyone prescribed prednisone or its equivalent. The recommendations serve as a starting point for evaluating your risk and establishing a management plan that may include prescription medicine for bone protection while taking steroids.

Group	Duration of Use or Anticipated Use	Daily Dose	Prescription Medicine Therapy
Premenopausal women or men younger than fifty with no history of fracture	Any duration	Any dose	Inadequate data for recommendation
Premenopausal women (child bearing potential) with history of fracture not due to trauma	1–3 months	Any dose	No recommendation
	3 months or longer	Less than 7.5 mg	No recommendation
		7.5 mg or more	Fosamax Actonel Reclast
Premenopausal women (not considering pregnancy) or men younger than fifty with history of fracture not due to trauma	1–3 months	5 mg or more	Fosamax Actonel
		If 7.5 mg or more	Also consider Reclast with Fosamax or Actonel
	3 months or longer	Any dose	Fosamax Actonel Reclast Forteo
Postmenopausal women or men older than fifty "low risk" (FRAX less than 10 percent)	3 months or longer	Less than 7.5mg	No prescription recommended
		7.5 mg or or more	Fosamax Actonel Reclast
Postmenopausal women or men older than fifty "medium risk" (FRAX 10 to to 20 percent)	3 months or longer	Less than 7.5 mg	Fosamax Actonel
		7.5 mg or more	Fosamax Actonel Reclast

			Fosamax
Postmenopausal women or men older than fifty "high risk" (FRAX 20 percent)	1 month or less	Less than 5 mg	Fosamax Actonel Reclast
		5 mg or more	Fosamax Actonel Reclast Forteo
	1 month or or longer	Any dose	Fosamax Actonel Reclast Forteo

These general recommendations serve as a starting point for helping you and your doctor to individualize your treatment plan based on your risk. A baseline DXA scan is recommended and a scan of the entire spine, called vertebral fracture assessment (VFA), may be considered as well. The identification of silent spine fractures would put you in a higher risk category.

If you are a postmenopausal woman or a man over age fifty, the guidelines recommend using the FRAX calculation to assess fracture risk. Using the ten-year probability of major osteoporotic fracture, three risk groups are identified: low, medium, and high. The "high-risk" group is the same as the National Osteoporosis Foundation classification of 20 percent or higher fracture probability. Therefore, individuals in this group should be considered for therapy even if they are not taking steroids. Those with a fracture probability less than 10 percent are categorized as "low risk," and those between 10 and 20 percent are categorized as "medium risk." The guidelines detail specific treatments based on risk category, duration or anticipated duration of use, and dose of steroids. Basically, prescription medicines are recommended for all risk levels and dosages. The exception is "low risk" individuals using less than 7.5 mg a day of prednisone or the equivalent dose of another steroid.

If you are premenopausal or a man younger than age fifty, the guidelines base risk assessment on your history of a fracture not related to trauma along with other risk factors. Recommendations for women in this age group depend on whether they are still interested in starting a family. Lack of research evidence limited the expert panel from making recommendations for some scenarios. Those without a history of fracture are at lower risk, and no recommendations are given for this group.

The guidelines do not address patients using inhaled steroids. However, patients with chronic lung disease who use steroid inhalers are at increased risk for fracture. Measurement of bone density would be appropriate along with evaluation of the overall risk-factor profile.

If you start bone-protective therapy, how long should you continue it? As a general rule, bone-protective therapy should be continued for the duration of steroid therapy. When steroids are stopped, bone density should be reassessed to determine whether further treatment is needed. For example, if you are a postmenopausal woman or a man older than fifty and are at high risk for fracture, you will most likely need to continue osteoporosis therapy to reduce your fracture risk.

The guidelines do not make specific recommendations on monitoring with DXA scans. Since large changes in bone density are possible in the first few months of therapy, bone density changes may be detectable within six months. In general, the standard practice is to recheck DXA after one year of therapy.

CHALLENGES

Other diseases are common if you are taking steroids. Juggling the concerns of "competing" illnesses and treatments can be quite complex and challenging for you and your doctors. Other side effects from steroids, such as difficulty sleeping, high blood pressure, and high blood sugar may receive more attention.

Don't forget about your bones! Dramatic bone losses may happen in a short period of time. Treatment with adequate calcium and vitamin D supplementation and bone-protective medicine, if indicated, can override the harmful bone effects of steroids.

The Bare Bones

- No dose of steroids is "safe" for bone health.
- If you receive a prescription for steroids, a second prescription for bone protection needs to be considered.
- When completely stopping steroids may not be possible, the lowest possible dose is desirable.
- Take adequate vitamin D supplements to maintain a blood level above 30 ng/ml and ensure adequate daily calcium intake.
- Exercise and take measures to prevent falls.

Rheumatoid Arthritis

Rheumatoid arthritis is an inflammatory type of arthritis that affects women more often than men. This type of arthritis is different from the common degenerative arthritis, called osteoarthritis, which occurs with aging or after injury. Each type of arthritis has distinct characteristics. You may think of rheumatoid arthritis as "sick joints" and osteoarthritis as "achy joints."

However, types of arthritis are often confused. When people are asked if they have rheumatoid arthritis, about 20 to 30 percent respond "yes" even though rheumatoid arthritis occurs in only about 1 percent of the population. This is a diagnosis made by a doctor, and it requires treatment that is quite different from osteoarthritis. Rheumatoid arthritis is an autoimmune disease, meaning the immune system attacks the body's own tissues, leading to inflammation in the joints and sometimes in other locations like the eyes or lungs.

Rheumatoid arthritis can involve any joint. It tends to be symmetrical, with pain and swelling affecting the same joint on both sides of the body. The most common joints affected are the knuckles and middle joints of the fingers, the wrist, the elbow, and the feet. In contrast, osteoarthritis of the hand affects joints at the end of the fingers next to the fingernail and the middle joints of the fingers. Osteoarthritis also affects the large joints of the hip and knee.

RHEUMATOID ARTHRITIS AND OSTEOPOROSIS: TWO SIDES OF THE SAME COIN

The inflammatory nature of rheumatoid arthritis not only causes local problems in the joints but also generalized bone loss. Both the disease itself and its treatments, particularly the use of steroids, increase bone loss. These observations led to the inclusion of rheumatoid arthritis as a major risk factor for osteoporosis and increased fracture risk. For example, rheumatoid arthritis is one of the criteria used in the fracture risk assessment tool, FRAX, to calculate the ten-year probability of fracture.

The inflammatory disease activity of rheumatoid arthritis and the amount of bone loss are related. Recent research has shed light on the possible mechanisms for these observations and has shown common links between the two processes. The inflammation associated with painful, swollen joints shifts the balance of bone turnover toward more bone breakdown. As a result of the increase in bone breakdown, there is acceleration of bone loss.

Bone breakdown also occurs locally in areas close to the inflamed joints. These lesions, called bone erosions, characterize the profound local effect of inflammation by rheumatoid arthritis on the joints. The local bone erosions may start early in the course of the disease. The bone-breakdown cells, osteoclasts, are responsible for these erosions. Osteoclasts are formed within the inflamed joint and are present in large numbers. However, few bone-forming cells, osteoblasts, are found in joints. Therefore, bone formation in rheumatoid arthritis is essentially absent at these localized sites of erosion. In contrast, osteoarthritis is characterized by the growth of bone protrusions or spurs due to too much bone formation. Bone erosions are not a feature of osteoarthritis.

The signal messenger (called RANKL), which controls the formation, function, and survival of osteoclasts, appears to be the key factor for local and generalized bone loss in rheumatoid arthritis. Inflammatory factors produced during periods of inflammation stimulate the production of more RANKL. Therefore, during increased disease activity, RANKL is increased locally in tissues surrounding the swollen joints and causes increased bone turnover.

TREATMENT TO PREVENT BONE LOSS

The disease course of rheumatoid arthritis tends to be characterized by flares and remissions. A flare is associated with inflammation with redness, pain, and swelling in the joints. General symptoms of fatigue and low-grade fever may also occur. When the inflammation disappears, the disease is inactive and in remission. The goal of therapy is to prevent and stop local bone damage and relieve pain and swelling. Treatment of rheumatoid arthritis usually includes multiple medicines to treat all aspects of the disease. Steroids are commonly used in combination with other medicines classified as "disease-modifying" that slow the progression of the disease. In addition, treatment often includes medicines referred to as "biologics," which target the immune system.

For generalized bone loss, treatment with medicine that blocks the breakdown of bone preserves overall bone mass and provides protection from bone loss. Therefore, bisphosphonates have been the mainstay of therapy to prevent bone loss in patients with rheumatoid arthritis, particularly those receiving treatment with steroids. The bisphosphonates—Fosamax, Actonel, and Reclast—are FDA-approved for treatment of patients on steroid therapy. If you are taking steroid medicine like prednisone, refer to the previous section titled "Steroid Use: Prednisone" for more details.

Because you may have to take multiple medications to treat rheumatoid arthritis, the once-a-year intravenous administration of Reclast may make it a more desirable option than pills, which require a specific dosing regimen. In addition, a small study suggested that Reclast may also be effective in decreasing local bone erosions.

Recent scientific evidence shows that decreasing RANKL protects against local bone erosions. Prolia, the osteoporosis medicine, works by inhibiting the RANKL messenger. Therefore, Prolia effectively increases bone density and decreases fracture risk. Prolia showed promising results in a small clinical trial in more than two hundred patients with rheumatoid arthritis. One year of therapy with Prolia 60 or 180 mg, given twice at six-month intervals in addition to ongoing use of methotrexate, showed reduction in bone erosions in comparison with the control group taking methotrexate alone. In addition, Prolia increased bone density at the hip and spine. However, Prolia did not have any direct effect on inflammation of the joints.

Future therapies for active rheumatoid arthritis may include Prolia in combination with anti-inflammatory medicines. The addition of Prolia may prove beneficial for preventing both generalized bone loss and local bone erosions. Additional research is underway.

The Bare Bones

- Patients with rheumatoid arthritis are at high risk for bone loss and fractures.
- Inflammation triggers both generalized bone loss and local bone erosions at joints typically of the hand, wrist, elbow, and feet.
- Bisphosphonates are often used to prevent generalized bone loss and lower the risk of fractures.
- Prolia may be useful for both protecting against local bone erosions and preventing generalized bone loss but is not yet approved for this indication.

Diabetes

Everyone seems to know someone with diabetes, or you may be diabetic yourself. More than 10 percent of adults in the US have diabetes. With more Americans becoming overweight and less active, the number of adults with diabetes is on the rise.

Diabetes mellitus is categorized into "Type 1" and "Type 2." Fewer than 10 percent of people with diabetes have type 1, which is usually diagnosed in children and young adults when their bodies stop making insulin. They require daily insulin treatment to survive.

The majority of diabetics have type 2 diabetes. Type 2 diabetics make plenty of insulin but their body tissues are resistant and don't properly respond to the action of insulin. Sometimes diet, weight loss, and exercise are able to control high blood sugars and even eliminate diabetes. Other times, the addition of medicines is required to bring blood sugars into the normal range.

You may be surprised to learn that diabetes is a risk factor for fractures. In recent years, an explosion of medical research has reported that diabetes and some of the agents used to treat it have adverse effects on bone health. *Both* type 1 and type 2 diabetes have negative effects on bone that result in an increased risk of fracture.

TYPE 1 DIABETES

Just a few weeks before her 55th birthday, then Supreme Court nominee Sonia Sotomayor tripped at the airport and fractured her right ankle. A few hours later, she was sporting a knee-high cast and walking on crutches to hearings in the Capitol that led up to her confirmation. Why should such a minor spill cause a fracture?

The media theorized that her fracture may have happened because she was older, worked indoors with little sunlight exposure, and had a sedentary profession. No one mentioned the connection to her history of diabetes, which I believe is the main contributing factor. I have neither the details of her fracture nor her medical history. However, Justice Sotomayor has openly talked about being diagnosed with type 1 diabetes at age eight and how she has been taking insulin ever since.

The problem is best characterized by the title of a commentary, "Sugar and Bone: A Not-So Sweet Story" by Dr. Clifford Rosen, an endocrinologist at the

Maine Medical Center. In an accompanying article, researchers from the University of Utah showed that high blood sugars are not good for the growing skeleton of adolescent girls. Therefore, girls with type 1 diabetes may not be able to reach their optimal peak bone mass, which results in smaller and weaker bones. A comparable study has not yet been done in boys.

Type 1 diabetics have low bone mass and an increased risk for adult osteoporosis and fractures. The mechanisms behind this observation are being actively investigated. High blood sugar may actually be toxic to bone. Various hormonal factors are also implicated. However, there is little doubt that diabetes itself causes problems in the skeleton. The propensity for fracture among type 1 diabetics is related to two factors: their bone density is lower than normal and their bones are more fragile. This is the result of a higher rate of bone turnover, with increased bone breakdown out of proportion to bone formation. If a fracture occurs, bone healing is slower and the new bone made could be of poorer quality.

Some but not all studies suggest that tighter control of diabetes may influence patient outcomes. Bone health may benefit from "tight control," which refers to the management of blood sugars in a narrow range rather than allowing large fluctuations. The better the control is, the stronger the bone will be. Lower bone mass is more likely if diabetes is diagnosed before puberty. It is also associated with the presence of other complications of diabetes. Osteoporosis and fractures must be added to the list of diabetes complications from long-term high blood sugars.

TYPE 2 DIABETES

In contrast, type 2 diabetics may have average or above average bone mineral density. Despite this, they still have an increased fracture risk—a paradox for sure! What's the reason for this inconsistency?

It is not clear, but diabetes is a complex disease that affects everything in your body, including bone. Bones of type 2 diabetics are more fragile. The reasons for the increased fragility are still being investigated but high blood sugars are thought to play an important role.

Studies show that diabetics may not make new bone well. Based on bone markers, type 2 diabetics have low bone turnover. The primary reason is reduced bone formation and not the increased bone breakdown that is typically seen in postmenopausal osteoporosis.

Other risk factors beyond bone mass may play a role. For example, diabetics have a greater risk of falling. This could be due to numbness or decreased feeling in the feet combined with balance and vision problems. Medicines that are taken for diabetes may also contribute to the increased fracture risk.

Over many years, physicians observed that diabetics had a disproportionate number of hip fractures. Diabetics have at least twice the risk of fracture compared to people with normal blood sugars. The increased risk includes fractures of the hip, upper arm (humerus), ankle, and foot.

Newly diagnosed diabetics are not at high risk for fracture. The increased fracture risk with type 2 diabetes is observed after five years or longer. Studies using DXA measurements shed some light on this observation. The actual bone density may be higher than average for age but type 2 diabetes is associated with more rapid bone loss.

In the Health, Aging, and Body Composition study or Health ABC study for short, a large group of men and women (3,075 subjects) ages seventy to seventy-nine was followed for four years. Older white women with diabetes had more rapid bone loss at the hip than women with normal blood sugars. However, bone loss in both men and black women with diabetes was no different than in those with normal blood sugars.

Similar findings were observed in the Study of Osteoporotic Fractures (SOF). Older women with diabetes had a higher rate of bone loss at the hip than those without diabetes. In contrast to Health ABC, a comparable effect was seen in older men who participated in the Study of Osteoporosis in Men (MrOS). Older men with diabetes had 60 percent greater loss of bone density at the hip than those older men who did not have diabetes.

The Study of Women's Health Across the Nation (SWAN) followed younger women who were going through menopause. Over three years of observation, bone loss at the hip was an astounding *ten times greater* among women with diabetes than among women without diabetes. In contrast, the rate of bone loss at the spine was not higher in diabetics. Diabetic women also had double the fracture rate of nondiabetic women.

More rapid bone loss, which causes a decrease in bone strength, increases the risk of fracture. On measurement of bone density in type 2 diabetics, using the usual T-score categories (normal, low bone mass, and osteoporosis) or calculated FRAX score may underestimate their fracture risk. All diabetics have a heightened risk of fracture regardless of their bone density.

Factors Leading to Fractures in Diabetes

Both types of diabetes are associated with an increased number of fractures. The factors leading to the higher risk of fractures are quite different.

Type 1 Diabetes	Type 2 Diabetes
Increased bone turnover due to increased bone breakdown	Low bone turnover due to decreased bone formation
Low bone mass	Normal to above normal bone mass
High blood sugar and growing skeleton	Rapid bone loss
Decreased adult bone density	Other factors beyond bone mass
	Treatment with TZDs

DIABETES MEDICINES

Thiazolidinediones, or "TZDs," are a class of oral diabetic drugs for people with type 2 diabetes. They are effective in lowering and controlling blood sugars. They help control blood sugar levels by making the cells of the body more sensitive to the action of insulin. Many times they are used in combination with other diabetic medicines. Unfortunately, these effective diabetes medicines may have a negative effect on your bone.

Drugs Called Thiazolidinediones: TZDs

Generic Name	Brand Name	Drug Company
pioglitazone	Actos®	Takeda Pharmaceuticals
pioglitazone in combination with other diabetes drugs	Actoplus Met®	Takeda Pharmaceuticals
	Duetact®	Takeda Pharmaceuticals
rosiglitazone	Avandia®	GlaxoSmithKline
rosiglitazone	Avandamet®	GlaxoSmithKline
in combination with other drugs	Avandaryl®	GlaxoSmithKline

Rezulin (generic name troglitazone), the first drug in the thiazolidine-diones (TZDs) class, was introduced in the late 1990s. It was withdrawn from the US market in 2000 due to a serious side effect (liver problems).

Avandia (rosiglitazone), which was approved in 1999, became widely used as an effective treatment for control of blood sugars in type 2 diabetics. Avandia's annual sales peaked at $2.2 billion in 2006 but have decreased markedly since because in 2007 new research found that Avandia had a potential for increased risk of heart problems and fractures. The FDA placed a "black box warning" on the label for heart failure and heart attacks.

The controversy about Avandia's effect on the heart continued, and some called for its removal from the market. After considerable review by the FDA, in September 2010 they instituted a "restricted program" for Avandia and its combination products to limit its use in new patients because of the risk of heart attack and stroke. These new safety measures will undoubtedly further decrease the use of Avandia. In addition, the patent for Avandia expires in 2012.

Avandia's "cousin" Actos (pioglitazone) has benefited, and its sales have increased. In 2010, Actos ranked number nine in US prescription medicine sales, generating $3.5 billion. The sales figures for Avandia and Actos mean that many, many diabetics are taking these medicines.

AVANDIA: FRACTURE IS AN UNEXPECTED CONSEQUENCE

In clinical trials of most new drugs, measures of bone health are not typically included in tests of safety. Researchers were surprised by a larger number of fractures found in a study of diabetes medicines.

The ADOPT study (A Diabetes Outcome Progression Trial) compared Avandia with two other diabetes medicines, Micronase (glyburide) and Glucophage (metformin). At the end of 2006, the researchers reported in the *New England Journal of Medicine* their four-year findings from treating more than four thousand diabetic men and women. At the conclusion of the paper, the researchers briefly added the unexpected finding of a higher rate of fractures, which had been identified in one of the three medicine groups prior to the article's publication. Women, but not men, who were treated with Avandia had more fractures than women in the other drug groups. The fractures were primarily of the upper arm, hand, and foot.

Because of the sites of fracture, debate has centered on whether these are osteoporotic fractures. The female subjects were in their midfifties and had been diagnosed with diabetes for two years or less. Hip and spine fractures are not typical for women in their fifties, so you would not expect those fractures; but arm and leg fractures are common. Later, other studies found similar rates of fracture.

Fractures are now listed on the Avandia prescribing information under *Warnings and Precautions*: "Increased incidence of bone fracture in female patients."

ACTOS IS ASSOCIATED WITH FRACTURES, TOO

Whether or not there was also a fracture problem with Actos was answered by the manufacturer's analysis of its clinical trial database of more than fifteen thousand patients. Women, but not men, receiving Actos (pioglitazone) had a higher number of fractures. The majority of the fractures were also in the arm or lower leg.

In March 2007, a letter to healthcare providers notified doctors of this new safety information. Increased fracture risk observed in women is now included in the Actos prescribing information under *Precautions*. The full prescribing label includes additional information about fractures that was gathered during the PROACTIVE study (Prospective Pioglitazone Clinical Trial in Macrovascular Events). Over an almost-three-year period, women with type 2 diabetes taking Actos had double the number of fractures compared to women on placebo.

MEN, TOO?

Overall, TZDs appear to have a less pronounced effect on bone in men than in women. However, the study period for the clinical trials using TZD drugs was short—four years or less. Over a longer term and with aging, would use of TZDs add additional risk on top of the increased risk from the diabetes itself?

Observational studies suggest that men may also be susceptible to bone loss associated with TZD therapy. One large British study suggested that older men and women are both at increased fracture risk as a result of taking TZDs. Although the FDA warnings and precautions for TZDs and fracture include only women, women *and* men with low bone mass and higher risk of fracture may want to use another type of diabetes medicine for control of their blood sugars.

TZDs: Mechanism of Action

Are the negative bone effects just a fluke observation? No, there is consistency across multiple studies. Scientists have explained the fracture findings based on the action of the TZDs. The mediator of the insulin-sensitizing effect of TZDs is found in numerous tissues, including bone. (The mediator is called the nuclear receptor peroxisome proliferator-activated receptor or PPAR-gamma for short.)

In the bone marrow, this mediator acts as a switch to determine whether certain stem cells become bone-building cells (osteoblasts) or fat cells. Once the mediator is turned on by the TZDs, more fat cells are produced and, as a result, fewer osteoblasts are made.

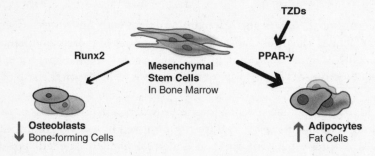

Adapted with permission from Adami, S. *Current Medical Research and Opinion* 2009; 25 (5): 1057–72. © 2009 Informa Healthcare.

In just a matter of a few months, these changes were measured indirectly with bone turnover markers in women. Their markers for building-bone osteoblasts were decreased while markers of bone breakdown were normal. After a short time (fourteen weeks), older, healthy women given Avandia had measurable bone loss at both the hip and spine. That is quick!

Another concern raised by decreased bone formation associated with TZDs is delay in fracture healing. This finding is based on lab mice, but further research in this important area is underway.

TREATMENT

Few data are available to guide treatment in diabetics beyond the use of the general measures: adequate calcium and vitamin D, good nutrition, and exercise. In a reanalysis of data from a Fosamax trial, it was determined that postmenopausal diabetic women tended to not gain as much bone density as nondiabetics taking Fosamax. Also of note, the diabetics in the placebo group lost bone more rapidly at the hip.

Research is needed to guide the design of strategies for improving diabetics' bone health. Since TZDs are effective in controlling blood sugars, are there ways to prevent the associated bone loss? Just like any new insights, new questions are raised that need answers.

At the present time, TZDs should not be used if you are at higher risk for fracture. If you are taking TZDs, monitor your bone density with regular DXA measurements every two years.

The Bare Bones

- Diabetics with either type 1 or type 2 are at higher risk for bone fractures.
- Bone health should be monitored in all diabetic patients.
- Actos and Avandia (TZDs) or related combinations may add to fracture risk.
- You should not take TZDs if you already have low bone density or osteoporosis.

Heartburn and Reflux: "GERD"

You may find that walking into a drugstore and buying a medicine to deal with a symptom is easier than scheduling an appointment to discuss what is going on with your doctor. It is! The challenge is to be a well-informed healthcare consumer. Sometimes you may plan on taking a medicine temporarily, but end up taking it long-term instead. You may forget to include the over-the-counter medicine in your list or bag of medicines when you do make it to the doctor.

Many people with heartburn or gastroesophageal reflux disease (GERD) medicate themselves with over-the-counter drugs. As you walk down the drugstore aisle, you have a variety of choices to battle stomach acid. You might choose antacids, such as Tums, or more powerful medicines such as Zantac®, Pepcid®, Prevacid, Prilosec, or Zegerid®. You may choose the generic store brand equivalents. The branded products are advertised widely, so the names may be familiar to you from your magazines or from television commercials. Zantac and Pepcid are classified as histamine2-receptor antagonists (H2 blockers); Prevacid, Prilosec, and Zegerid are proton pump inhibitors (PPIs).

Why am I making the distinction? Because recent major research studies have connected the use of PPIs to an increased risk of fractures, especially hip fractures. Both H2 blockers and PPIs work by reducing stomach acid secretion. The H2 blockers affect the first step of acid secretion by blocking the histamine of the acid-producing cells and about 70 percent of stomach acid production. Proton pump inhibitors block the proton pump, which is the last step of acid production by the stomach. As a result, PPIs suppress up to 99 percent of stomach acid and are more potent than the H2 blockers. Therefore, PPIs are prescribed more often than the older, less effective H2 blockers.

The availability of PPIs on the drugstore shelves is growing as well. Lower dose formulations of Prilosec, Prevacid, and Zegerid are available over-the-counter (OTC) without a prescription. The FDA approved these OTC treatments for frequent heartburn. In addition, one prescription pain reliever, Vimovo®, now contains esomeprazole in combination with naproxen, a nonsteroidal anti-inflammatory drug (NSAID), to lessen the risk of stomach upset or ulcers.

Proton Pump Inhibitors "PPIs"

Brand Name	Generic Name
Aciphex®	rabeprazole
Dexilant™ (formerly Kapidex®; name changed 2010)	dexlansoprazole
Nexium®	esomeprazole
Prevacid®	lansoprazole
Prilosec®	omeprazole
Protonix®	pantoprazole
Zegerid® (brand production for prescription strength stopped in 2010 when patents were ruled invalid. A lower strength generic is available OTC.)	omeprazole

PPIs are now among the most widely prescribed class of medicines. In 2010, PPIs ranked eighth in number of prescriptions written in the US. The brand Nexium was number two in sales of all prescription drugs, generating $6.3 billion—just behind the cholesterol-lowering drug Lipitor.®

Millions of Americans are taking PPIs as prescription and OTC medicines.

PPIs AND FRACTURE RISK

Two research groups first reported the link between PPIs and fracture risk in 2006. Examining the British General Practice Research Database of more than 1.7 million persons, researchers reported that PPI therapy was associated with an increased risk (44 percent higher) of hip fractures. Risk increased with longer duration of use, and the highest risk was seen among those receiving high-dose PPI therapy. A large Danish study reported a similar magnitude of risk increase for hip fracture and a small increase (18 percent) in risk for all fractures.

Subsequent studies found similar results. A database analysis from the Canadian province of Manitoba observed that residents who suffered an osteoporosis-related fracture were almost twice as likely to have used a PPI for at least seven years. For hip fracture, there was an increased risk of fracture after five or more years of use. Using PPIs for fewer years was not linked to increased fracture risk.

In the US, researchers from the Osteoporotic Fractures in Men Study

(MrOS) and the Study of Osteoporotic Fractures (SOF) found that use of PPIs in older women, as well as in older men with low daily calcium intake, was associated with an increased risk of nonspine fractures. Based on the women's results, the SOF researchers estimated that one extra nonspine fracture would be expected for every ten women treated for five years with a PPI. While this represents a small individual risk, given the widespread use of these medicines, the numbers for the US population as a whole are large.

The link between long-term use of proton pump inhibitors and greater likelihood of osteoporosis-related fractures of the hip, wrist, or spine is based on observational studies. This type of study describes the association but does not prove cause and effect. A clinical trial would be needed to establish causality without a doubt. In the future, it is unlikely such trials will be undertaken to try to show a harmful outcome.

POOR CALCIUM ABSORPTION

One plausible explanation for the link between PPIs and increased fracture risk is that PPIs may affect calcium balance by decreasing calcium absorption in the small intestine. Hydrochloric acid is needed for the absorption of calcium in the small intestine. Since proton pump inhibitors inhibit the production and secretion of hydrochloric acid in the stomach, calcium may not be dissolved or adequately absorbed from food or supplements. Because users of PPIs tend to take them for a long time, this could lead to a negative whole-body calcium balance, resulting in higher rates of bone loss and a greater risk of fractures.

If this is true, could adequate amounts of calcium intake diminish the observed adverse bone effects of PPI use? It is not known. However, you should be vigilant to ensure that your daily diet and supplements contain 1,000 to 1,200 mg of calcium. It is also important to remember that adequate vitamin D intake is necessary for maintaining a blood level of 30 ng/ml or greater for your body's ability to absorb calcium.

CALCIUM SUPPLEMENTATION: DOES IT MATTER?

Calcium Carbonate versus Calcium Citrate

I usually recommend taking calcium citrate when you are taking medicine to suppress acid, but studies to fully address the choice of a calcium supplement if you are taking long-term PPI therapy have not been done.

Calcium carbonate requires acid for dissolving while calcium citrate does not. Usually, you take calcium carbonate with or after a meal, but the timing of calcium citrate does not matter.

When older women volunteers who used Prilosec 20 mg daily for two weeks took calcium carbonate on an empty stomach after fasting overnight, calcium absorption was significantly decreased. It is unclear whether absorption is normal if calcium carbonate is taken with a meal, which is when it should be taken. Calcium carbonate and calcium citrate have not been compared when taken with a meal in people receiving PPI therapy.

Some experts base their recommendations for calcium on indirect evidence from studies in patients who do not produce acid. These patients can absorb calcium carbonate when taken with a meal. This suggests that taking calcium carbonate during meals should work.

However, my interpretation, based on the best available evidence regarding the choice of a calcium supplement, is that you should take calcium citrate at mealtime for good measure along with increasing calcium in your diet.

BALANCE BENEFITS OF PPIs AND RISK OF FRACTURE

Based on fracture risk alone, I would not recommend stopping a PPI if you need it. However, your risk of fracture should be assessed in conjunction with the "whole picture" of all other risk factors. If you already have low bone mass, you should talk with your doctor about strategies to lower your fracture risk. Reassess with your doctor the indication for taking the medicine and reason for continuing its use. You may consider:

- lowering your dose of PPI medicine
- changing to another non-PPI medicine
- temporarily stopping the PPI medicine to see if you still need it
- using PPI medicine only when symptoms occur

In addition, make sure you are taking an absorbable calcium supplement and adequate vitamin D.

The Bare Bones

- Higher fracture risk is an unexpected consequence of use of proton pump inhibitors (PPIs).
- Fracture risk increases with long-term use and higher doses of PPIs.
- If possible, try to decrease or stop your use of PPIs.
- Eat a diet rich in calcium and use calcium citrate as a calcium supplement, if needed.

Depression

This topic found its way into an unlikely place—a *Luann* comic strip (April 1, 2009). Luann, the teenage main character, asks her high school friend, Gunther, why he is blaming himself for his mother's fracture. He replies, "Well, I read that depression may weaken bones...." He blames his mother's depression on the hardships in raising him as a single mother.

Depression and Osteoporosis: A Cause or an Effect?

Depression itself has been shown to be associated with hip fracture in older women, a finding not entirely explained by falls. Is depression a cause of osteoporosis? Or does depression only develop after osteoporosis and fractures? Certainly, depression is a common complication after one suffers a life-altering hip fracture. However, the answers are complex and seem to lead to more questions. Another relevant question is, does the treatment of depression cause fractures?

Multiple studies have reported that women and men diagnosed with major depression or even depressed mood had lower bone mass. However, not all studies have agreed on this finding. The association between depression and bone density and fractures has been inconsistent. Many reasons may explain the conflicting results, including differences in the study populations, differences in the tools used to assess depressive symptoms and to make the diagnosis of depression, and the effects of different medicines.

Study results indicate that the association between depression and bone density was similar in the spine, hip, and forearm. The effect was stronger in women than in men and it was stronger in postmenopausal women, who are at highest risk of bone loss and fracture, than in premenopausal women.

Low bone density among those with depression is not site dependent. This suggests a general process effect rather than one related to falls or inactivity. Researchers have suggested several plausible mechanisms for the link between depression and bone health. For example, depression is associated with higher levels of the "stress" hormone called cortisol.

Elevated levels of cortisol rev up bone metabolism so that bone breaks down faster. Over a long period of time, this would add up to more bone loss than expected. Indeed, studies measuring bone turnover show higher levels of bone breakdown in depressed patients. What is not known is whether the increased cortisol levels in depressed patients are high enough to cause this. Proteins that cause inflammation, called cytokines, have also been implicated. The evidence for these theories is inconclusive.

Behaviors associated with depression and depressed mood may indirectly influence bone health. For example, smoking, alcohol use, and decreased physical activity could contribute to bone loss and lower bone density. Higher risk of falls and weight loss may also be factors.

Is it the disease itself or does this observed risk apply only to those who take antidepressant medicines? The older antidepressants in the tricyclic class (named for their chemical structure) may increase fracture due to falls. Side effects of the tricyclic antidepressants, such as difficulty with balance, increased heart rate, and decreased blood pressure, particularly on standing, increase the risk of falls.

These side effects are usually not associated with the class of medicines called selective serotonin reuptake inhibitors, referred to as SSRIs. Recent major research studies have connected the use of SSRIs with a direct effect on the bone, which causes an increased risk of bone loss and fractures. While studies evaluating the association between depression and bone density are mixed, studies on SSRIs are more consistent.

SSRIs

SSRIs are the most commonly prescribed antidepressants. Although they are classified for treatment of depression, they are prescribed for many other problems. Because they are used so extensively, you might think "SSRIs are good for everything." A frequent reason for postmenopausal women to receive prescriptions for SSRIs is to relieve hot flashes and night sweats.

Selective Serotonin Reuptake Inhibitors: SSRIs

Depression is linked to an imbalance of the brain's chemicals that allow brain nerve cells to communicate. These chemicals are called neurotransmitters. They send messages back and forth between nerve cells. After the neurotransmitter sends its message, it is absorbed back into the brain nerve cell. This process is called "reuptake." One of the neurotransmitters is a chemical known as serotonin. The serotonin transporter regulates its uptake.

Selective serotonin reuptake inhibitors (SSRIs) work by blocking the reuptake process in brain nerve cells. SSRIs inhibit the serotonin transporter so that the serotonin is not taken up in the nerve cells. By increasing the amount of serotonin in between the nerve cells, the proper chemical balance is restored, and this may resolve the depression.

Brand Name	Generic Name
Celexa®	citalopram
Lexapro®	escitalopram
Luvox®	fluvoxamine
Paxil® Pexeva®	paroxetine
Prozac® Rapiflux® Sarafem® Selfemra®	fluoxetine
Zoloft®	sertraline

Starting in the late 1980s with Prozac, SSRI agents for the treatment of depression entered the marketplace. Over the years, their use has expanded to many other ailments. SSRIs remain a popular choice for treatment of depression. Antidepressants that include SSRIs and other products, called SNRIs, including Savella®, Cymbalta®, and Effexor®, rank second among the top therapeutic classes of medicines by number of prescriptions written in 2010. This equated to US sales of $11.6 billion, just behind the $11.9 billion spent for proton pump inhibitors. Of the SSRIs, Lexapro has the largest share of the market.

Most, but not all, studies in large populations of individuals taking SSRIs have shown harmful bone effects. However, the large number of men and women examined had an association that was consistent among studies. Those on SSRIs had lower bone density at all sites, and over time had an increased rate of bone loss. SSRIs were associated with increased risk of hip, spine, nonspine, and forearm fractures. Daily SSRI use in adults aged fifty years and older was associated with an increase in fracture risk of 50 to 100 percent. In addition, higher doses and longer duration of use increased the negative effect on bone density and risk of fracture.

Researchers from the Osteoporotic Fractures in Men Study (MrOS) found that the use of SSRIs in older men over the age of sixty-five was associated with lower bone density. No bone density differences were observed for other types of antidepressants. The MrOS researchers reported that the observed difference in bone density for SSRIs was similar to that of steroid use, such as prednisone. After examining fractures in other populations, investigators have also concluded that the magnitude of fracture risk is similar to steroid use.

However, the link between long-term use of SSRIs and greater likelihood of osteoporosis-related fractures is based on observational studies. Observational studies describe the association, but unlike clinical trials, they do not prove cause and effect.

Like SSRIs, serotonin norepinephrine reuptake inhibitors (SNRIs) work in part by blocking reuptake of serotonin. Antidepressants in this class share some common characteristics with SSRIs. However, these newer medicines, like Cymbalta, Savella, and Effexor, have not been systematically studied in terms of bone effects.

The Serotonin Connection: Brain, Bone, and Gut

SSRIs may increase the risk of bone loss and fracture through a mechanism that has recently been discovered—the serotonin connection of the brain, bone, and gut. This new research in bone biology may potentially explain the bone effects observed in patients using SSRIs. As it turns out, all the bone cells—osteoclasts, osteoblasts, and osteocytes—have serotonin receptors. Bone cells take up serotonin like nerve cells through a serotonin transporter. SSRIs inhibit the serotonin transporter in the bone cells in a process similar to one in the nerve cells of the brain. An amazing discovery, but what does it mean?

The serotonin produced in the brain does not cross into the circulation of the body due to a barrier membrane, called the blood-brain barrier. So where does the serotonin come from that is used by the bone cells? The source of this serotonin was a total mystery until 2008, when a team of researchers led by Dr. Gerard Karsenty, professor and chair of genetics and development at Columbia University Medical Center, cracked the code. They found that serotonin produced in the gut circulates to the bone cells to activate the serotonin receptors.

Serotonin made by the gut can directly control bone formation. The researchers found that as more serotonin reached the bone, more bone was lost. On the other hand, lower levels of serotonin resulted in denser, stronger bones. They were able to prevent bone loss in mice by slowing the production of serotonin in the gut.

However, the negative bone effects produced by circulating serotonin do not fully explain the bone effects of SSRIs. Instead, the serotonin transporters in bone cells may have a role in determining bone mass and structure. It is still too early to understand all of the ramifications of this exciting discovery in bone biology, since not all of the mechanisms operating in the bone-brain-gut connection have been defined.

Observations thus far suggest that this connection may be very important. It could even lead to development of new medicines for treating osteoporosis. In addition, perhaps a "new SSRI" will be developed that targets the brain's serotonin transporters without affecting the serotonin transporters in the rest of the body.

Balancing Benefits of SSRIs and Risk of Fracture

I am certainly not going to tell you to stop taking your SSRIs. They are effective medicines for depression and other problems. Discuss your bone health in light of this information with your doctor. I believe that the evidence and possible biologic reasons for the action of SSRIs on bone are strong enough to consider these medicines a significant risk factor for osteoporosis and fractures. Your risk of fracture should be assessed in conjunction with the "whole picture" of all other risk factors.

Pay special attention to the general measures for bone health, including adequate calcium intake and vitamin D supplementation, exercise, and fall prevention. Clinical trials have not been done to address any special considerations beyond the usual options for prescription medicine therapy for osteoporosis.

Use of SSRIs in children and teenagers is largely unexplored. What effect SSRIs may have on bone during the growth phase is not known at this time. Because of the potential for harmful bone effects, it would be prudent to minimize use of this class of medicines in this age group.

Whether the disease, depression, itself also "weakens bones," as the comic strip character, Gunther, told Luann, is not clear. New insights from bone biology discoveries will hopefully provide answers in the near future.

The Bare Bones

- Depression by itself is associated with lower bone density and higher fracture risk. However, explanations and evidence are conflicting.
- SSRIs are associated with an increase in the risk of all fractures and with lower bone density.
- Fracture risk increases with higher doses of SSRIs and long-term use.
- If you need treatment with an antidepressant and are at high risk of fracture, the choice of medicine should take into account the risk of fractures associated with SSRIs.

Breast Cancer

For many years, women with breast cancer were considered to be safe from osteoporosis. The two diseases were thought to exist at opposite poles according to estrogen status: too much estrogen equaled breast cancer; too little estrogen equaled osteoporosis. As you might expect, that is not the case. Both are common problems, and there is a large overlap.

Low bone mass and an increased risk of fractures are common in women with breast cancer. This may be due to the effects of both the cancer itself and the drugs used to treat it. Management of bone health has emerged as an important part of comprehensive breast cancer care. As a result, many medical oncologists have expanded their role to include assessment of bone health as part of your care.

BONE DENSITY AND FRACTURES

Bone density measured in breast cancer survivors may be lower than normal and fracture risk is higher. This may be a consequence of treatment for breast cancer. Bone mass tends to be higher in breast cancer patients prior to treatment, but that is not always the case. Low bone density may be present before any treatment as well.

Dr. Donna Kritz-Silverstein, a colleague of mine at the University of California, San Diego, and I compared the bone density of postmenopausal women with newly diagnosed breast cancer, prior to any therapy, with age-matched normal controls. We observed little difference in bone density between women with and without breast cancer. Women were remarkably similar in all aspects of lifestyle and risk factors for osteoporosis and breast cancer. The only differing characteristic was that women with breast cancer had more body fat at their waists, a place we would all like to be trimmer!

The bottom line is that a DXA scan of your hip and spine is needed to find out your baseline bone density prior to treatment. This information will help guide management over the long-term. If one was not done as part of your initial battery of tests, don't worry. At any point in time, the bone density will be useful. If you have not had a bone density scan yet, get one at your earliest convenience.

TREATMENTS

Chemotherapy

Chemotherapy and its consequence on bone health is primarily a concern for premenopausal and perimenopausal women. Chemotherapy causes early menopause in over half of premenopausal or perimenopausal women. The abrupt loss of estrogen causes rapid bone loss, particularly in the spine. The bone in the spine responds dramatically to the lack of hormone by revving up its metabolism and breaking down bone fast. This creates a higher risk of spine fractures in later life.

This same response occurs in postmenopausal women who stop taking estrogen when breast cancer is diagnosed.

A direct harmful effect of chemotherapy on bone has been suggested but not proven. Chemotherapy given for breast cancer usually consists of a "cocktail" of ingredients. With multiple drugs, it is difficult to identify exactly which drug may be a culprit. Methotrexate, a common agent used in different chemotherapy regimens, may have a direct toxic effect on bone-formation cells, resulting in bone loss.

Radiation Therapy

Newer techniques and types of equipment used for radiation therapy do not affect the bone.

Hormonal Therapy

Not to be confused with estrogen therapy or "hormone replacement therapy," hormonal therapy is actually antiestrogen therapy. It is usually prescribed for a five-year course after the initial breast cancer treatments.

Tamoxifen

Tamoxifen has long been the breast cancer "insurance drug" that is used for five years to prevent the reccurrence of breast cancer. Tamoxifen is a "designer estrogen." In some parts of the body, it acts like estrogen, while in others it works as an antiestrogen. Technically, tamoxifen is called a selective estrogen receptor modulator, or "SERM" for short. In the bone, it mimics the effect of estrogen and protects against bone loss. In contrast, estrogen is blocked in the breast tissue, and breast tumor growth is prevented.

For postmenopausal women, a newer type of drug called an aromatase inhibitor is more effective than tamoxifen in preventing return of breast cancer. Since aromatase inhibitors (AIs) were adopted as standard therapy for postmenopausal women with hormone-sensitive early breast cancer, the use of tamoxifen has declined. However, because of high cost and/or inability to tolerate aromatase inhibitors, tamoxifen is still commonly used.

Tamoxifen remains the standard of care in premenopausal women with regular menstrual periods who are still making their own estrogen. In contrast to postmenopausal women, bone may be lost at an accelerated rate in premenopausal women rather than being preserved. This paradoxical effect is not completely understood. Therefore, premenopausal women using tamoxifen should have regular bone density scans every two years.

Aromatase Inhibitors

Rather than blocking estrogen's activity like tamoxifen, aromatase inhibitors actually prevent the body from making estrogen. These potent medicines dramatically reduce circulating estrogen by about 90 percent. As you might expect, this is not good for bone. Bone loss with an increased risk of fracture is the main problem with use of aromatase inhibitors.

What Are Aromatase Inhibitors?

Once your ovaries shut down with menopause, your body still produces some estrogen. The adrenal glands that sit on top of the kidneys produce androgens, the precursor to estrogen. An enzyme called aromatase is in tissues such as fat, muscle, liver, and breast. It converts the adrenal androgen to an aromatic state that is estrogen. Aromatase inhibitors (AIs) prevent the body from making this conversion to estrogen, hence the name.

Three different aromatase inhibitors are available:

Brand	Generic Name
Arimidex®	anastrozole
Aromasin®	exemestane
Femara®	letrozole

The different modes of action of aromatase inhibitors and tamoxifen explain their effects on bone. This was demonstrated in the bone substudy of the Arimidex, Tamoxifen, Alone or in Combination (ATAC) trial. After five years, the

Arimidex-treated women lost bone in the lumbar spine (-6 percent) and total hip (-7 percent). In contrast, those on tamoxifen had stable bone density at the total hip and a modest increase at the lumbar spine (+3 percent).

In addition, the early high rate of bone loss with Arimidex at the spine appeared to slow after the second year of treatment. However, the rate of bone loss at the hip was consistent over the five years. Early postmenopausal women (within four years of their last menstrual period) had the highest rate of loss at the lumbar spine, at -11 percent after five years. No one who started with normal bone density became osteoporotic while on Arimidex. That should be reassuring; however, women with low bone mass (T-scores between -1 and -2.5) did develop osteoporosis during the five-year treatment period.

Even so, it is important to point out that the majority of fractures occur in women with low bone mass (T-scores between -1 and -2.5) who are prescribed aromatase inhibitors. In the overall ATAC trial, fractures were more common in the Arimidex-only group. Similar findings were observed in trials using the other aromatase inhibitors, Aromasin and Femara. Prevention of aromatase inhibitor–associated bone loss is key to reducing risk of low bone density and fractures.

Prevention of Aromatase Inhibitor Bone Loss

First of all, the general principles of a bone-healthy lifestyle, along with adequate calcium and vitamin D, are essential but not enough. Additional bone-protection strategies are required for women treated with aromatase inhibitors. Multiple studies have been done and more are underway with different bisphosphonates and the new "first in class drug" Prolia. The acronyms abound: BIG, AZURE, HALT, IBIS, SABRE, Z-FAST, ZO-FAST, to name a few of the trials.

In the bisphosphonate class, Actonel, Boniva, Zometa, and a drug not available in the US (clodronate) have been evaluated separately, but there are no head-to-head comparison trials. All prevent bone loss and provide good bone protection in women taking aromatase inhibitors. The bulk of the studies have been with Zometa. Note that Zometa is zoledronic acid given in a 4 mg dose intravenously (by vein), which is the same drug marketed in a 5 mg dose as Reclast, which is indicated for postmenopausal osteoporosis. The frequency of Zometa use varied in the trials. A typical course was Zometa administered intravenously every six months.

Overall, Zometa is well tolerated and takes only fifteen minutes to be given by vein. Mild flu-like symptoms may occur in the first three days after the dose. Taking two acetaminophen (Tylenol) tablets beforehand may prevent or lessen these symptoms. Some protocols may specify more extensive use of acetaminophen, such as two tablets every six hours starting the day before the infusion and continuing for two to three days. Damage to the jawbone, called "osteonecrosis of the jaw," is a potential problem, but it is uncommon. You may lower your risk with good dental hygiene and by avoiding dental procedures that involve the bone.

Prolia (denosumab) is first in a new class of drugs designed to inhibit proteins that activate bone-destroying osteoclast cells. In the HALT (Hormone Ablation Therapy) Breast Cancer study, women with low bone mass (T-score between -1 and -2.5) who were taking aromatase inhibitors received either Prolia or placebo. Prolia 60 mg was given by a simple injection just under the skin (subcutaneous) every six months for two years. The Prolia group gained bone mass at the spine and hip and the placebo group lost bone.

Bone loss due to aromatase inhibitors is manageable with preventive therapy using bisphosphonates or Prolia. Therefore, the potential detrimental effects of aromatase inhibitors on the bone need not influence their use, which is needed to prevent breast cancer recurrence.

Other Benefits of Bone-Active Drugs: Weakening Cancer?

Exciting results show that the benefits of bisphosphonates and Prolia may extend beyond preserving bone and preventing fractures. Bone is the most frequent site of cancer relapse beyond the breast itself, called metastases.

Early studies with clodronate in Europe suggested that bisphosphonates may prevent spread of breast cancer to the bone. Bisphosphonates and Prolia create a "hostile" environment for cancer cells so they will not be attracted to the bone surface and grow. The recent data with Prolia and the potent bisphosphonate Zometa suggest that bone-targeted treatments may indeed prevent metastasis to the bone.

These potent bone drugs may also have direct effects on tumor cell growth, which modify the course of the disease. In one trial with the aromatase inhibitor Femara, Zometa was given immediately and every six months over five years or was started later for treatment of rapid bone loss or fracture. Not only was beginning treatment immediately with Zometa superior for bone protection, but fewer women had recurrence of their cancer at *any site, not just the bone*. The immediate versus delayed results suggest a direct antitumor effect of Zometa.

Similar results were found in the Austrian Breast Cancer Study Group (ABCSG XII), a large study of premenopausal women who took medicine to suppress estrogen produced from their ovaries. They were divided into groups that received either tamoxifen or the aromatase inhibitor Arimidex, and each of these groups was subdivided into groups that either did or did not take Zometa every six months for three years. Those receiving Zometa had 35 percent fewer distant and local recurrences. Zometa now has an FDA indication for use along with standard cancer therapies in women who have bone metastases from breast cancer. However, Zometa may not be used in patients with reduced kidney function.

Prolia (denosumab), through a different mechanism, may provide bone protection. Cancer cells appear to stimulate production of the messenger protein (RANK ligand, or RANKL) that increases osteoclast activity, resulting in local bone breakdown and skeletal complications. Prolia works by binding to the messenger protein and inhibiting its actions. Based on the bone biology, use of Prolia should counteract the effect of cancer cells and may also have a direct antitumor effect.

In studies of patients with bone metastases from solid tumors, a dose of 120 mg of denosumab was administered every four weeks. Upon FDA-approval for the prevention of skeletal-related events in patients with bone metastases from solid tumors, the brand name given for this dose of denosumab and frequency of use was "Xgeva," which distinguishes the new formulation from the lower dose and twice-yearly administration of Prolia.

In a large study of 2,046 women with advanced breast cancer and bone metastasis, the subjects were randomized to receive Xgeva 120 mg or Zometa 4 mg every four weeks. The study monitored for "bone-related events," which included fracture due to cancer, spinal cord compression, or need for radiation therapy or surgery to bone. Xgeva prevented more bone-related events than Zometa. Xgeva also delayed development to first bone-related events by 18 percent compared with Zometa. Although Xgeva was superior to Zometa in delaying or preventing bone-related events, overall survival, disease progression, and rates of side effects were similar between groups. In contrast to Zometa, Xgeva can be given to patients with reduced kidney function.

These results are encouraging; stay tuned for more in the near future, as current trials report their findings. Use of potent osteoporosis drugs for prevention of complications from breast cancer would be a welcome added benefit. To think they may prevent or delay the onset of metastases to other sites beyond bone and even prolong survival is mind-boggling.

GENERAL GUIDELINES

Increased awareness of the impact of breast cancer on bone health has led to increased use of preventive measures. Bone-specific therapies may play a role not only for prevention of bone loss and maintenance of bone mass but also for the added benefit of anticancer properties.

Osteoporosis medicines are being utilized more and more as part of comprehensive breast cancer care. The use of aromatase inhibitors for five years after the initial treatment of breast cancer requires careful evaluation of osteoporosis risk factors and management to prevent bone loss. Several bisphosphonates and Prolia are being evaluated for the indication of prevention of bone loss for women receiving aromatase inhibitors for breast cancer treatment.

For those breast cancer survivors who are at high risk of fracture, the options for lowering fracture risk are the same as those for women with post-menopausal osteoporosis. However, there are several cautionary notes. Estrogen should not be used at all. If you have used tamoxifen, do not use its "cousin" Evista because it could actually fuel breast cancer growth. Because of concerns about osteosarcoma, a cancer of the bone, Forteo should not be used if you have received radiation therapy.

Zometa and Xgeva (denosumab 120 mg) given every four weeks have FDA-approval for use in women with bone metastases from breast cancer. Additional effects of these medicines, such as actual antitumor effects, are under investigation.

Medicine	First Five Years While Receiving Aromatase Inhibitors	Breast Cancer Survivors with High Risk of Fractures
Bisphosphonates	Prevents aromatase inhibitor bone loss	
Actonel (risedronate)	Reduces bone loss	Effective
Boniva (ibandronate)	Trials with oral and intraveneous dosing	Effective
Fosamax or generic alendronate	Little data	Effective
Zometa 4 mg or Reclast 5 mg (zoledronic acid)	Zometa 4 mg prevents bone loss and improves bone density	Effective Usually given as Reclast 5 mg once yearly for osteoporosis indications
Calcitonin	No applicable studies	Low potency
Estrogen	Not suitable	Not suitable
Evista (raloxifene)	In same class of drugs as tamoxifen; do not use in combination with aromatase inhibitors	Do not use after tamoxifen
Forteo (teriparatide)	No data	Do not use if you have received radiation therapy
Prolia (denosumab)	Prevents bone loss and improves density	Effective

The Bare Bones

Bone health evaluation is an essential part of comprehensive breast cancer care. Women with breast cancer at higher risk for bone loss and fractures include:

- Those age sixty-five years and older
- Those ages sixty to sixty-four with risk factors for fracture
- All women receiving aromatase inhibitors; bone loss is highest in early postmenopause (within four years of the last menstrual period)
- Premenopausal women on therapies that cause premature menopause
- Premenopausal women taking tamoxifen

Optimize your bone health with general measures. Discuss with your physician regular monitoring of bone density and whether use of bone-specific medicines is needed.

Prostate Cancer

More than two million American men alive today have been diagnosed with prostate cancer at some point in time. After skin cancer, prostate cancer is the most common cancer in men. The number of men battling prostate cancer is staggering. According to the latest statistics from the American Cancer Society, an estimated 217,730 new cases were diagnosed in 2010. The good news hidden here is that the number of prostate cancer deaths continues to decline. They report a nearly 100 percent, five-year chance of survival for prostate cancer found in the prostate only or spread from the prostate to nearby areas.

This means that for most men prostate cancer is a chronic disease. Since men with prostate cancer are living longer, they may be receiving treatment for longer periods of time. It is now recognized that some therapies may increase bone loss and the risk of fractures. As a result, doctors are more attuned to the importance of bone health in their patients treated for prostate cancer.

Why Are Men with Prostate Cancer at Risk for Bone Loss and Fracture?

In the same way that hormonal (antiestrogen) therapy for women with breast cancer increases the risk of bone loss and fracture, hormonal therapy for prostate cancer boosts the risk of bone loss and fracture in men. In prostate cancer treatment, the hormones being suppressed or blocked are the male hormones, called androgens, including testosterone. You may see the term "androgen deprivation therapy" or ADT. That abbreviation always makes me think of the home security company. You can think of the treatment as a way to keep the body secure and safe from the growth of prostate cancer cells.

Initially, androgen deprivation therapy was used to treat advanced prostate cancer. Now it has much wider use in earlier stages, such as in men with prostate-specific antigen (PSA) levels that are creeping up after their initial cancer therapy. It is estimated that one-third of the two million prostate cancer survivors in the US are on hormonal therapy. Unfortunately, this treatment comes with some difficult side effects. Recent reports of increased heart disease risk and death may change how commonly these drugs are prescribed.

With hormonal therapy, blood levels of testosterone drop by more than 95 percent and estrogen decreases by about 80 percent. As a result, rapid bone loss is a particular problem in the first year of therapy. The rate of bone loss during initial androgen deprivation therapy may be similar or even higher than the rate of loss seen in women at menopause. Initially, the average bone loss at the hip and spine is 2 to 4 percent per year. The loss of bone may be greatest at the forearm. Most studies report a steady decline of bone density that continues throughout long-term therapy.

What Is Hormonal Therapy?

Hormonal (androgen deprivation) therapy takes away the "fuel" needed for prostate cancer cells to prosper by decreasing testosterone. Until medicines were developed, the only way to reduce male hormones was by surgically removing both testicles. Fortunately, medicines offer another option. Even so, due to other health considerations, surgery may still be necessary and may be used in combination with medicines.

The most common medicines block production of testosterone by tricking the body into thinking there is already enough testosterone. These medicines are called luteinizing hormone-releasing hormone (LHRH) agonists, or you may see them referred to as gonadotropin-releasing hormone (GnRH) agonists. These are given by injection or by small implants placed under the skin that may last up to one year.

Brand	Generic Name
Eligard® Lupron® Viadur®	leuprolide
Trelstar®	triptorelin
Vantas®	histrelin
Zoladex®	goserelin

One drug that is similar to LHRH agonists, Firmagon® (generic degarelix), is an LHRH antagonist given once a month by injection. Instead of "trickery," it directly blocks the pituitary secretion of the hormones that stimulate the production of testosterone. This drug is given either for a short time at the beginning of hormonal therapy before starting the LHRH agonists or on a regular, long-term basis.

It may be necessary to add other drugs to the above treatments from the "anti-androgens" class to further lower testosterone. The preferred anti-androgen is Casodex® (generic bicalutamide). Others include Eulexin® (generic flutamide) or Nilandron® (nilutamide).

Not surprisingly, this translates into lower bone mass and increased fracture rates for men on hormonal therapy. A recent analysis of multiple studies reported that androgen deprivation therapy increased the risk for overall fracture by 23 percent compared with men with prostate cancer not undergoing treatment. Older age and other chronic problems boosted the risk even higher.

Other factors may also contribute to fracture risk. Androgen deprivation therapy also decreases muscle bulk. Low vitamin D was often found in study participants, even in places with abundant sunshine such as south Texas. Loss of muscle mass and low vitamin D contribute to weakness and increased risk of falls, particularly in older men.

What Bone-Related Evaluation Should Be Done If You Are Starting Hormonal Therapy?

Talk with your doctor. Basically, the same general bone health assessment done for women can be applied to men with prostate cancer. You want to try to avoid other risk factors like smoking, too much alcohol (more than two drinks a day), and other bone "unhealthy" medicines.

Lab tests should include a test of your vitamin D level. Make sure your vitamin D is above the minimum level of 30 ng/ml.

A bone density scan is essential. In addition to the routine hip and spine scans, many centers are also including a forearm scan and vertebral fracture assessment. A repeat scan is recommended in one year if you start out low and in two years if you start in the normal range.

What Can You Do to Minimize Bone Loss Caused by Hormonal Therapy?

The key is to start by minimizing risk factors. Ensure that you are taking in 1,200 mg of calcium between your diet and supplements each day. The amount of vitamin D needed to achieve a level above 30 ng/ml will vary from individual to individual. The majority will reach that target with supplements of 800 IU to 2,000 IU daily. Regular physical exercise may help lessen the loss not only of bone but of muscle as well.

No specific drugs are approved by the FDA for preventing or treating osteoporosis in men who are taking hormonal therapy for prostate cancer. Treatment options for preventing bone loss associated with prostate cancer therapies are similar to the treatment options for osteoporosis in men without prostate cancer. Bisphosphonates have been the mainstay in reducing bone loss. In addition to oral Fosamax (generic alendronate), two bisphosphonates given by vein and commonly used in cancer patients are Aredia® (pamidronate) and Zometa (4 mg of zoledronic acid, same medicine as Reclast). These show success in preventing bone loss and even increasing bone density in men receiving hormonal therapy for prostate cancer.

Since estrogens also play a key role in men's bone metabolism, "designer" estrogens, called selective estrogen-receptor modulators or SERMS, may be used. The drugs Evista (raloxifene) and Fareston® (toremifene) increase bone density at the hip and spine as well. Common side effects of these medicines, like hot flashes, possible breast growth, and tendency to develop blood clots, make these drugs a less desirable option.

In a recent randomized controlled trial of over 1,400 men with prostate cancer who were on androgen deprivation therapy, Prolia 60 mg given every six months demonstrated gains in bone density over three years at the spine, hip, and forearm. In contrast, those in the placebo group lost bone. In addition, Prolia accounted for a 62 percent lower risk in new spine fractures at three years compared with placebo. Based on this study, its manufacturer, Amgen, is hoping for FDA approval of Prolia for the treatment and prevention of bone loss in men undergoing hormonal therapy for prostate cancer. Of note, neither bisphosphonates nor SERMS in other similar studies showed gains at the forearm measurement site.

Another strategy includes intermittent administration of hormonal therapy. A "drug-free" period may stop bone loss. However, the risk and benefits of this management approach are still being evaluated for effectiveness in treating prostate cancer.

At present, intravenous bisphosphonates (Aredia and Zometa) are the medicines most commonly used to prevent and treat bone loss in men on hormonal therapy for prostate cancer. With the recent robust results using the new osteoporosis drug Prolia, there will be more use of this agent in the future.

Does Everyone Need to Take a Bone-Specific Drug to Counter the Hormonal Therapy?

An assessment of your bone health with your doctor is going to answer that question. If your bone density is normal and you don't have other risk factors for fracture, bone-specific drugs to counter bone loss with hormonal therapy are not initially needed. You will need to optimize your calcium and vitamin D and improve your nutrition and exercise habits. In addition, you will need careful monitoring of your bone density, with a repeat DXA scan after two years of therapy and on regular intervals after that.

On the other hand, if you start out with low bone density, you do not have bone to lose. You need to maintain every bit you have. In addition to the general bone-health measures, talk with your doctor about bisphosphonates and Prolia as options for preserving or even building up your bone mass to prevent fractures.

Bone is the most likely place for prostate cancer to spread. Just as in breast cancer, bisphosphonates and Prolia may counteract the effect of prostate cancer cells on the bone.

Zometa and a double dose of Prolia (denosumab) formulation, called Xgeva 120 mg, are FDA-approved for use every four weeks to decrease bone complications from prostate cancer that has spread to the bone. In one comparison study of these two agents, Xgeva 120 mg was superior to Zometa 4 mg in prevention of bone-related complications in patients with prostate cancer and bone metastases that progressed despite hormonal therapy. Additional studies are underway to investigate the efficacy of osteoporosis medicines for preventing bone metastases. Others are focused on men with advanced prostate cancer.

The Bare Bones

Hormonal therapy given to some men with prostate cancer causes bone loss and increased fracture risk. Extra measures are needed to protect your bone health:

- Measure your bone density with a DXA scan of the hip, spine, and forearm. Get regular one- to two-year follow-up scans.
- Optimize your lifestyle: stop smoking, moderate your alcohol use, and get regular exercise.
- Ensure dietary and supplemental calcium totaling 1,200 mg daily and maintain adequate vitamin D levels year round.
- Consider bisphosphonates or Prolia to prevent bone loss when using hormonal therapy.

Long-Term Care Setting: Assisted Living and Nursing Facilities

A dults older than age eighty-five are the fastest growing segment of our population. You may have a parent or loved one who is fortunate enough to be part of this long-lived group. Along with this population boom, senior residential living communities and facilities are growing in number by leaps and bounds. Many of these communities offer a range of options from independent living through skilled-care nursing homes. In addition, "boomerang seniors" are another growing phenomenon; that is, aging parents moving in with their adult children.

Residents in assisted living and nursing homes have the highest risk for fracture of anyone. Unfortunately, this risk is frequently not addressed even if your parent changed residence to one of these facilities specifically because of a fracture. The bone connection is often overlooked. It may be up to you to bring up the topic and work with the staff and your parent's doctor to reduce the risk of falls and fractures.

ASSISTED LIVING

Assisted living is "housing with supportive services" that fills the niche between living in your own home and living in a nursing home. These facilities can be an attractive option for people who no longer are able to live independently but do not need the medical care provided in a nursing home. The average assisted living resident walks with the assistance of a cane or walker and receives help with some of their daily activities, such as bathing and dressing.

Residents in the assisted living facilities usually require additional assistance and services over time. In all likelihood, with a lower level of physical or mental functioning, the resident would no longer meet the facilities' entry criteria. But most facilities try to keep their residents as long as possible before moving them to a higher level of support—the skilled nursing home. Plus, the staff bonds with your parent, and their goal is to have 100 percent occupancy.

One of the common reasons for discharge from the assisted living facility is a fall with injury. The most common serious injury is *hip fracture*. Surveys of residents in assisted living show that they do not perceive osteoporosis to be as important or urgent as other health concerns. In the context of their overall health, they see osteoporosis as neither disabling nor immediately life threatening.

From a national survey, three-quarters of women older than eighty are estimated to have osteoporosis. These high numbers refer to women living independently in the community. Since women residing in assisted living tend to be frailer, the percentage is probably even higher. No matter how you look at it, residents in assisted living are at extremely high risk of devastating, life-altering or fatal fractures.

Assisted living residents maintain their regular doctors and leave the facility to go to their doctor visits. They need to talk with their doctor about lowering their risk of falls and fractures. Vitamin D blood levels may need to be checked to ensure that supplementation is adequate to maintain a level above 30 ng/ml. This simple measure may help reduce falls and fractures and improve muscle strength.

The facility itself should have a protocol in place for fall prevention. At the present time, assisted living facilities are not federally regulated but are under state law. It is up to each facility or its parent company to set up and implement procedures to decrease falls and fractures. Find out about the fall prevention measures in place at the facility your loved one resides in or may be considering. The facility staff members want to keep everyone safe and minimize their liability as well.

NURSING HOMES: SKILLED NURSING FACILITIES

With aging, maintenance of independence is a major goal. Sometimes, due to unforeseen circumstances or multiple problems of aging, independence is not possible. Injuries from falls account for 40 percent of all nursing home admissions. Nursing homes provide the medical care and support needed for those with physical and mental limitations.

Osteoporosis is common. Osteoporosis is estimated to be present in approximately 90 percent of women and 50 percent of men living in nursing homes. Fractures are all too common. In a study of nearly 1,500 Caucasian women living in nursing homes in Maryland, about one in nine residents had a fracture each year. They happen more often among those who are able to walk or move from bed to chair and are not common among bed-bound residents. If one is up and moving, the risk of falls with injury is high. Hip fractures are the most common fracture.

About one-fifth of all hip fractures in the US occur in women residing in nursing homes. Low bone mass predicts osteoporotic fracture. However, among frail nursing home residents, association of low bone mass to fracture risk is less clear. Nursing home residents have many additional risk factors for fracture in addition to low bone density, such as unsteady walking, poor memory and confusion, and the use of multiple medicines, all of which lead to an increased risk of falls.

Osteoporosis is often ignored. Nursing home residents may have other competing illnesses and more "immediate" problems. Adding to an already long list of medicines, osteoporosis medicines, which require special dosing instructions, can prove cumbersome. Even adding calcium and vitamin D is challenging. History of falls and fractures is not correlated with who is diagnosed and treated in nursing homes.

Nursing home residents are provided with medical care in the facility. Doctors and often their staff, a nurse practitioner or physician assistant, may oversee the residents' care. In addition to complex and competing problems, doctors cite short stays at facilities, medicine costs, and reimbursement issues as barriers to treating high-risk patients, even those who have already fractured.

Another common reason for not treating osteoporosis in the nursing home is the perception that "it is no use," due to the limited amount of time a frail, older person may have to live. However, high-risk patients *do benefit* from treatment. In addition, the osteoporosis medicines decrease fracture risk quickly, with significant reductions within the first year of therapy.

It is never too late to treat osteoporosis in order to decrease fracture risk and improve quality of life. However, few nursing home residents are currently receiving treatment for osteoporosis despite elevated fracture risk or even a recent fracture. Many patients slip between the cracks after sustaining a major fracture. The continuity of their care is often lost amid transfers from hospital care to rehabilitation to a new permanent residence. Even though a fracture may have started the cascade of events, an "osteoporosis" diagnosis does not end up on their list of problems. Therefore, it is not appropriately addressed and treated.

OSTEOPOROSIS TREATMENT

Treatment in this high-risk group encompasses the same general measures and medicines as in younger adults with an emphasis on fall prevention.

Fall Prevention

Strategies to prevent falls are a critical part of osteoporosis management. All nursing homes should have programs in place for fall and fracture prevention.

Research shows that the simple strategy of identifying those at high risk for falls may decrease the number of falls per person by nearly half. An evaluation of thigh muscle (quadriceps) strength, which is an independent risk factor for falls and fracture, is essential. These muscles are key for standing up, sitting, making transfers from bed to chair, and walking. Therapy to strengthen quadriceps muscle and training to safely transfer and walk are helpful.

Evidence from randomized clinical trials shows that up to half of falls in older people can be prevented. The trials used either a single intervention strategy (such as exercise) or programs that focus on reducing risk factors. Based on the consistency of results, the most effective interventions for the prevention of falls and fractures include the use of strength and balance training, followed by reducing the number and dosage of medicines, and adding supplementation of vitamin D and calcium.

Hip Protectors

In theory, wearing an external hip protector that absorbs the energy of a fall or diverts it away from the bone makes sense as a way to prevent a broken hip during falls. It is as if you have an air bag on your hip to cushion the blow. Unfortunately, hip protectors have not been effective in practice. Residents find they are difficult to put on and are bulky under their clothes, so they do not wear them.

Results from the latest well-designed clinical trial in nursing home residents showed that the specific protector it tested failed to prevent hip fractures. The study subjects did wear the hip protector; they just did not work. More research is needed in this area before recommending the use of hip protectors.

Calcium and Vitamin D

Previously, the moderate protective effect of vitamin D on fracture risk was attributed primarily to changes in bone mineral density. However, vitamin D may directly improve muscle strength and reduce fracture risk through fall prevention.

There is some dispute as to whether the effects are the result of vitamin D alone or only vitamin D in combination with calcium. Usually, one of the nine or more medicines on the resident's daily list is a calcium tablet combined with vitamin D. This adequately supplies daily calcium. Additional vitamin D is usually in the daily multivitamin. However, those two sources together are usually not enough to support a vitamin D blood level over 30 ng/ml.

In this population, adequate vitamin D supplementation decreases falls and fractures and improves muscle strength. *Vitamin D is important*. Make sure that your parent's vitamin D level is checked and that appropriate amounts of supplement are given to maintain levels above 30 ng/ml.

Medicines

Ideally, the medicines for osteoporosis treatment should be tested for safety and effectiveness in this older population of individuals who reside in long-term care facilities. However, clinical trials with high-risk patients are challenging in this setting. Reclast is the only osteoporosis medication for which a large fracture trial has been done with individuals who sustained a hip fracture. These individuals usually received rehabilitation services in a nursing home after hospital discharge. Fosamax was evaluated for bone density changes and safety among female residents of long-term care facilities.

Beyond Reclast, Fosamax, calcium, and vitamin D, no other studies have been designed to look at older individuals in this living situation. Little data is available from similar age groups who are healthier and living in the community setting. Actonel was evaluated in a large fracture trial of high-risk older individuals. Other large pivotal fracture trials recruited "healthy" women who met entry criteria up to age cutoffs of eighty, eighty-five, and more recently ninety years old.

Several medicines may be easier to use in these settings. Administration by shots under the skin or infusions by vein may have appeal for residents on multiple oral medicines, or those with digestive diseases or concern about intolerability or absorption. These methods guarantee delivery to the bone.

The extended release formulation of Actonel, called Atelvia, which is given after breakfast once weekly, avoids the fasting requirements of Fosamax, Actonel, and Boniva. However, Atelvia still requires remaining upright for thirty minutes after taking the medicine.

The once-a-year dosing of Reclast has a distinct advantage over other medicines. The intravenous administration bypasses any concerns about digestive side effects from pills or cumbersome dosing. Use of Reclast ensures that individuals are actually getting the medicine. The most common limitation on use of Reclast in this high-risk group is reduced kidney function.

The advantage of Prolia, a shot given once every six months, is that it can be used in those with reduced kidney function. Because of its unique mechanism of action, Prolia is a potent alternative to other antiresorptives. Forteo is also an effective option, since it causes bone formation and improvement of the microstructure of bone. Sometimes the staff of a long-term care facility will be a little reticent to use this medicine because it is a daily injection. However, the prefilled syringe is easy to use and lasts twenty-eight days.

Medicine	Taken by	Studies in Long-term Care
Reclast	Infusion in vein given once a year.	New hip fracture patients treated in first ninety days after surgery had 35 percent fewer fractures and the number of deaths were reduced by 28 percent over two years.
Fosamax (alendronate)	Pill 70 mg once a week on empty stomach. One must stay upright for thirty minutes before eating or taking other medicines. Only water is allowed.	Randomized clinical trial in long-term care facilities showed that bone density increases to the same degree as in younger women over two years.
Actonel	Pill 35 mg once weekly or 150 mg once monthly on empty stomach. One must stay upright for thirty minutes before eating or taking other medicines. Only water is allowed.	Subjects who participated in a clinical trial and required long-term care had bone density improvements. No formal study has been designed specifically for long-term care setting.
Atelvia	Extended release pill is given after breakfast. One must stay upright for thirty minutes.	Same medicine as Actonel.
Boniva	Pill 150 mg once a month on empty stomach. One must stay upright for sixty minutes before eating or taking other medicines. Only water is allowed. May also be given by intravenous infusion every three months.	No data
Calcitonin	Nasal spray each day or daily shot under the skin.	No data
Prolia	Shot twice a year under the skin.	No data
Forteo	Shot daily under the skin using prefilled pen for up to twenty-four months.	No data

The Bare Bones

- Residents in long-term care facilities are likely to have osteoporosis and are at high risk for fractures, especially hip fractures.
- Osteoporosis is often overlooked and not treated in these settings.
- Residents in long-term care facilities are likely to have low vitamin D levels. Separate vitamin D supplements are often needed to keep vitamin D levels above 30 ng/ml.
- Fall prevention and effective medicines are part of a comprehensive program to lower risk of fractures.

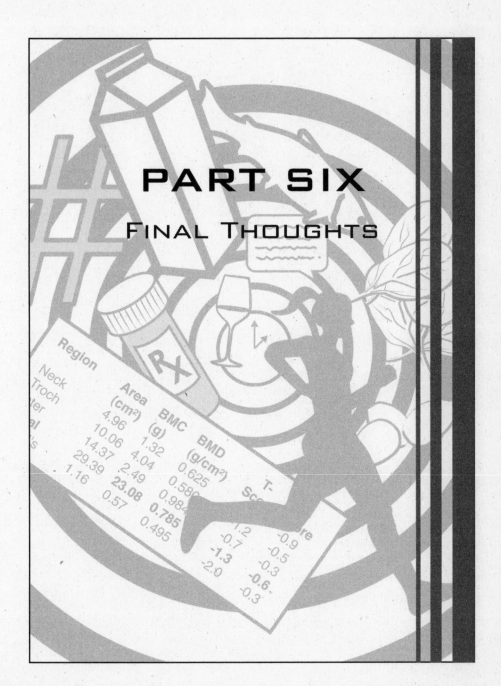

PART SIX

Final Thoughts

The Bone Health Top Ten

If you have read some of the sections of this book before getting to this one, you will find familiar topics. If you have browsed your way to this section, it is a sneak preview of what is in store. The condensed, take-home messages in this top ten summary represent a snapshot of broader information. You are encouraged to delve deeper in the earlier sections for more detail.

10. Not just for women

Bone health is important for boys and girls, men and women of all shapes, sizes, races, and ethnicities. Although Caucasian and thin Asian women are at highest risk, anyone can develop osteoporosis. Men account for about 30 percent of all fractures. Even though African American men and women are at lowest risk and Hispanics are intermediate risk, the numbers of non-Caucasians sustaining fractures are projected to markedly increase.

9. Family history

Genes make a difference. If your mother or father or grandparents had a hip fracture or other fractures, your risk of fracture is increased. However, you can change your "bone destiny." Genes are influenced by your lifestyle. Lower your risk by making healthy choices.

8. Hormones

The goal is to build the skeleton as strong and as sturdy as possible during childhood and young adulthood, then minimize bone loss throughout adulthood to prevent fractures in later life. Estrogen and testosterone are the main hormonal support for growth and maintenance of bone. Peak bone growth occurs around the time of puberty. Any disruption of hormones will result in failure to achieve peak bone mass or, in adults, loss of bone. For women, the loss of estrogen with transition to menopause causes acceleration of bone loss.

7. Fracture risk

If you have factors associated with increased fracture risk, bone density testing is recommended for the perimenopausal and early postmenopausal time frame. Also, adults who have had a fracture after age fifty, all women sixty-five and older, and men over seventy, regardless of risk factors, should have a bone density scan. Results from your bone density, measured by dual energy x-ray absorptiometry (DXA), and your risk factors are used to calculate your personal ten-year probability of major fractures and hip fracture.

6. Common health problems and medicines

Your bone health is part of your overall health. Keep your doctor in the loop. Many common illnesses and medicines used to treat them are associated with harmful effects on your bones. Talk with your doctor about possible bone connections and minimize your risks. If you have a fracture between your office visits, don't forget to report that fact to your primary care doctor. Additional evaluation for contributing causes may be indicated.

5. Bone-healthy diet

Just as your mother said, "Eat your vegetables," especially green leafy vegetables such as kale and bok choy. Almonds, halibut, wild salmon, tuna fish, cheese, and white beans are other bone-healthy foods for your grocery cart. Eat and drink everything in moderation and maintain a healthy weight.

4. Exercise

Get thirty to sixty minutes of physical activity more days a week than not. A comprehensive workout program, including weight-bearing, cardio, and muscle-strengthening exercises along with balance training, is best. Move more during the day. Try a pedometer to keep track of your steps, and aim for 10,000 steps each day.

3. Calcium

Calcium recommendations for daily intake are based on your age. It is difficult to get enough calcium from your diet each day, but try to choose calcium-rich foods. If not, you may need to add calcium supplements to meet your daily requirements.

2. Vitamin D

Unless you are taking a vitamin D supplement, it is highly likely that you have low vitamin D. Few foods supply natural or added vitamin D and you cannot count on sunlight exposure most months of the year. Vitamin D is needed for efficient absorption of calcium and is required for many other functions in the body. You need to get *enough* vitamin D to maintain a minimum vitamin D blood level of 30 ng/ml. The amount of supplementation required to reach that target varies from individual to individual, but the usual range is 800 to 2,000 IU a day.

1. It is never too late...

It is never too late to get started on good measures for your bone health. You can prevent fractures, even if you have already had one. For high-risk individuals, the basic bone-healthy measures are very important, but you may need the help of prescription osteoporosis therapies to lower your fracture risk.

Putting It All Together: Tips for the Whole Family

W hen I began writing this book, I did not know how the final section would "put it all together." Along the way, I received many questions and requests for information about what to do for the whole family. As a result, this final section provides tips for you and your family by age or stage of life. Many of these points will be useful throughout your life. They are good not only for your bone health but for your overall health and longevity. Talk with your doctor about bone health during your and your family's regular check-ups. Staying bone healthy is a lifetime endeavor.

EXPECTANT MOTHERS

Amid all the planning and excitement of anticipating your baby's birth, osteoporosis and hip fractures are unlikely to be on your mind. However, during your pregnancy is a good time to start thinking about prevention of those later-life problems that may be impacted by what happens in the womb.

Optimize calcium intake. The total requirement for calcium during pregnancy is 1,000 mg daily. Check the label of your prenatal vitamins. Most brands contain 200 to 300 mg of calcium. Figure out how much calcium is in your typical diet. If it does not provide enough calcium, either add to your dietary sources or take a calcium supplement to meet the 1,000 mg goal.

Measure your vitamin D level. Prenatal vitamins alone do not supply enough vitamin D. Most brands contain only 200 to 400 IU. Additional supplementation is often needed to maintain an adequate vitamin D blood level above 30 ng/ml. The only accurate way to know how much vitamin D you should be taking is by knowing your blood level. Talk with your doctor to arrange a blood test.

NEW MOTHERS

Add vitamin D with breastfeeding. Your baby needs vitamin D supplements each day if you are breastfeeding. As a new mother, life is hectic and it is easy to forget to give the vitamin drops to your baby. Set up a system to help you remember, and do not forget your vitamin D either. If you are using both formula and breast milk, you will still need to supplement. A total of 400 IU is the daily vitamin D dose for your infant. Bottle-fed babies are supplied with enough vitamin D from the fortified formula.

Continue to optimize your calcium intake. During breastfeeding you tend to lose bone even when you take sufficient calcium. The loss is temporary and bone will be regained after weaning. Maintain your daily calcium intake of 1,000 mg through your diet and supplements. Continue this amount each day until menopause, when your total calcium intake increases to 1,200 mg daily.

YOUR CHILDREN

The first two decades of life are the window of opportunity to establish the strongest bones possible. Think of osteoporosis as a childhood disease that is manifested in late life with fractures. It is hard to maintain focus on such a distant horizon, but it may help to remember that the payoff is not only in years to come but also in the short term, as good bone health will decrease the chances of childhood fractures. Getting a healthy start is key to strong bones and establishing healthy lifelong habits.

Toddlers (ages 1–3)

Start healthy eating habits. Introduce healthy foods into the diet. Stay away from fast foods that are high in calories, fat, and salt.

Eat calcium rich foods. Dairy foods are rich in calcium and protein for growing bones. About two eight-ounce glasses of milk or the equivalent will supply the recommended 700 mg of daily calcium.

Kids (ages 4–8)

Educate about healthy choices. Teaching your kids how to make good nutritional choices is key to establishing good lifelong habits. Start the morning with a bone-healthy breakfast of yogurt and fruit. The recommended dietary allowance for calcium for kids in this age group increases to 1,000 mg a day, which is about three glasses of milk or its equivalent.

Limit soft drinks. Soft drinks tend to displace milk drinking. Kids lose the bone-building benefits of calcium, vitamin D, and protein from milk. Other drinks, like juices and fruit drinks, need to be limited, too. Offer water as an alternative choice after their daily calcium intake has been met.

Play outdoors. Spending time outdoors each day encourages physical activity. Sunshine during the summer months gives some bonus vitamin D.

Tweens (ages 9–13)

Increase calcium in the diet. This is when the growth spurt starts. More than 40 percent of children's eventual adult bone mass is attained from about age nine to thirteen in girls and nine to fourteen in boys. More calcium is needed to support their bone growth. About four glasses of milk or the equivalent is needed to meet the goal of 1,300 mg of calcium a day.

Jump. Jumping activities increase bone density more than the typical physical exercises in gym class. Weight-bearing exercises, which put a mechanical load on bones, are the best bone builders. Encourage activities that involve jumping up and down or running.

Participate in team sports. Team sports help maintain fitness. Working as part of a team provides great lessons and discipline for life.

Limit television and electronics time. The sedentary activities of television, computers, and video games take away from physical activity time. Encourage physical activity during the day and limit electronics to a few hours in the evening.

Teens

Encourage healthy habits. The teen years are the most difficult time for parental influence. Peer pressure and independent thinking may trump healthy habits. Take advantage of the influence you still have by providing healthy choices in the home.

Keep up calcium intake. Calcium is essential for growing bones. Teens tend to substitute soft drinks or other noncalcium-containing beverages for milk. If drinking milk is not their thing, substitute yogurt or nondairy sources to get 1,300 mg of calcium a day.

Consider a vitamin D supplement. If your teens are not drinking milk, they may not be getting enough vitamin D. As a fat-soluble vitamin, it does not have to be taken every day. Once a week will suffice. They may be able to skip the supplement during the summer months if they are spending time outdoors.

Maintain a healthy weight. Weight is a balance between too little and too much. Neither being underweight nor being overweight is healthy for bones. Maintaining a healthy weight is essential for girls to have regular menstrual periods and the estrogen support needed for growing bones.

Don't start smoking. Cigarette smoking may seem "cool," but it is addictive. Cigarettes are expensive, not only to buy, but for healthcare in the long run. Help your teens avoid this risk.

YOUR 20s

During this time, a person gains a small amount of bone in the range of 5 to 10 percent. This is the "consolidation" phase, which ends with the achievement of peak bone mass by the end of your twenties. As you embark on your career or further training, you must make time to take care of yourself. The demands of a new job or school may be overwhelming but don't let your healthy lifestyle lapse.

Limit alcohol. Finally, you hit the legal drinking age, although there is a good chance you already have been imbibing. Despite reports that beer is good for your bones, do not overdo it. Limit the number of alcoholic beverages to no more than one or two a day, if you drink at all.

Exercise regularly. Establishing a regular exercise regimen is key. Figure out how to fit daily exercise into your job or school schedule. Put exercise on your calendar just like meetings or appointments.

Eat your vegetables. Meals "on the go" tend to be high in protein and fat and scant on vegetables. Avoid fast foods. They tend to be loaded with hidden salt. Your mother's advice was right, of course.

Find out about your family history. Connect the dots. Talk with your parents and grandparents about their health histories and the histories of other family members. Ask specifically about fractures and falls. Knowing about your grandfather's slip on the ice and hip fracture is important for your health. Being aware of your family history can help reinforce your healthy habits. By making the right choices to optimize your health you decrease the chances of having the same problems that affected your parents or grandparents.

YOUR 30s

Your peak bone mass has been established. Now it is vital to hang on to what you have. A healthy lifestyle has never been more crucial. Juggling your career and family may have you stressed out. You cannot forget about taking care of yourself.

Avoid yo-yo dieting. The battle of the bulge may be a problem. Pregnancy or a lapse in your physical activity may have added a few unwanted pounds. Weight loss of even a few pounds can cause bone loss. Try to maintain a stable healthy weight.

Counter caffeine with calcium. Gourmet coffee shops are ubiquitous. They tempt us with supersized cups of coffee that deliver big jolts of caffeine. Some of the specialty drinks are loaded with calories as well. Drinking coffee and other caffeine-containing drinks tends to promote loss of calcium through your urine, particularly if you have a low calcium intake. Add some milk or order a latte to help compensate.

Look for hidden salt. These days, the salt shaker is not the main source of salt in your diet. Unfortunately, prepared and packaged foods are. You can get a couple days worth of salt in one Chinese take-out dish. Less obvious sources of hidden salt are tomato juice, canned beans, and pepperoni pizza. Identify sources of salt in your diet. Read the nutrition facts on the labels of foods to identify the sodium content before you purchase. Consume less than 2,300 mg a day of dietary sodium.

YOUR 40s

Estrogen upheaval is looming. About half of women will transition to menopause during this decade. Menopausal transition is typically from your late forties to early fifties. Perimenopause may be symptomatic for some of you. Waking up with soaking night sweats is no fun. Hang on for the hormone roller coaster; it can be a wild ride or not bad at all.

Get a DXA bone density scan. Once you are perimenopausal or early post-menopausal, a baseline bone density measurement is recommended if you have risk factors for osteoporosis. The "DXA" scan should include both your hip and spine. Talk with your doctor about when it is time to arrange for this quick and painless test.

Assess your fracture risk. Your fracture risk is assessed in concert with your bone density results. A fracture assessment questionnaire, called FRAX, is a helpful tool for determining your risk of major osteoporotic and hip fractures in the next ten years. Important risk factors, along with the results from your bone density, go into the calculation. The results serve as a starting point for discussion with your doctor. Guidelines from the National Osteoporosis Foundation define the characteristics of higher risk individuals who should consider treatment with bone-specific medicines.

Measure your height. Have your height measured every year at your doctor's office when you have your annual exam. A loss of one inch for men or two inches for women may be a sign of silent spine fractures.

YOUR 50s

In postmenopause, the goal is to reduce the loss of bone associated with loss of estrogen. Bone loss may slow after early menopause. Decrease your fracture risk with general measures of nutrition, calcium, vitamin D, and exercise. Consider bone-specific medicines when general bone measures are not enough.

Increase your daily calcium. The recommendation for daily calcium increases to 1,200 mg for women over fifty. It is difficult to achieve that goal with diet alone, but do not overdo it either. The total of dietary *plus* supplemental calcium intake should be 1,200 mg.

Reassess your vitamin D intake. As you increase your calcium, you should add up how much vitamin D you are taking each day. Most calcium supplements have vitamin D added. Check the supplement facts on the back of your calcium and vitamin supplements. Having a blood test for vitamin D is the most accurate way to know if you are taking enough to maintain adequate levels.

Increase physical activity. With loss of estrogen, your metabolism resets. More exercise is needed to burn calories and keep toned. Schedule your exercise for at least sixty minutes, six days a week. Work on under-challenged muscles in your upper body to help prevent rounding of your shoulders. A combination of weight resistance and weight-bearing cardio activities is the best regimen. Keep changing your routine to optimize the effects of exercise on the bone.

Consider low-dose estrogen. If your hot flashes and night sweats are too much to handle, think about short-term use of estrogen. Estrogen is now available in lower doses. You can start with the lowest dose and gradually increase as needed. Low-dose estrogen prevents bone loss.

YOUR 60s

Schedule a DXA bone density scan. For women, a bone density measurement of your hip and spine is recommended at age sixty-five, if you haven't already had one. In addition, a scan of your entire spine to look for silent spine fractures can be done on most DXA machines. It is important to know if you have had a spine fracture so that you can take measures to prevent another one. Ask your doctor to include a "vertebral fracture assessment" or "VFA" as part of your bone density testing.

Consider osteoporosis medicines. If you have a fracture, your chance of another fracture within the next couple of years is high. The goal is to prevent fractures and stay fit. Effective medicines are available to help decrease your risk of fractures as part of your overall treatment plan. Discuss your options for osteoporosis medicines with your doctor.

Tell your children. Do not keep the results of your bone density secret. If your bone density is low or you start on osteoporosis medicines, share your medical information with your children. It is important for them to know their risk and it may motivate them to stay more attuned to their bone health.

Watch your medicines. Some prescription medicines or even over-the-counter medicines can play havoc and counteract all your other good bone-healthy habits. Take all your medicines, vitamins, and supplements with you to each visit with your doctor so he can review everything you are using.

Consider other health problems. Be aware of other problems that may have a bone impact. Virtually any disease or illness has the potential for affecting your bones. New connections with bone are being discovered in the research labs all the time.

Stay active. Staying active is more important than ever before. Regular exercise is the closest thing you have to a fountain of youth. Adopt "painless" habits, such as parking at the far end of the shopping mall or grocery store rather than trying to get the closest parking space.

YOUR 70s AND OLDER

These tips are important for all seniors in their seventies, eighties, and nineties. To avoid repetition, they are combined into a single group. Ninety percent of fractures are associated with a fall. Regardless of your bone density, fractures are unlikely to happen if you don't fall.

Limit your cocktail hour. You should have only one or two drinks at most each day. Not only is more alcohol bad for your bones, it affects your brain more than when you were younger. Drinking increases your risks for falls and injury.

Prevent falls. Fall-proof your home to lessen the chances of falling. Your home can be the most dangerous place for fractures. Work on balance and increasing strength in your core and leg muscles. Enlisting the help of a personal trainer is good way to start, or you might consider joining a class in a local fitness center.

Recheck your vitamin D. Vitamin D supports not only your bones but also your muscles. The simple measure of having an adequate vitamin D blood level lessens your chances of falls and supports your muscle strength.

Use it or lose it. Muscle loss is a major problem for those in this age range. Stay as physically active as possible. If you are unable to continue strength-building activities, watch for the availability of a low-level, high frequency vibration platform to help maintain your bone density. If further research results are positive, standing on the low-intensity vibration platform for just minutes a day in your home may benefit your bones.

FOR MEN ONLY

Bone matters for men, too. Thirty percent of all fractures occur in men, including one-quarter of hip fractures. Men do not do well after sustaining hip fractures. In fact, one-third of men die within one year of having a hip fracture. Few diseases cause such high death rates. The same general principles for good bone health apply. Since men start out with more bone mass, it takes longer to become fragile. However, men are more likely to have habits that are harmful to bone, such as smoking and drinking.

Schedule a bone density scan. The National Osteoporosis Foundation recommends screening for all men at age seventy. You will need a DXA scan earlier if you have risk factors, medical problems, or medicines that increase your risk. For example, prostate cancer is a common chronic disease with aging. The treatments for prostate cancer may accelerate bone loss. Osteoporosis medicines may help prevent the associated bone loss.

FINAL WORDS

Achieving good bone health is simple but it's also hard work. If lifestyle changes were easy, everyone would be in tip-top shape. A few simple changes to your lifestyle will pay off in the long run. Start small and make gradual incremental changes. You do not need to do it all at once. Even some changes are better than none. Small changes can make a huge difference.

These bone-healthy measures do not exist in a vacuum. A bone-healthy lifestyle goes hand-in-hand with good health practices for lowering the risk of other major health problems like heart disease, breast cancer, and diabetes. Good bone health practices help achieve overall optimal health. However, it is also important to recognize when lifestyle changes are not enough.

New risk assessment tools integrate risk factors with bone density to estimate your fracture risk. If you have low bone density or "osteopenia," these valuable tools help as a starting point for your decision-making discussions with your doctor. Osteoporosis medicines should be reserved for use when your risk for fracture is high or you have already fractured.

Although there is no "cure" for osteoporosis, more treatment options are available than ever before. Bone-specific medicines help decrease your risk of fractures but they do not eliminate it. These medicines are a portion of your overall treatment. You still need to do your part with nutrition, calcium, vitamin D, exercise, and fall prevention.

Please share what you have learned with your family and friends. Set a good example for them. It is never too early or too late to take care of your bone health—and your family's bone health.

Many questions remain unanswered and still more remain to be discovered. Further research is needed to clarify current controversies, and new controversies are sure to emerge. Stay up-to-date with the latest developments in bone health at *4BoneHealth.org*. I look forward to continuing the dialogue with you there.

The Bare Bones
Tips for boosting bone health over your lifetime:

- Eat a healthy diet and maintain a healthy weight.
- Get thirty to sixty minutes of physical activity more days than not.
- Eat calcium-rich foods and, if that is still not enough, add a supplement.
- Maintain an optimal vitamin D level.
- Avoid tobacco and limit alcohol.
- After menopause, assess your fracture risk. Consider medicines, if needed.

Bone Healthy Shopping List

Produce
Bok Choy
Broccoli
Kale
Turnip Greens
Citrus Fruits
Figs

Dairy
Yogurt
Milk
Cheeses
Cottage Cheese

Miscellaneous
Dried or Canned Beans
Black-eyed Peas
Tea, Green or Black
Pudding

Frozen
Ice Cream
Frozen Yogurt
Vegetables, if not fresh

Breads & Cereals
Fortified Products

Fish
Halibut
Salmon, Wild
Trout
Tuna
Sardines

Staples
Enriched Flour
Enriched Rice
Enriched Cornmeal
Molasses, Blackstrap

Snacks
Unsalted Almonds
Soy Nuts
Trail Mix

Refrigerator Case
OJ-Calcium Fortified
Eggs

Check Nutrition Facts

Big Words: Medical Terms Broken Down

These are common words associated with bone health. If the word you are looking for is not listed, check the index for pages where you can find additional information.

Anabolics: medicines that turn on the bone-builder cells (osteoblasts) to promote formation of new bone. Forteo is the sole member of the anabolic group.

Antiresorptives: medicines that target the bone-breakdown cells (osteoclasts). These include the bisphosphonate class of medicines (Actonel, Atelvia, Boniva, Fosamax, generic alendronate, and Reclast), as well as calcitonin, estrogens, Evista, and Prolia. Decreasing bone breakdown results in slowing bone loss and improving bone density.

Bone Mineral: the crystalline component of bone made up of calcium and phosphorus in the form of hydroxyapatite.

BMD (Bone Mineral Density): bone mass is quantified by measurement of bone mineral. Bone mineral density predicts fracture risk.

Bone densitometry or bone density scan: the measurement of bone mass; the current gold standard device is the DXA machine, which quantifies bone mineral density of various skeletal sites, including the lower (lumbar) spine, hip, and forearm.

Bone scan: In contrast to a bone density scan, a bone scan is a nuclear medicine study. Any area of bone that has increased metabolic activity (fracture, tumor, or infection) will show increased uptake of the radioisotope.

Bone formation: the building of bone mass by cells called osteoblasts.

Bone remodeling: the continual process of bone-breakdown cells and bone-formation cells working in concert to keep bone repaired. An imbalance in bone remodeling causes problems. When bone breakdown exceeds new bone formation, such as with loss of estrogen in the menopause transition, bone loss occurs.

Bisphosphonates: synthetic compounds of the natural phosphorus that binds to the bone mineral. The name refers to the chemical structure of these phosphorus compounds: two phosphonate groups linked by a carbon atom. The structure of the side chains that branch from the carbon atom differentiates the various bisphosphonates. Fosamax, generic alendronate, Actonel, Atelvia, Boniva, and Reclast make up this class. Bisphosphonates block the breakdown of the bone by physically interfering with the bone-breakdown cells, or osteoclasts.

Cancellous bone: the spongy or trabecular bone tissue of the inner parts of the bones found in the vertebrae (spine), pelvis, and end sections of the long bones. This type of bone resembles a rigid sponge with a plate-like meshwork of beams. The plates within this kind of bone are called "trabeculae." These act like cross braces that support and prevent collapse of the structure.

Compact bone or cortical bone: the hard, dense bone tissue of the shafts of the long bones of the arms and legs and the outer shell of all bones in the body. It comprises about 80 percent of the skeleton.

DXA (dual-energy x-ray absorptiometry): the full name is descriptive of the technique. The dual-energy x-ray part of the name accounts for the use of two different energy levels of x-ray. Absorptiometry refers to radiation passing through various body tissues that have different patterns of absorption. The differences in the two beams of radiation that pass through the body's tissues allow subtraction of the bone measurement from the measurement of the surrounding tissues. The results are usually reported as bone mineral density (BMD), which is a calculated measure in grams per square centimeter (g/cm^2). Diagnosis is based on standardized T-scores or Z-scores, depending on age and sex.

Femoral neck or neck of femur: the narrowest portion of the hip; located between the femur's ball head and shaft. This area is a common site of hip fracture.

Femur: thighbone; the bone between the hip and knee joints.

Fracture: broken bone; the structural failure of bone.

FRAX: the fracture risk calculator developed by the World Health Organization. The FRAX tool incorporates results of the hip (femoral neck) bone density with personal risk factors to calculate your ten-year fracture probability. Treatment guidelines use the results of the ten-year probability of fracture for individuals with low bone mass or "osteopenia."

Kyphoplasty: a technique for treatment of an acute painful spine fracture. A balloon is inflated inside the bone (vertebral body) to create a space and then cement is injected to stabilize the fracture.

NHANES (National Health and Nutrition Examination Survey): a program of studies designed to assess the health and nutritional status of adults and children in the US by studying representative samples from different parts of the country.

Nonvertebral fracture: a fracture that occurs in bones other than the spine.

Osteoblasts: cells that form new bone in the bone remodeling cycle.

Osteoclasts: cells that break down bone in the bone remodeling cycle.

Osteocytes: cells within the structure of the bone that form an interconnected network.

Osteomalacia: a disease that means "soft bones." A very low vitamin D level, generally 15 ng/ml or less, is the most common cause. This results in an inadequate supply of calcium and phosphorus, both of which are essential for maintaining the hardness and strength of bone through a process called mineralization. If new bone does not mineralize, it is soft and rubbery.

Osteopenia: low bone mass; the World Health Organization criteria define osteopenia as bone mineral density T-scores between -1 and -2.5 measured at the lumbar spine, total hip, femoral neck, or forearm. "Low bone mass" is now the preferred name for this range of bone density.

Osteoporosis: a disease characterized by progressive and silent loss of bone that makes your bones thinner and weaker so that they are more likely to fracture or break. The World Health Organization criteria define osteoporosis as bone mineral density T-scores of -2.5 or less measured at the lumbar spine, total hip, femoral neck, or forearm.

Parathyroid and parathyroid hormone (PTH): the parathyroid consists of four small glands that are located in the neck, usually on the backside of the thyroid. The parathyroid's sole role is to regulate calcium in the body by producing parathyroid hormone.

RANKL (receptor-activating nuclear factor [kappa]B ligand): the intermediary messenger that regulates the bone remodeling cycle. Produced by osteoblasts, RANKL regulates the creation of osteoclasts and their activity by binding to receptor sites (RANK) on the surface of the precursor cells of osteoclasts and immature osteoclasts.

Resorption: the breakdown of bone by osteoclasts; this is followed by bone formation in the bone remodeling cycle.

SERM (Selective Estrogen Receptor Modulator): also called an Estrogen Agonist/Antagonist (EAA); this "designer estrogen" has a split personality. In some tissues it works like estrogen and in other tissues it has the opposite effect. Evista is the only SERM approved by the FDA for prevention and treatment of osteoporosis.

Trabecular bone: the spongy bone tissue of the inner parts of the pelvis, the end sections of the long bones, and the bones found in the vertebrae (spine). This bone, also referred to as cancellous bone, resembles a rigid sponge with a plate-like meshwork of beams. The plates within this kind of bone are called "trabeculae." These act like cross-braces to support and prevent collapse of the structure.

T-score: the standardized measurement of bone mineral density; compares an individual's measured bone mineral density with a reference database of same-sex young adults whose average scores are representative of peak bone mass. T-scores are applicable for diagnosis in postmenopausal women and men over the age of fifty.

Vertebra (Vertebrae, plural): the individual bone in the spine. Each level is comprised of a central portion called the vertebral body, a bony arch that goes around the spinal cord, and several projections for attachment of muscles.

Vertebral fracture: a structural failure of the vertebral body. Vertebral fractures may either be "silent" (not associated with any symptoms; usually identified by x-ray) or "clinical" (painful; usually diagnosed by a doctor).

Vertebral Fracture Assessment (VFA): a DXA scan of the upper and lower areas of the spine to detect vertebral fractures.

Vertebroplasty: a procedure for treatment of an acute painful spine fracture. Cement is injected inside the vertebral body to stabilize the fracture.

Z-score: standardized comparison of an individual's measured bone mineral density with same-age individuals from a reference database. Z-scores are used to diagnose low bone mass in younger adults, premenopausal women, men under the age of fifty, and children.

Internet Resources: Click on It

Various organizations, government agencies, and pharmaceutical companies provide resources online that focus on bone health. These educational materials are not intended to substitute for an evaluation by your doctor but are designed to help you become better informed. Be sure to bookmark your favorite websites.

ORGANIZATIONS

National Osteoporosis Foundation (NOF)

http://www.nof.org

The National Osteoporosis Foundation (NOF) is dedicated to the prevention of osteoporosis and broken bones through programs of public and clinician awareness, education, advocacy, and research. A section titled "Get the Facts on Osteoporosis" provides educational resources for the public and links to community and online support groups sponsored by the NOF.

International Osteoporosis Foundation (IOF)

http://www.iofbonehealth.org

The International Osteoporosis Foundation promotes prevention, diagnosis, and treatment of osteoporosis worldwide. Click on the "Patients & Public" tab for relevant information.

International Society for Clinical Densitometry (ISCD)

http://www.iscd.org

This professional organization promotes excellence in the assessment of skeletal health, including bone densitometry or measurement of bone density. Click on the "Patient Information" sidebar for a general overview of bone density testing and Vertebral Fracture Assessment. In addition, you may search for technologists and clinicians in your area who have special certification in bone densitometry.

National Bone Health Alliance (NBHA)

http://www.nationalbonehealthalliance.org

The National Bone Health Alliance brings together the expertise and resources of the bone health community. Select the "Consumers" tab for their newsletter and special offers.

American Academy of Orthopaedic Surgeons (AAOS)
http://www.orthoinfo.org
Provided by the American Academy of Orthopaedic Surgeons, *Your Orthopaedic Connection* is a patient-oriented website that deals with orthopaedic issues and surgeries. The website includes a patient education library and relevant current news.

American Orthopaedic Association's Own the Bone Program
http://www.ownthebone.org
The goal of the Own the Bone program is to close the treatment gap between the repair of an osteoporotic fracture and the prevention of future fractures. If you have had a fracture, click on the "Patients" tab to learn about steps you can take to prevent another fracture.

American Physical Therapy Association (APTA)
http://www.moveforwardpt.com
The website of the American Physical Therapy Association contains useful consumer information. By clicking on the "Find a PT" tab, you will be able to search for a physical therapist in your area who is right for your specific needs.

American College of Rheumatology (ACR)
http://www.rheumatology.org/practice/clinical/patients/index.asp
Handy patient information sheets are available about rheumatic diseases, including osteoporosis; types of healthcare professionals who treat patients with rheumatic conditions; several common medicines used to treat rheumatic diseases; and topics related to treatment, such as jaw problems (osteonecrosis of the jaw).

GrassrootsHealth
http://www.grassrootshealth.org
GrassrootsHealth focuses on vitamin D education and raising awareness about high rates of deficiency by, among other things, hosting public forums across the US and Canada. Testing of vitamin D levels is available through participation in their D*action study.

The Hormone Foundation
http://www.hormone.org
The Hormone Foundation is the patient education affiliate of the

Endocrine Society. Information on endocrine disorders and treatments, including osteoporosis and bone health, is available on the website. You may also search for an endocrinologist by zip code.

North American Menopause Society (NAMS)

http://www.menopause.org

Resources focused on menopause for midlife women are available by clicking on the "For Consumers" tab. If you are looking for healthcare providers with expertise in menopause management, you can search for a NAMS-certified menopause practitioner in your area.

United States Bone and Joint Initiative

http://www.usbjd.org

The Bone and Joint Initiative is the continuation of a ten-year program that targets the care of people with bone and joint disorders. Public education programs conducted by healthcare professionals are available for your community group by request. These include "Fit to a T," which refers to bone density T-score and "PB & J," which educates teenagers about prevention of bone and joint disorders.

American Bone Health

http://www.americanbonehealth.org

American Bone Health is an organization in the San Francisco Bay area that expanded from a research organization, the Foundation for Osteoporosis Research and Education (FORE). Sign up for their consumer newsletter, BoneSense.

4BoneHealth

http://www.4bonehealth.org

Bone health information for the whole family. Includes dynamic entries based on bone health in the news and recent research publications.

GOVERNMENT-SPONSORED

Best Bones Forever!

http://www.bestbonesforever.gov

A bone-health campaign sponsored by the US Department of Health and Human Services for girls and their best friends to "grow strong together and stay strong forever!" The goal is to increase calcium and vitamin D consumption and physical activity by encouraging girls to get active and choose bone-healthy foods. The site also contains sections for parents and educators.

Clinical Trials Resource

http://www.clinicaltrials.gov
Search for any clinical trials that are recruiting patients or are in progress. This is a service of the National Institutes of Health (NIH).

MedlinePlus

http://medlineplus.gov
MedlinePlus, the National Institutes of Health's website for consumers, is produced by the world's largest medical library, the National Library of Medicine. You can use MedlinePlus to learn about diseases, medicines, and wellness issues. You can also get links to the latest medical research on your topic or look up a medical word.

National Center for Complementary and Alternative Medicine

http://nccam.nih.gov
This NIH center provides resources and general guidance about complementary and alternative medicine.

NIH Osteoporosis and Related Bone Diseases National Resource Center

http://www.osteo.org
The National Resource Center for osteoporosis and related bone diseases covers the prevention, early detection, and treatment of osteoporosis and related bone diseases. A link is provided for the *2004 Surgeon General's Report on Bone Health and Osteoporosis: What It Means to You.*

NIHSeniorHealth

http://nihseniorhealth.gov
This site includes basic health and wellness information developed for older adults by the NIH. It also features an application that allows users to hear the text read aloud. The category titled "Bones and Joints" includes the topics of falls and osteoporosis.

OTHER RESOURCES

FRAX Calculator

http://www.shef.ac.uk/FRAX
Calculate your fracture risk using this calculator.

WebMD

http://www.webmd.com/osteoporosis
WebMD covers osteoporosis and many other diseases and conditions.

PHARMACEUTICAL COMPANY SPONSORED

Each medicine has a website with specific information on the product.
Type in the brand name then ".com" to access the product information
using your Web browser. For example, Actonel's website is at
http://www.actonel.com.

Some of the other pharmaceutical-sponsored websites have helpful general information as well as links to additional websites:

Know My Bones

http://www.knowmybones.com

Acknowledgements

The Complete Book of Bone Health would not have been possible without the assistance of numerous individuals. Dr. Julie Silver, assistant professor at Harvard Medical School and chief editor of books at Harvard Health Publications, kickstarted the process. In October 2008, she taught me the nuts and bolts of publishing in her course called Medical Non-Fiction Writing for Physicians. As part of the same conference, which was produced by SEAK, Inc., I was fortunate to meet my agent Katharine Sands of Sarah Jane Freymann Literary Agency, who has shepherded me through the entire publication process. The hard work of editor-in-chief Steven L. Mitchell and his staff at Prometheus Books has made this up-to-date and evidence-based resource on bone health a reality.

I am especially grateful to Dr. Sally Ride for writing an insightful foreword. We share a vision of education for boosting bone health. Her endeavors through Sally Ride Science are inspiring and important for educating a new generation of girls and boys in the areas of science, math, and technology.

Friends, colleagues, and new friends gained in the process all contributed to the making of this book. Four readers were constantly ready at their computers to receive and review each chapter one by one. Dr. Mary Barry, Luanne Kittle, Sarah Wagner, and Joy Ward generously provided hours and hours of labor, advice, and encouragement. Talented Tim Gunther meticulously produced all the professional illustrations.

In an incredibly short period of time, professional editor Julie Ward exercised her skill to help me meet the word count. Sports journalist and author Jill Lieber Steeg edited line by line and did an incredible job of fact checking in a subject area far afield from sports. Julie and Amy Beattie painstakingly reviewed printed copies of the manuscript.

Numerous colleagues were generous with their time in taking my phone calls, e-mails, and questions. Special kudos are in order for Dr. Robert Heaney, Diane Claflin, Dr. Elliott Schwartz, Dr. Robert Marcus, Dr. Susan Lupo, Dr. Silvina Levis, Dr. Michael Kleerekoper, Dr. Vera Barile, Winnie Arnn, Peggy King, Janet Alexander, Dee Steinberg, and Dr. Elizabeth Barrett-Connor.

Last but most important has been the unwavering support and love provided by my husband, Dave Grundies, and my family.

Diane L. Schneider, MD
May 2011

References

INTRODUCTION:
To Your Bone-Healthy Life

US Department of Health and Human Services. *Bone Health and Osteoporosis: A Report of the Surgeon General*. Rockville, MD: US Department of Health and Human Services Office of the Surgeon General, 2004.

PART ONE: BONE HEALTH BASICS
Building Perfect Bones: Timing Is Everything

Cooper, C., J.G. Eriksson, T. Forsén, et al. "Maternal Height, Childhood Growth, and Risk of Hip Fracture in Later Life: A Longitudinal Study." *Osteoporosis International* 12 (2001): 623–29.

Davies, J.H., B.A.J. Evans, and J.W. Gregory. "Bone Mass Acquisition in Healthy Children." *Archives of Disease in Childhood* 90 (2005): 373–78.

Esterle, L., M. Nguyen, O. Walrant-Debray, et al. "Adverse Interaction of Low-Calcium Diet and Low 25(OH)D Levels on Lumbar Spine Mineralization in Late-Pubertal Girls." *Journal of Bone and Mineral Research* 25 (2011): 2392–98.

Heaney, R.P., S. Abrams, B. Dawson-Hughes, et al. "Peak Bone Mass." *Osteoporosis International* 11 (2000): 985–1009.

Hernandez, C.J., G.S. Beaupré, and D.R. Carter. "A Theoretical Analysis of the Relative Influences of Peak BMD, Age-Related Bone Loss, and Menopause on the Development of Osteoporosis." *Osteoporosis International* 14 (2003): 843–47.

Leunissen, R.W.J., T. Stijnen, A.C.S. Hokken-Koelega, et al. "Influence of Birth Size and Body Composition on Bone Mineral Density in Early Adulthood: The Program Study." *Clinical Endocrinology* 69 (2008): 386–92.

MacKelvie, K.J., K.M. Khan, and H.A. McKay. "Is There a Critical Period for Bone Response to Weight-Bearing Exercise in Children and Adolescents? A Systematic Review." *British Journal of Sports Medicine* 36 (2002): 250–57.

Pollock, N. K., P. J. Bernard, K. Wenger, et al. "Lower Bone Mass in Prepubertal Overweight Children with Prediabetes." *Journal of Bone and Mineral Research* 25 (2010): 2760–69.

Recker, R., J. Lappe, K. Davies, and R. Heaney. "Characterization of Perimenopausal Bone Loss: A Prospective Study." *Journal of Bone and Mineral Research* 15 (2000): 1965–73.

Recker, R., J. Lappe, K.M. Davies, and R. Heaney. "Bone Remodeling Increases Substantially in the Years after Menopause and Remains Increased in Older Osteoporosis Patients." *Journal of Bone and Mineral Research* 19 (2004): 1628–33.

Sayers, A., and J.H. Tobias. "Estimated Maternal Ultraviolet B Exposure Levels in Pregnancy Influence Skeletal Development of the Child." *Journal of Clinical Endocrinology & Metabolism* 94 (2009): 765–71.

Viljakainen, H. T., M. Pekkinen, E. Saarnio, et al. "Dual Effect of Adipose Tissue on Bone Health During Growth." *Bone* 48 (2011): 212–17.

Wang, Q., S. Cheng, and M. Alén. "Bone's Structural Diversity in Adult Females Is Established Before Puberty." *Journal of Clinical Endocrinology & Metabolism* 94 (2009): 1555–61.

Yarborough, D.E., E. Barrett-Connor, and D.J. Morton. "Birth Weight as a Predictor of Adult Bone Mass in Postmenopausal Women: The Rancho Bernardo Study." *Osteoporosis International* 11 (2000): 626–30.

Zamora, S.A., D.C. Belli, R. Rizzoli, D.O. Slosman, and J.P. Bonjour. "Lower Femoral Neck Bone Mineral Density in Prepubertal Former Preterm Girls." *Bone* 29 (2001): 424–27.

Fracture Facts: One Tough Break Leads to Another

Barrett-Connor, E., C.M. Nielson, E. Orwoll, et al. for The Osteoporotic Fractures in Men (MrOS) Study Group. "Epidemiology of Rib Fractures in Older Men: Osteoporotic Fractures in Men (MrOS) Prospective Cohort Study." *British Medical Journal* 340 (2010): c1069.

Barrett-Connor, E., S.G. Sajjan, E.S. Siris, et al. "Wrist Fracture as a Predictor of Future Fractures in Younger Versus Older Postmenopausal Women: Results from the National Osteoporosis Risk Assessment (NORA)." *Osteoporosis International* 19 (2008): 607–13.

Bliuc, D., N.D. Nguyen, V.E. Milch, et al. "Mortality Risk Associated with Low-Trauma Osteoporotic Fracture and Subsequent Fracture in Men and Women." *Journal of the American Medical Association* 301 (2009): 513–21.

Brauer, C.A., M. Coca-Perraillon, D.M. Cutler, and A.B. Rosen. "Incidence and Mortality of Hip Fractures in the United States." *Journal of the American Medical Association* 302 (2009): 1573–79.

Brenneman, S.K., E. Barrett-Connor, S. Sajjan, et al. "Impact of Recent Fracture on Health-Related Quality of Life in Postmenopausal Women." *Journal of Bone and Mineral Research* 21 (2006): 809–16.

Burge, R., B. Dawson-Hughes, D.H. Solomon, et al. "Incidence and Economic Burden of Osteoporosis-Related Fractures in the United States, 2005–2025." *Journal of Bone and Mineral Research* 22 (2007): 465–75.

Center, J.R., D. Bliuc, T.V. Nguyen, and J.A. Eisman. "Risk of Subsequent Fracture after Low-Trauma Fracture in Men and Women." *Journal of the American Medical Association* 297 (2007): 387–94.

Center, J.R., T.V. Nguyen, D. Schneider, et al. "Mortality after All Major Types of Osteoporotic Fracture in Men and Women: An Observational Study." *Lancet* 353 (1999): 878–82.

Edwards, B.J., J. Song, D.D. Dunlop, et al. "Functional Decline after Incident Wrist Fractures—Study of Osteoporotic Fractures: Prospective Cohort Study." *British Medical Journal* 341 (2010): c3324.

Haentjens, P., J. Magaziner, C. S. Colón-Emeric, et al. "Meta-Analysis: Excess Mortality after Hip Fracture among Older Women and Men." *Annals of Internal Medicine* 152 (2010): 380–90.

Ioannidis, G., A. Papaioannou, W.M. Hopman, et al. "Relation between Fractures and Mortality: Results from the Canadian Multicentre Osteoporosis Study." *Canadian Medical Association Journal* 181 (2009): 265–71.

Kirmani, S., D. Christen, P. Fischer, et al. "Bone Structure at the Distal Radius during Adolescent Growth." *Journal of Bone and Mineral Research* 24 (2009): 1033–42.

Mackey, D.C., L.Y. Lui, P.M. Cawthon, et al. "High-Trauma Fractures and Low Bone Mineral Density in Older Women and Men." *Journal of the American Medical Association* 298 (2007): 2381–88.

Melton, L.J., A.W. Lane, C. Cooper, et al. "Prevalence and Incidence of Vertebral Deformities." *Osteoporosis International* 3 (1993): 113–19.

Pasco, J.A., E. Seeman, M.J. Henry, et al. "The Population Burden of Fractures Originates in Women with Osteopenia, Not Osteoporosis." *Osteoporosis International* 17 (2006): 1404–09.

Siris, E.S., S. Gehlbach, J.D. Adachi, et al. "Failure to Perceive Increased Risk of Fracture in Women 55 Years and Older: The Global Longitudinal Study of Osteoporosis in Women (GLOW)." *Osteoporosis International* 22 (2011): 27–35.

Wainwright, S.A., L.M. Marshall, K.E. Ensrud, et al. "Hip Fracture in Women without Osteoporosis." *Journal of Clinical Endocrinology & Metabolism* 90 (2005): 2787–93.

Challenges and Choices: What You Can and Cannot Change

Bakhireva, L.N., E. Barrett-Connor, D. Kritz-Silverstein, and D.J. Morton. "Modifiable Predictors of Bone Loss in Older Men: A Prospective Study." *American Journal of Preventive Medicine* 26 (2004): 436–42.

Beck, T.J., M.A. Petit, G. Wu, et al. "Does Obesity Really Make the Femur Stronger? BMD, Geometry, and Fracture Incidence in the Women's Health Initiative-Observational Study." *Journal of Bone and Mineral Research* 24 (2009): 1369–79.

Burger, H., C. de Laet, P. Van Daele, et al. "Risk Factors for Increased Bone Loss in an Elderly Population." *American Journal of Epidemiology* 147 (1998): 871–79.

Cummings, S.R., M.C. Nevitt, W.S. Browner, et al. "Risk Factors for Hip Fracture in White Women. Study of Osteoporotic Fractures Research Group." *New England Journal of Medicine* 332 (1995): 767–73.

Holbrook, T.L., and E. Barrett-Connor. "A Prospective Study of Alcohol Consumption and Bone Mineral Density." *British Medical Journal* 306 (1993): 1506–09.

Kanis, J.A., H. Johansson, A. Oden, et al. "A Family History of Fracture and Fracture Risk: A Meta-Analysis." *Bone* 35 (2004): 1029–37.

Kanis, J.A., H. Johansson, O. Johnell, et al. "Alcohol Intake as a Risk Factor for Fracture." *Osteoporosis International* 16 (2005): 737–42.

Kanis, J.A., O. Johnell, A. Oden, et al. "Smoking and Fracture Risk: A Meta-Analysis." *Osteoporosis International* 16 (2005): 155–62.

Kanis, J.A., O. Johnell, C. De Laet, et al. "A Meta-Analysis of Previous Fracture and Subsequent Fracture Risk." *Bone* 35 (2004): 375–82.

Laet, C.D., J.A. Kanis, H. Johanson, et al. "Body Mass Index as a Predictor of Fracture Risk: A Meta-Analysis." *Osteoporosis International* 16 (2005): 1330–38.

Lewis, C.E., S.K. Ewing, B.C. Taylor, et al. "Predictors of Non-Spine Fracture in Elderly Men: The MrOS Study." *Journal of Bone and Mineral Research* 22 (2007): 211–19.

Looker, A.C., H.W. Wahner, W.L. Dunn, et al. "Updated Data on Proximal Femur Bone Mineral Levels of US Adults." *Osteoporosis International* 8 (1998): 468–89.

Morton, D.J., E. Barrett-Connor, D. Kritz-Silverstein, D.L. Wingard, and D.L. Schneider. "Bone Mineral Density in Postmenopausal Caucasian, Filipina, and Hispanic Women." *International Journal of Epidemiology* 32 (2003): 150–56.

Oncken, C., K. Prestwood, A. Kleppinger, et al. "Impact of Smoking Cessation on Bone Mineral Density in Postmenopausal Women." *Journal of Women's Health* 15 (2006): 1141–50.

Richards, J.B., F.K. Kavvoura, F. Rivadeneira, et al. "Collaborative Meta-Analysis: Associations of 150 Candidate Genes with Osteoporosis and Osteoporotic Fracture." *Annals of Internal Medicine* 151 (2009): 528–37.

Siris, E.S., S.K. Brenneman, E. Barrett-Connor, et al. "The Effect of Age and Bone Mineral Density on the Absolute, Excess, and Relative Risk of Fracture in Postmenopausal Women Aged 50–99: Results from the National Osteoporosis Risk Assessment (NORA)." *Osteoporosis International* 17 (2006): 565–74.

The Bone Cycle: Cruise Control and Overdrive

Boyle, W.J., W.S. Simone, and D.L. Lacey. "Osteoclast Differentiation and Activation." *Nature* 423 (2003): 337–42.

Eghbali-Fatourechi, G., S. Khosla, A. Sanyal, et al. "Role of RANK Ligand in Mediating; Increased Bone Resorption in Early Postmenopausal Women." *Journal of Clinical Investigation* 111 (2003): 1221–30.

Lee, T.C., A. Staines, and D. Taylor. "Bone Adaptation to Load: Microdamage as a Stimulus for Bone Remodeling." *Journal of Anatomy* 201 (2002): 437–46.

Matsuo, K., and N. Irie. "Osteoclast-Osteoblast Communication." *Archives of Biochemistry and Biophysics* 473 (2008): 201–209.

Theoleyre, S., Y. Wittrant, S.K. Kwan Tat, et al. "The Molecular Triad OPG/RANK/RANKL: Involvement in the Orchestration of Pathophysiological Bone Remodeling." *Cytokine & Growth Factor Reviews* 15 (2004): 457–75.

Väänänen, H.K., and T. Laitala-Leinonen. "Osteoclast Lineage and Function." *Archives of Biochemistry and Biophysics* 473 (2008): 132–38.

Yadav, V.K., J.H. Ryu, N. Suda, et al. "Lrp5 Controls Bone Formation by Inhibiting Serotonin Synthesis in the Duodenum." *Cell* 135 (2008): 825–37.

PART TWO: ASSESSMENT OF BONE HEALTH

General Evaluation: Visiting with Your Doctor

Dawson-Hughes, B., A.N.A. Tosteson, L.J. Melton, et al. "Implications of Absolute Fracture Risk Assessment for Osteoporosis Practice Guidelines in the USA." *Osteoporosis International* 19 (2008): 449–58.

Nguyen, T., P. Sambrook, P. Kelly, et al. "Prediction of Osteoporotic Fractures by Postural Instability and Bone Density." *British Medical Journal* 307 (1993): 1111–15.

Nicholson, P.H.F., M.J. Haddaway, M.W.J. Davie, and S.F. Evans. "Vertebral Deformity, Bone Mineral Density, Back Pain, and Height Loss in Unscreened Women over 50 Years." *Osteoporosis International* 3 (1993): 300–307.

US Preventive Services Task Force. "Screening for Osteoporosis: US Preventive Services Task Force Recommendation Statement." *Annals of Internal Medicine* 154 (2011): 356–364.

Bone Density Scan: DXA 101

Baim S., M.B. Leonard, M.L. Bianchi, et al. "Official Positions of the International Society for Clinical Densitometry and Executive Summary of the 2007 ISCD Pediatric Position Development Conference." *Journal of Clinical Densitometry* 11 (2008): 6–21.

Baim, S., N. Binkley, J.P. Bilezikian, et al. "Official Positions of the International Society for Clinical Densitometry and Executive Summary of the 2007 ISCD Position Development Conference." *Journal of Clinical Densitometry* 11 (2008): 75–91.

Blake, G.M., and I. Fogelman. "The Clinical Role of Dual Energy X-Ray Absorptiometry." *European Journal of Radiology* 71 (2009): 406–14.

Dawson-Hughes, B., A.C. Looker, A.N.A. Tosteson, et al. "The Potential Impact of New National Osteoporosis Foundation Guidance on Treatment Patterns." *Osteoporosis International* 21 (2010): 41–52.

Johnell, O., J.A. Kanis, A. Oden, et al. "Predictive Value of BMD for Hip and Other Fractures." *Journal of Bone and Mineral Research* 20 (2005): 1185–94.

Kanis, J.A., A. Oden, O. Johnell, et al. "The Use of Clinical Risk Factors Enhances the Performance of BMD in the Prediction of Hip and Osteoporotic Fractures in Men and Women." *Osteoporosis International* 18 (2007): 1033–46.

National Osteoporosis Foundation. *Clinician's Guide to Prevention and Treatment of Osteoporosis*. Washington, DC: National Osteoporosis Foundation, 2008.

Pasco, J.A., E. Seeman, M.J. Henry, et al. "The Population Burden of Fractures Originates in Women with Osteopenia, Not Osteoporosis." *Osteoporosis International* 17 (2006): 1404–09.

Schneider, D.L., R. Bettencourt, and E. Barrett-Connor. "Clinical Utility of Spine Bone Density in Elderly Women." *Journal of Clinical Densitometry* 9 (2006): 255–60.

Siris, E.S., P.D. Miller, E. Barrett-Connor, et al. "Identification and Fracture Outcomes of Undiagnosed Low Bone Mineral Density in Postmenopausal Women: Results from the National Osteoporosis Risk Assessment." *Journal of the American Medical Association* 286 (2001): 2815–22.

Tosteson, A.N.A., L.J. Melton, B. Dawson-Hughes, et al. "Cost-Effective Osteoporosis Treatment Thresholds: The United States Perspective." *Osteoporosis International* 19 (2008): 437–47.

US Preventive Services Task Force. "Screening for Osteoporosis: US Preventive Services Task Force Recommendation Statement." *Annals of Internal Medicine* 154 (2011): 356–64.

Watts, N.B., E.S. Siris, S.R. Cummings, and D.C. Bauer. "Filtering FRAX." *Osteoporosis International* 21 (2010): 537–41.

Other Measurements: The Alphabet Soup of Imaging

Bauer, J.S., and T.M. Link. "Advances in Osteoporosis Imaging." *European Journal of Radiology* 71 (2009): 440–49.

Boutroy, S., B. Van Rietbergen, E. Sornay-Rendu, et al. "Finite Element Analysis Based on In Vivo HR-PQCT Images of the Distal Radius Is Associated with Wrist Fracture in Postmenopausal Women." *Journal of Bone and Mineral Research* 23 (2008): 392–99.

Cohen, A., D.W. Dempster, R. Muller, et al. "Assessment of Trabecular and Cortical Architecture and Mechanical Competence of Bone by High-Resolution Peripheral Computed Tomography: Comparison with Transiliac Bone Biopsy." *Osteoporosis International* 21 (2010): 263–73.

Genant, H.K., K. Engelke, and S. Prevrhal. "Advanced CT Bone Imaging in Osteoporosis." *Rheumatology (Oxford)* 47, supplement 4 (2008): iv9–iv16.

Kazakia, G.J., B. Hyun, A.J. Burghardt, et al. "In Vivo Determination of Bone Structure in Postmenopausal Women: A Comparison of HR-PQCT and High-Field MR Imaging." *Journal of Bone and Mineral Research* 23 (2008): 463–74.

Nayak, S., I. Olkin, H. Liu, et al. "Meta-Analysis: Accuracy of Quantitative Ultrasound for Identifying Patients with Osteoporosis." *Annals of Internal Medicine* 144 (2006): 832–41.

Orwoll, E. S., L. M. Marshall, C. M. Nielson, et al. "Finite Element Analysis of the Proximal Femur and Hip Fracture Risk in Older Men." *Journal of Bone and Mineral Research* 24 (2009): 475–83.

Stein, E. M., X. S. Liu, T. L. Nickolas, et al. "Abnormal Microarchitecture and Reduced Stiffness at the Radius and Tibia in Postmenopausal Women with Fractures." *Journal of Bone and Mineral Research* 25 (2010): 2572–81.

Bone Turnover Markers: Dynamic Assessment

Delmas, P.D., R. Eastell, P. Garnero, et al. "The Use of Biochemical Markers of Bone Turnover on Osteoporosis." *Osteoporosis International* 6 (2000): S2–S17.

Garnero, P., E. Sornay-Rendu, M.C. Chapuy, and P.D. Delmas. "Increased Bone Turnover in Late Postmenopausal Women Is a Major Determinant of Osteoporosis." *Journal of Bone and Mineral Research* 11 (1996): 337–49.

Garnero, P., P. Vergnaud, and N. Hoyle. "Evaluation of a Fully Automated Serum Assay for Total N-Terminal Propeptide of Type I Collagen in Postmenopausal Osteoporosis." *Clinical Chemistry* 54 (2008): 188–96.

Gerdhem, P., K.K. Ivaska, S.L. Alatalo, et al. "Biochemical Markers of Bone Metabolism and Prediction of Fracture in Elderly Women." *Journal of Bone and Mineral Research* 19 (2004): 386–93.

Johnell, O., A. Odén, C. De Laet, et al. "Biochemical Indices of Bone Turnover and the Assessment of Fracture Probability." *Osteoporosis International* 13 (2002): 523–26.

Lenora, J., K.K. Ivaska, K.J. Obrant, and P. Gerdhem. "Prediction of Bone Loss Using Biochemical Markers of Bone Turnover." *Osteoporosis International* 18 (2007): 1297–305.

Melton, L.J., C.S. Crowson, W.M. O'Fallon, et al. "Relative Contributions of Bone Density, Bone Turnover, and Clinical Risk Factors to Long-Term Fracture Prediction." *Journal of Bone and Mineral Research* 18 (2003): 312–18.

Monitoring with Follow-Up DXAs: NOT One and Done

Clowes, J.A., N.F.A. Peel, and R. Eastell. "The Impact of Monitoring on Adherence and Persistence with Antiresorptive Treatment for Postmenopausal Osteoporosis: A Randomized Controlled Trial Part Three: General Measures for Bone Health." *The Journal of Clinical Endocrinology & Metabolism* 89 (2004): 1117–23.

Hayen, A., J. Craig, D.C. Bauer, et al. "Value of Routine Monitoring of Bone Mineral Density after Starting Bisphosphonate Treatment: Secondary Analysis of Trial Data." *British Medical Journal* 338 (2009): b2266.

Lewiecki, E.M., and N.B. Watts. "Assessing Response to Osteoporosis Therapy." *Osteoporosis International* 19 (2008): 1363–68.

PART THREE: GENERAL MEASURES FOR BONE HEALTH

Exercise: On Your Mark, Get Set, GO!

Baxter-Jones, A.D.G., S.A. Kontulainen, R.A. Faulkner, and D.A. Bailey. "A Longitudinal Study of the Relationship of Physical Activity to Bone Mineral Accrual from Adolescence to Young Adulthood." *Bone* 43 (2008): 1101–07.

Bouxsein, M.L., E.R. Myers, and W.C. Hayes. "Biomechanics of Age-Related Fractures." In *Osteoporosis*, edited by R. Marcus, D. Feldman, and J. Kelsey, 373–93. San Diego: Academic Press, 1996.

Bouxsein, M.L., J. Melton, III, B.L. Riggs, et al. "Age- and Sex-Specific Differences in the Factor of Risk for Vertebral Fracture: A Population-Based Study Using QCT." *Journal of Bone and Mineral Research* 21 (2006): 1475–82.

Daly, R.M., L. Saxon, C.H. Turner, et al. "The Relationship Between Muscle Size and Bone Geometry during Growth and in Response to Exercise." *Bone* 34 (2004): 281–87.

Engelke, K., W. Kemmler, D. Lauber, et al. "Exercise Maintains Bone Density at Spine and Hip EFOPS: A 3-Year Longitudinal Study in Early Postmenopausal Women." *Osteoporosis International* 17 (2006): 133–42.

Feskanich, D., W. Willett, and G. Colditz. "Walking and Leisure Time Activity and Risk of Hip Fracture in Postmenopausal Women." *Journal of the American Medical Association* 288 (2002): 2300–2306.

Going, S., T. Lohman, L. Houtkooper, et al. "Effects of Exercise on Bone Mineral Density in Calcium-Replete Postmenopausal Women with and without Hormone Replacement Therapy." *Osteoporosis International* 8 (2003): 637–44.

Haudenschild, A.K., A.H. Hsieh, S. Kapila, and J.C. Lotz. "Pressure and Distortion Regulate Human Mesenchymal Stem Cell Gene Expression." *Annals Biomedical Engineering* 37 (2009): 492–502.

Iuliano-Burns, S., L. Saxon, G. Naughton, et al. "Regional Specificity of Exercise and Calcium during Skeletal Growth in Girls: A Randomized Controlled Trial." *Journal of Bone and Mineral Research* 18 (2003): 156–62.

Kontulainen, S., H. Sievänen, P. Kannus, et al. "Effect of Long-Term Impact-Loading on Mass, Size, and Estimated Strength of Humerus and Radius of Female Racquet-Sports Players: A Peripheral Quantitative Computed Tomography Study Between Young and Old Starters and Controls." *Journal of Bone and Mineral Research* 17 (2002): 2281–89.

Ma, H., T. Leskinen, M. Alen, et al. "Long-Term Leisure Time Physical Activity and Properties of Bone: A Twin Study." *Journal of Bone and Mineral Research* 24 (2009): 1427–33.

Nader, P.R., R.H. Bradley, R.M. Houts, et al. "Moderate-to-Vigorous Physical Activity from Ages 9 to 15 Years." *Journal of the American Medical Association* 300 (2008): 295–305.

Papaioannou, A., J.D. Adachi, K. Winegard, et al. "Efficacy of Home-Based Exercise for Improving Quality of Life among Elderly Women with Symptomatic Osteoporosis-Related Vertebral Fracture." *Osteoporosis International* 14 (2003): 677–82.

Scott, D., L. Blizzard, J. Fell, and G. Jones. "Ambulatory Activity, Body Composition, and Lower-Limb Muscle Strength in Older Adults." *Medicine & Science in Sports & Exercise* 41 (2009): 383–89.

Sen, B., Z. Xie, N. Case, et al. "Mechanical Strain Inhibits Adipogenesis in Mesenchymal Stem Cells by Stimulating a Durable Beta-Catenin Signal." *Endocrinology* 149 (2008): 6065–75.

Sinaki, M., J.C. Canvin, B.E. Phillip, et al. "Site Specificity of Regular Health Club Exercise on Muscle Strength, Fitness, and Bone Density in Women Aged 29 to 45 Years." *Mayo Clinic Proceedings* 79 (2004): 639–44.

Warden, S.J., R.K. Fuchs, A.B. Castillo, et al. "Exercise When Young Provides Lifelong Benefits to Bone Structure and Strength." *Journal of Bone and Mineral Research* 22 (2007): 251–59.

Weeks, B.K., C.M. Young, and B.R. Beck. "Eight Months of Regular In-School Jumping Improves Indices of Bone Strength in Adolescent Boys and Girls: The Power PE Study." *Journal of Bone and Mineral Research* 23 (2008): 1002–11.

Fall Prevention: Fall-Proof Yourself and Your Home

Delbaere, K., J.C.T. Close, H. Brodaty, et al. "Determinants of Disparities between Perceived and Physiological Risk of Falling among Elderly People: Cohort Study." *British Medical Journal* 341 (2010): c4165.

Faulkner, K., J. Cauley, S. Studenski, et al. "Lifestyle Predicts Falls Independent of Physical Risk Factors." *Osteoporosis International* 20 (2009): 2025–34.

Formiga, F., M. Navarro, E. Duaso, et al. "Factors Associated with Hip-Fracture Related Falls among Patients with a History of Recurrent Falling." *Bone* 43 (2008): 941–44.

Groen, B.E., E. Smulders, J. Duysens, et al. "Martial Arts Fall Training to Prevent Hip Fractures in the Elderly." *Osteoporosis International* 21 (2010): 215–21.

Kalyani, R.R., B. Stein, R. Valiyil, et al. "Vitamin D Treatment for the Prevention of Falls in Older Adults: Systematic Review and Meta-Analysis." *Journal of the American Geriatrics Society* 58 (2010): 1299–1310.

Luukinen, H., M. Herala, K. Koski, et al. "Fracture Risk Associated with a Fall according to Type of Fall among the Elderly." *Osteoporosis International* 1 (2000): 361–64.

Mulle, M., D.L. Knol, S.A. Danner, et al. "Multifactorial Intervention to Reduce Falls in Older People at High Risk of Recurrent Falls." *Archives of Internal Medicine* 170 (2010): 1110–17.

National Center for Injury Prevention and Control, Center for Disease Control. "Unintentional Fall Nonfatal Injuries and Rates per 100,000, 2008." Web–Based Injury Statistics Query and Reporting System (WISQARS). http://www.cdc.gov/injury/wisqars/.

Peeters, G., N.M. Schoor, and P. Lips. "Fall Risk: The Clinical Relevance of Falls and How to Integrate Fall Risk with Fracture Risk." *Best Practice and Research Clinical Rheumatology* 3 (2009): 797–804.

Schwartz, A.V., M.C. Nevitt, B.W. Brown, et al. "Increased Falling as a Risk Factor among Older Women: The Study of Osteoporotic Fractures." *American Journal of Epidemiology* 161 (2005): 180–85.

Sherrington, C., J.C. Whitney, S.R. Lord, et al. "Effective Exercise for the Prevention of Falls: A Systematic Review and Meta-Analysis." *Journal of the American Geriatric Society* 56 (2008): 2234–43.

Nutrition: Take a Bite out of Your Fracture Risk

Binkley, N.C., J. Harke, D. Krueger, et al. "Vitamin K Treatment Reduces Undercarboxylated Osteocalcin but Does Not Alter Bone Turnover, Density, or Geometry in Healthy Postmenopausal North American Women." *Journal of Bone and Mineral Research* 24 (2009): 983–91.

Booth, S.L., G. Dallal, M.K. Shea, et al. "Effect of Vitamin K Supplementation on Bone Loss in Elderly Men and Women." *The Journal of Clinical Endocrinology & Metabolism* 93 (2008): 1217–23.

Cabrera, C., R. Artacho, and R. Giménez. "Beneficial Effects of Green Tea—A Review." *Journal of the American College of Nutrition* 25 (2006): 79–99.

Dargent-Molina, P., S. Sabia, M. Touvier, et al. "Proteins, Dietary Acid Load, and Calcium and Risk of Postmenopausal Fractures in the E3N French Women Prospective Study." *Journal of Bone and Mineral Research* 23 (2008): 1915–22.

Darling, A.L., D.J. Millward, D.J. Torgerson, et al. "Dietary Protein and Bone Health: A Systematic Review and Meta-Analysis." *American Journal of Clinical Nutrition* 90 (2009): 1674–92.

Devine, A., J.M. Hodgson, I.M. Dick, and R.L. Prince. "Tea Drinking Is Associated with Benefits on Bone Density in Older Women." *American Journal of Clinical Nutrition* 86 (2007): 1243–47.

Fenton, T.R., A.W. Lyon, M. Eliasziw, S.C. Tough, and D.A. Hanley. "Meta-Analysis of the Effect of the Acid-Ash Hypothesis of Osteoporosis on Calcium Balance." *Journal of Bone and Mineral Research* 24 (2009): 1835–40.

Food and Nutrition Board, Institute of Medicine of the National Academies. *Dietary Reference Intakes for Energy, Carbohydrate. Fiber, Fat, Fatty Acids, Cholesterol, Protein, and Amino Acids (2002/2005)*. Washington, DC: National Academies Press.

Food and Nutrition Board, Institute of Medicine of the National Academies. *Dietary Reference Intakes for Vitamin A, Vitamin K, Arsenic, Boron, Chromium, Copper, Iodine, Iron, Manganese, Molybdenum, Nickel, Silicon, Vanadium, and Zinc (2001)*. Washington, DC: National Academies Press.

Hegarty, V.M., H.M. May, and K.T. Khaw. "Tea Drinking and Bone Mineral Density in Older Women." *American Journal of Clinical Nutrition* 71 (2000): 1003–1007.

Jensen, C., L. Holloway, G. Black. "Long-Term Effects of Nutrient Intervention or Markers of Bone Remodeling and Calciotropic Hormones in Late-Postmenopausal Women." *American Journal of Clinical Nutrition* 75 (2002): 1114–20

Lim, L.S., L.J. Harnack, D. Lazovich, et al. "Vitamin A Intake and the Risk of Hip Fracture in Postmenopausal Women: The Iowa Women's Health Study." *Osteoporosis International* 15 (2004): 552–59.

McLean, R.R., P.F. Jacques, J. Selhub, et al. "Homocysteine as a Predictive Factor for Hip Fracture in Older Persons." *New England Journal of Medicine* 350 (2004): 2042–49.

Melhus, H., K. Michaelsson, A. Kindmark, et al. "Excessive Dietary Intake of Vitamin A Is Associated with Reduced Bone Mineral Density and Increased Risk for Hip Fracture." *Annals of Internal Medicine* 129 (1998): 770–78.

Michaelsson, K., H. Lithell, B. Vessby, and H. Melhus. "Serum Retinol Levels and the Risk of Fracture." *New England Journal of Medicine* 348 (2003): 287–94.

Misra, D., S.D. Berry, K.E. Broe, et al. "Does Dietary Protein Reduce Hip Fracture Risk in Elders? The Framingham Osteoporosis Study." *Osteoporosis International* 22 (2011): 345–49.

Morton, D., E. Barrett-Connor, and D.L. Schneider. "Vitamin C Supplement Use and Bone Mineral Density in Postmenopausal Women." *Journal of Bone and Mineral Research* 16 (2001): 135–40.

Promislow, J.H., D. Goodman-Gruen, D.J. Slymen, and E. Barrett-Connor. "Protein Consumption and Bone Mineral Density in the Elderly." *American Journal of Epidemiology* 155 (2002): 636–44.

Promislow, J.H., D. Goodman-Gruen, D.J. Slymen, and E. Barrett-Connor. "Retinol Intake and Bone Mineral Density in the Elderly: The Rancho Bernardo Study." *Journal of Bone and Mineral Research* 17 (2002): 1311–20.

Rude, R.K., F.R. Singer, and H.E. Gruber. "Skeletal and Hormonal Effects of Magnesium Deficiency." *Journal of the American College of Nutrition* 28 (2009): 131–41.

Sahni, S., L. A. Cupples, R. R. McLean, et al. "Protective Effect of High Protein and Calcium Intake on the Risk of Hip Fracture in the Framingham Offspring Cohort." *Journal of Bone and Mineral Research* 25 (2010): 2770–76.

Sahni, S., M.T. Hannan, D. Gagnon, et al. "Protective Effect of Total and Supplemental Vitamin C Intake on the Risk of Hip Fracture—A 17-Year Follow-Up from the Framingham Osteoporosis Study." *Osteoporosis International* 20 (2009): 1853–61.

Tucker, K.L., D.P. Kiel, J.J. Powell, et al. "Dietary Silicon and Bone Mineral Density: The Framingham Study." *Journal of Bone and Mineral Research* 19 (2001): 276–81.

US Department of Agriculture, Agricultural Research Service. "USDA National Nutrient Database for Standard Reference, Release 22 Nutrient Lists" (2010). Nutrient Data Laboratory Home Page. http://www.ars.usda.gov/ba/bhnrc/ndl.

Van Meurs, J.B., R.A. Dhonukshe-Rutten, S.M. Pluijm, et al. "Homocysteine Levels and the Risk of Osteoporotic Fracture." *New England Journal of Medicine* 350 (2004): 2033–41.

Von Muhlen, D., S. Safii, S.K. Jassal, et al. "Associations between the Metabolic Syndrome and Bone Health in Older Men and Women: The Rancho Bernardo Study." *Osteoporosis International* 18 (2007): 1337–44.

Weaver, C.M., W.R. Proulx, and R. Heaney. "Choices for Achieving Adequate Dietary Calcium with a Vegetarian Diet." *American Journal of Clinical Nutrition* 70 (1999): 543S–548S.

Weiss, L.A., E. Barrett-Connor, and D. von Muhlen. "Ratio of N-6 to N-3 Fatty Acids and Bone Mineral Density in Older Adults: The Rancho Bernardo Study." *American Journal of Clinical Nutrition* 81 (2005): 934–38.

Wu, C.H., Y.C. Yang, W.J. Yao, et al. "Epidemiological Evidence of Increased Bone Mineral Density in Habitual Tea Drinkers." *Archives of Internal Medicine* 162 (2002): 1001–1006.

Calcium: It Is Essential

Bailey, R.L., K.W. Dodd, and J.A. Goldman. "Estimation of Total Usual Calcium and Vitamin D Intakes in the United States." *Journal of Nutrition* 140 (2010): 817–22.

Barrett-Connor, E., J.C. Chang, and S.L. Edelstein. "Coffee-Associated Osteoporosis Offset by Daily Milk Consumption. The Rancho Bernardo Study." *Journal of the American Medical Association* 271 (1994): 280–83.

Bischoff-Ferrari, H.A., B. Dawson-Hughes, J.A. Baron, et al. "Milk Intake and Risk of Hip Fracture in Men and Women: A Meta-Analysis of Prospective Cohort Studies." *Journal of Bone and Mineral Research* 26 (2011): 833–39.

Black, R.E., S.M. Williams, I.E. Jones, and A. Goulding. "Children Who Avoid Drinking Cow Milk Have Low Dietary Calcium Intakes and Poor Bone Health." *American Journal of Clinical Nutrition* 76 (2002): 675–80.

Bolland, M.J., A. Avenell, J.A. Baron, et al. "Effect of Calcium Supplements on Risk of Myocardial Infarction and Cardiovascular Events: Meta-Analysis." *British Medical Journal* 341 (2010): c3691.

Committee to Review Dietary Reference Intakes for Vitamin D and Calcium, Food and Nutrition Board, Institute of Medicine. *Dietary Reference Intakes for Calcium and Vitamin D*. Washington, DC: National Academy Press, 2010.

French, S.A., B.H. Lin, and J.F. Guthrie. "National Trends in Soft Drink Consumption among Children and Adolescents Aged 6–17 Years: Prevalence, Amounts and Sources, 1977/78 Through 1994/98." *Journal of the American Dietetic Association* 103 (2003): 1326–31.

Gonnelli, S., M.S. Campagna, A. Montagnani, et al. "Calcium Bioavailability from a New Calcium-Fortified Orange Beverage, Compared with Milk in Healthy Volunteers." *International Journal for Vitamin and Nutrition Research* 77 (2007): 249–54.

Greendale, G.A., E. Barrett-Connor, S.L. Edelstein, S. Ingles, and R. Haile. "Dietary Sodium and Bone Mineral Density: Results of a 16-Year Follow-Up Study." *Journal of the American Geriatric Society* 42 (1994): 1050–55.

Heaney, R.P., M.S. Dowell, J. Bierman, et al. "Absorbability and Cost Effectiveness in Calcium Supplementation." *Journal of the American College of Nutrition* 20 (2001): 239–46.

Huncharek, M., J. Muscat, and B. Kupelnick. "Impact of Dairy Products and Dietary Calcium on Bone-Mineral Content in Children: Results of a Meta-Analysis." *Bone* 43 (2008): 312–21.

Lanou, A.J., S.E. Berkow, and N.D. Barnard. "Calcium, Dairy Products, and Bone Health in Children and Young Adults: A Reevaluation of the Evidence." *Pediatrics* 115 (2005): 736–43.

Lewis J.R., J. Calver, K. Zhu, et al. "Calcium Supplementation and the Risks of Atherosclerotic Vascular Disease in Older Women: Results of a 5-Year RCT and a 4.5-Year Follow-Up." *Journal of Bone and Mineral Research* 26 (2011): 35–41.

Rafferty, K., R.P. Heaney, M.S. Dowell, et al. "Bioavailability of the Calcium in Fortified Soy Imitation Milk, with Some Observations on Method." *American Journal of Clinical Nutrition* 71 (2000): 1166–69.

Soroko, S., T.L. Holbrook, S.L. Edelstein, and E. Barrett-Connor. "Lifetime Milk Consumption and Bone Mineral Density in Older Women." *American Journal of Public Health* 84 (1994): 1319–22.

US Department of Agriculture and US Department of Health and Human Services. Dietary Guidelines for Americans, 2010. 7th Edition, Washington, DC: US Government Printing Office, December 2010.

Vanselow, M.S., M.A. Pereira, D. Neumark-Sztainer, and S.K. Raatz. "Adolescent Beverage Habits and Changes in Weight over Time: Findings from Project EAT." *American Journal of Clinical Nutrition* 90 (2009): 1489–95.

Weaver, C.M., W.R. Proulx, and R. Heaney. "Choices for Achieving Adequate Dietary Calcium with a Vegetarian Diet." *American Journal of Clinical Nutrition* 70 (1999): 543S–548S.

Weaver, C.M., E. Janle, B. Martin, et al. "Dairy Versus Calcium Carbonate in Promoting Peak Bone Mass and Bone Maintenance during Subsequent Calcium Deficiency." *Journal of Bone and Mineral Research* 24 (2009): 1411–19.

Whiting, S.J., A. Healey, S. Psiuka, and R. Mirwald. "Relationship between Carbonated and Other Low Nutrient Dense Beverages and Bone Mineral Content of Adolescents." *Nutrition Research* 21 (2001): 1107–1115

Winzenberg, T., K. Shaw, J. Fryer, and G. Jones. "Effects of Calcium Supplementation on Bone Density in Healthy Children: Meta-Analysis of Randomized Controlled Trials." *British Medical Journal* 333 (2006): 775.

Vitamin D: Are You Getting Enough of the Sunshine Vitamin?

Binkley, N., D. Gemar, J. Engelke, et al. "Evaluation of Ergocalciferol or Cholecalciferol Dosing, 1,600 IU Daily or 50,000 IU Monthly in Older Adults." *Journal of Clinical Endocrinology & Metabolism* 96 (2011): 981-88.

Bischoff-Ferrari, H.A. "Optimal Serum 25-Hydroxyvitamin D Levels for Multiple Health Outcomes." *Advances in Experimental Medicine and Biology* 624 (2008): 55–71.

Bischoff-Ferrari, H. A., B. Dawson-Hughes, W. C. Willett, et al. "Effect of Vitamin D on Falls: A Meta-Analysis." *Journal of the American Medical Association* 291 (2004): 1999–2006.

Bischoff-Ferrari, H.A., T. Dietrich, E.J. Orav, and B. Dawson-Hughes. "Positive Association between 25-Hydroxy Vitamin D Levels and Bone Mineral Density: A Population-Based Study of Younger and Older Adults." *American Journal of Medicine* 116 (2004): 634–39.

Bischoff-Ferrari, H.A., E. Giovannucci, W.C. Willett, et al. "Estimation of Optimal Serum Concentrations of 25-Hydroxyvitamin D for Multiple Health Outcomes." *American Journal of Clinical Nutrition* 84 (2006): 18–28.

Bisehoff-Ferrari, H.A., A. Shao, B. Dawson-Hughes, et al. "Benefit–Risk Assessment of Vitamin D Supplementation." *Osteoperosis International* 21 (2010): 1121–32

Bischoff-Ferrari, H.A., W.C. Willett, J.B. Wong, et al. "Fracture Prevention with Vitamin D Supplementation: A Meta-analysis of Randomized Controlled Trials." *Journal of the American Medical Association* 293 (2005): 2257–64.

Committee to Review Dietary Reference Intakes for Vitamin D and Calcium, Food and Nutrition Board, Institute of Medicine. *Dietary Reference Intakes for Calcium and Vitamin D*. Washington, DC: National Academy Press, 2010.

Dawson-Hughes, B., A. Mithal, J.P. Bonjour, et al. "IOF Position Statement: Vitamin D Recommendations for Older Adults." *Osteoporosis International* 21 (2010): 1151–54.

Dawson-Hughes, B., and H.A. Bischoff-Ferrari. "Therapy of Osteoporosis with Calcium and Vitamin D." *Journal of Bone and Mineral Research* 65 (2007): 501–506.

DIPART (Vitamin D Individual Patient Analysis of Randomized Trials) Group. "Patient Level Pooled Analysis of 68,500 Patients from Seven Major Vitamin D Fracture Trials in US and Europe." *British Medical Journal* 340 (2010): b5463.

Garland, C., and F. Garland. "Do Sunlight and Vitamin D Reduce the Likelihood of Colon Cancer?" *International Journal of Epidemiology* 9 (1980): 227–31.

Ginde, A.A., M.C. Liu, and C.A. Camargo Jr. "Demographic Differences and Trends in Vitamin D Insufficiency in the US Population, 1988–2004." *Archives of Internal Medicine* 169 (2009): 626–32.

Heaney, R. P., and M. F. Holick. "Why the IOM Recommendations for Vitamin D Are Deficient." *Journal of Bone and Mineral Research* 26 (2011): 455–57.

Holick, M.F. "High Prevalence of Vitamin D Inadequacy and Implications for Health." *Mayo Clinic Proceedings* 81 (2006): 353–73.

Holick, M.F. "Vitamin D Deficiency." *New England Journal of Medicine* 357 (2007): 266–81.

Holick, M.F., E.S. Siris, N. Binkley, et al. "Prevalence of Vitamin D Inadequacy among Postmenopausal North American Women Receiving Osteoporosis Therapy." *Journal of Clinical Endocrinology & Metabolism* 90 (2005): 3215–24.

Kimball, S., G.E. Fuleihan, R. Vieth, et al. "Vitamin D: A Growing Perspective." *Critical Reviews in Clinical Laboratory Sciences* 45 (2008): 339–414.

Kuchuk, N.O., S.M.F. Pluijm, N.M. van Schoor, et al. "Relationships of Serum 25-Hydroxyvitamin D to Bone Mineral Density and Serum Parathyroid Hormone and Markers of Bone Turnover in Older Persons." *Journal of Clinical Endocrinology & Metabolism* 94 (2009): 1244–50.

Kumar, J., P. Muntner, F. Kaskel, et al. "Prevalence and Associations of 25-Hydroxyvitamin D Deficiency in US Children: NHANES 2001–2004." *Pediatrics* 124 (2009): e362–70.

Levis, S., A. Gomez, C. Jimenez, et al. "Vitamin D Deficiency and Seasonal Variation in an Adult South Florida Population." *Journal of Clinical Endocrinology & Metabolism* 90 (2005): 1557–62.

Mansbach, J.M., A.A. Ginde, C.A. Camargo Jr. "Serum 25-Hydroxyvitamin D Levels among US Children Aged 1 to 11 Years: Do Children Need More Vitamin D?" *Pediatrics* 124 (2009): 1404–10.

Molgaard, C., K.F. Michaelsen. "Vitamin D and Bone Health in Early Life." *Proceedings of the Nutrition Society* 62 (2003): 823–28.

Moore, C.E., M.M. Murphy, M.F. Holick. "Vitamin D Intakes by Children and Adults in the United States Differ among Ethnic Groups." *Journal of Nutrition* 135 (2005): 2478–85.

Orwoll, E., C.M. Nielson, L.M. Marshall, et al. "Vitamin D Deficiency in Older Men." *Journal of Clinical Endocrinology & Metabolism* 94 (2009): 1214–22.

Pasco, J.A., M.J. Henry, M.A. Kotowicz, et al. "Seasonal Periodicity of Serum Vitamin D and Parathyroid Hormone, Bone Resorption, and Fractures: The Geelong Osteoporosis Study." *Journal of Bone and Mineral Research* 19 (2004): 752–58.

Reid, I. R., and A. Avenell. "Evidence-Based Policy on Dietary Calcium and Vitamin D." *Journal of Bone and Mineral Research* 26 (2011): 452–54.

Reinehr, T., G. de Sousa, U. Alexy, et al. "Vitamin D Status and Parathyroid Hormone in Obese Children before and after Weight Loss." *European Journal of Endocrinology* 157 (2007): 225–32.

Rosen, C.J., C.R. Kessenich, D. Vereault, D. Schneider, M.F. Holick, and T. Chen. "Mechanisms of Seasonal Bone Loss in Elderly Postmenopausal Women." In *Biologic Effects of Light 1995*, edited by M.F. Holick and T. Chen, 56–63. New York: Walter de Gruyer, 1996.

Souberbielle, J.C., J.J. Body, J.M. Lappe, et al. "Vitamin D and Musculoskeletal Health, Cardiovascular Disease, "Autoimmunity and Cancer: Recommendations for Clinical Practice." *Autoimmunity Reviews* 9 (2010): 709–15.

Tylavsky, F.A., K.A. Ryder, S. Cheng, et al. "Vitamin D, Parathyroid Hormone, and Bone Mass in Adolescents." *Journal of Nutrition* 135 (2005): 2735S–38S.

Ward, K.A., G. Das, J.L. Berry, et al. "Vitamin D Status and Muscle Function in Post-Menarchal Adolescent Girls." *Journal of Clinical Endocrinology & Metabolism* 94 (2009): 559–63.

Wicherts, I.S., N.M. van Schoor, A.J. Boeke, et al. "Vitamin D Status Predicts Physical Performance and Its Decline in Older Persons." *Journal of Clinical Endocrinology & Metabolism* 92 (2007): 2058–65.

PART FOUR: THERAPIES FOR PREVENTION AND TREATMEMT OF OSTEOPOROSIS

FDA-Approved Medicines: Introduction

Dawson-Hughes, B., A.C. Looker, A.N.A. Tosteson, et al. "The Potential Impact of New National Osteoporosis Foundation Guidance on Treatment Patterns." *Osteoporosis International* 21 (2010): 41–52.

Seeman, E., J. Compston, J. Adachi, et al. "Non-Compliance: The Achilles' Heel of Anti-Fracture Efficacy." *Osteoporosis International* 18 (2007): 711–19.

Silverman, S. L., and D. T. Gold. "Healthy Users, Healthy Adherers, and Healthy Behaviors?" *Journal of Bone and Mineral Research* 26 (2011): 681-82.

Fosamax (and Generic Alendronate): The First Kid on the Block

Black, D.M., A.V. Schwartz, K.E. Ensrud, et al. "Effects of Continuing or Stopping Alendronate after 5 Years of Treatment: The Fracture Intervention Trial Long-Term Extension (FLEX): A Randomized Trial." *Journal of the American Medical Association* 296 (2006): 2927–38.

Black, D.M., S.R. Cummings, D.B. Karpf, et al. "Randomized Trial of Effect of Alendronate on Risk of Fracture in Women with Existing Vertebral Fractures." *Lancet* 348 (1996): 1535–41.

Bone, H.G., D. Hosking, J.P. Devogelaer, et al. "Ten Years Experience with Alendronate for Osteoporosis in Postmenopausal Women." *New England Journal of Medicine* 350 (2004): 1189–99.

Cummings, S.R., D.M. Black, D.E. Thompson, et al. "For the Fracture Intervention Trial Research Group: Effects of Alendronate on Risk of Fracture in Women with Low Bone Density but without Vertebral Fractures." *Journal of the American Medical Association* 280 (1998): 2077–82.

Liberman, U.A., S.R. Weiss, J. Broll, et al. "Effect of Oral Alendronate on Bone Mineral Density and the Incidence of Fractures in Postmenopausal Osteoporosis." *New England Journal of Medicine* 333 (1995): 1437–43.

Ringe, J.D., A. Dorst, H. Faber, et al. "Alendronate Treatment of Established Primary Osteoporosis in Men: 3-Year Results of a Prospective, Comparative, Two-Arm Study." *Rheumatology International* 24 (2004): 110–13.

Rodan, G., A. Reszka, E. Golub, and R. Rizzoli. "Bone Safety of Long-Term Bisphosphonate Treatment." *Current Medical Research and Opinion* 20 (2004): 1291–1300.

Schnitzer, T., H.G. Bone, S. Crepaldi, et al. "Therapeutic Equivalence of Alendronate 70 mg Once Weekly and Alendronate 10 mg in the Treatment of Osteoporosis." *Aging Clinical and Experimental Research* 12 (2000): 1–12.

Schwartz, A.V., D.C. Bauer, S.R. Cummings, et al. "Efficacy of Continued Alendronate for Fractures in Women with and without Prevalent Vertebral Fracture: The FLEX Trial." *Journal of Bone and Mineral Research* 25 (2010): 976–82.

Seeman, E. "To Stop or Not to Stop, That Is the Question." *Osteoporosis International* 20 (2009): 187–95.

Wysowski, D.K., and J.T. Chang. "Alendronate and Risedronate: Reports of Severe Bone, Joint, and Muscle Pain." *Archives of Internal Medicine* 165 (2005): 346–47.

Actonel [Risedronate]: Me, Too?

Brown, J.P., D.L. Kendler, M.R. McClung, et al. "The Efficacy and Tolerability of Risedronate Once a Week For the Treatment of Postmenopausal Osteoporosis." *Calcified Tissue International* 71 (2002): 103–111.

Delmas, P., M.R. McClung, J.R. Zanchetta, et al. "Efficacy and Safety of Risedronate 150 mg Once a Month in the Treatment of Postmenopausal Osteoporosis." *Bone* 42 (2008): 36–42.

Harris, S.T., N.B. Watts, H.K. Genant, et al. "Effects of Risedronate Treatment on Vertebral and Nonvertebral Fractures in Women with Postmenopausal Osteoporosis: A Randomized Controlled Trial." *Journal of the American Medical Association* 282 (1999): 1344–52.

McClung, M.R., P. Geusens, P.D. Miller, et al. "Effect of Risedronate on the Risk of Hip Fracture in Elderly Women. Hip Intervention Program Study Group." *New England Journal of Medicine* 344 (2001): 333–40.

Mellstrom, D.D., O.H. Sorensen, S. Goemaere, et al. "Seven Years of Treatment with Risedronate in Women with Postmenopausal Osteoporosis." *Calcified Tissue International* 75 (2004): 462–68.

Reginster, J., H.W. Minne, O.H. Sorensen, et al. "Randomized Trial of the Effects of Risedronate on Vertebral Fractures in Women with Established Postmenopausal Osteoporosis." *Osteoporosis International* 11 (2000): 83–91.

Sorensen, O., G.M. Crawford, H. Mulder, et al. "Long-Term Efficacy of Risedronate: A 5-Year Placebo-Controlled Clinical Experience." *Bone* 32 (2003): 120–26.

Boniva [Ibandronate]: "The Sally Field Drug"

Chesnut, C.H. III, A. Skag, C. Christiansen, et al. "Effects of Oral Ibandronate Administered Daily or Intermittently on Fracture Risk in Postmenopausal Osteoporosis." *Journal of Bone and Mineral Research* 19 (2004): 1241–49.

Delmas, P.D., R.R. Recker, C.H. Chesnut III, et al. "Daily and Intermittent Oral Ibandronate Normalize Bone Turnover and Provide Significant Reduction in Vertebral Fracture Risk: Results From the BONE Study." *Osteoporosis International* 15 (2004): 792–98.

Eisman, J.A., R. Civitelli, S. Adami, et al. "Efficacy and Tolerability of Intravenous Ibandronate Injections in Postmenopausal Osteoporosis: 2-Year Results From the DIVA Study." *Journal of Rheumatology* 35 (2008): 488–97.

McClung, M.R., M.A. Bolognese, F. Sedarati, et al. "Efficacy and Safety of Monthly Oral Ibandronate in the Prevention of Postmenopausal Bone Loss." *Bone* 44 (2009): 418–22.

Miller, P.D., M.R. McClung, L. Macovei, et al. "Monthly Oral Ibandronate Therapy in Postmenopausal Osteoporosis: 1-Year Results from the MOBILE Study." *Journal of Bone and Mineral Research* 20 (2005): 1315–22.

Reginster, J.Y., S. Adami, P. Lakatos, et al. "Efficacy and Tolerability of Once-Monthly Oral Ibandronate in Postmenopausal Osteoporosis: 2-Year Results from the MOBILE Study." *Annals of the Rheumatic Diseases* 65 (2006): 654–61.

Stakkestad, J.A., P. Lakatos, R. Lorenc, et al. "Monthly Oral Ibandronate Is Effective and Well Tolerated after 3 Years: The MOBILE Long-Term Extension." *Clinical Rheumatology* 27 (2008): 955–60.

Reclast [Zoledronic Acid]: Just Once a Year

Black, D.M., P.D. Delmas, R. Eastell, et al. "Once-Yearly Zoledronic Acid for Treatment of Postmenopausal Osteoporosis." *New England Journal of Medicine* 356 (2007): 1809–22.

Colón-Emeric, C.S., P. Mesenbrink, K.W. Lyles, et al. "Potential Mediators of the Mortality Reduction with Zoledronic Acid after Hip Fracture." *Journal of Bone and Mineral Research* 25 (2010): 91–97.

Eriksen, E.F., K.W. Lyles, C.S. Colón-Emeric, et al. "Antifracture Efficacy and Reduction of Mortality in Relation to Timing of the First Dose of Zoledronic Acid after Hip Fracture." *Journal of Bone and Mineral Research* 24 (2009): 1308–13.

Lyles, K.W., C.S. Colón-Emeric, J.S. Magaziner, et al. "Zoledronic Acid in Reducing Clinical Fracture and Mortality after Hip Fracture." *New England Journal of Medicine* 357 (2007): 1799–1809.

Estrogens: Effects on Bone

Anderson, G.L., M. Limacher, A.R. Assaf, et al. "Effects of Conjugated Equine Estrogen in Postmenopausal Women with Hysterectomy: The Women's Health Initiative Randomized Controlled Trial." *Journal of the American Medical Association* 291 (2004): 1701–12.

Barrett-Connor, E., L.E. Wehren, E.S. Siris, et al. "Recency and Duration of Postmenopausal Hormone Therapy: Effects on Bone Mineral Density and Fracture Risk in the National Osteoporosis Risk Assessment (NORA) Study." *Menopause* 10 (2003): 412–19.

Cauley, J.A., J. Robbins, Z. Chen, et al. "Effects of Estrogen plus Progestin on Risk of Fracture and Bone Mineral Density: The Women's Health Initiative Randomized Trial." *Journal of the American Medical Association* 290 (2003): 1729–38.

Jackson, R.D., J. Wactawski-Wende, A.Z. LaCroix, et al. "Effects of Conjugated Equine Estrogen on Risk of Fractures and BMD in Postmenopausal Women with Hysterectomy: Results from the Women's Health Initiative Randomized Trial." *Journal of Bone and Mineral Research* 21 (2006): 817–28.

Lindsay, R., J.C. Gallagher, M. Kleerekoper, et al. "Effect of Lower Doses of Conjugated Equine Estrogens with and without Medroxyprogesterone Acetate on Bone in Early Postmenopausal Women." *Journal of the American Medical Association* 287 (2002): 2668–76.

Prestwood, K.M., A.M. Kenny, A. Kleppinger, et al. "Ultralow-Dose Micronized 17β-Estradiol and Bone Density and Bone Metabolism in Older Women—A Randomized Controlled Trial." *Journal of the American Medical Association* 290 (2003): 1042–48.

Rossouw, J.E., G.L. Anderson, R.L. Prentice, et al. "Risks and Benefits of Estrogen plus Progestin in Healthy Postmenopausal Women." *Journal of the American Medical Association* 288 (2002): 321–30.

Yates, J., E. Barrett-Connor, S. Barlas, et al. "Rapid Loss of Hip Fracture Protection after Estrogen Cessation: Evidence from the National Osteoporosis Risk Assessment." *Obstetrics Gynecology* 103 (2004): 440–46.

Evista [Raloxifene]: The Designer Estrogen or "SERM"

Black, L.J., M. Sato, E.R. Rowley, et al. "Raloxifene (LY139481 HCI) Prevents Bone Loss and Reduces Serum Cholesterol without Causing Uterine Hypertrophy in Ovariectomized Rats." *Journal of Clinical Investigation* 93 (1994): 63–69.

Delmas, P.D., K.E. Ensrud, J.D. Adachi, et al. "Efficacy of Raloxifene on Vertebral Fracture Risk Reduction in Postmenopausal Women with Osteoporosis: Four-Year Results from a Randomized Clinical Trial." *Journal of Clinical Endocrinology & Metabolism* 87 (2002): 3609–3617.

Ensrud, K., A.R. Genazzani, M.J. Geiger, et al. "Effect of Raloxifene on Cardiovascular Adverse Events in Postmenopausal Women with Osteoporosis." *American Journal of Cardiology* 97 (2006): 520–27.

Ensrud, K.E., J.L. Stock, E. Barrett-Connor, et al. "Fracture Risk in Postmenopausal Women: The Raloxifene Use for the Heart Trial." *Journal of Bone and Mineral Research* 23 (2008): 112–20.

Ettinger, B., D.M. Black, B.H. Mitlak, et al. "Reduction of Vertebral Fracture Risk in Postmenopausal Women with Osteoporosis Treated with Raloxifene: Results from a 3-Year Randomized Clinical Trial." *Journal of the American Medical Association* 282 (1999): 637–45.

Martino, S., J.A. Cauley, E. Barrett-Connor, et al. "Continuing Outcomes Relevant to Evista: Breast Cancer Incidence in Postmenopausal Osteoporotic Women in a Randomized Trial of Raloxifene." *Journal of the National Cancer Institute* 96 (2004): 1751–61.

Siris, E.S., S.T. Harris, E. Eastell, et al. "Skeletal Effects of Raloxifene after 8 Years: Results from the Continuing Outcomes Relevant to Evista (CORE) Study." *Journal of Bone and Mineral Research* 20 (2005): 1514–24.

Calcitonin—Miacalcin, Fortical: The Nasal Sprays

Chestnut, C.H. III, S. Silverman, A. Kim, et al. "A Randomized Trial of Nasal Spray Salmon Calcitonin in Postmenopausal Women with Established Osteoporosis: The Prevent Recurrence of Osteoporotic Fractures Study." *American Journal of Medicine* 109 (2000): 267–76.

Cummings, S. "What PROOF Proves about Calcitonin and Clinical Trials." *American Journal Medicine* 109 (2000): 330–31.

Knopp, J.A., B.M. Diner, M. Blitz, et al. "Calcitonin for Treating Acute Pain of Osteoporotic Vertebral Compression Fractures: A Systematic Review of Randomized, Controlled Trials." *Osteoporosis International* 16 (2005): 1281–90.

Overgaard, K., R. Lindsay, and C. Christiansen. "Patient Responsiveness to Calcitonin

Salmon Nasal Spray: A Subanalysis of a 2-Year Study." *Clinical Therapeutics* 17 (1995): 680–85.

Forteo [Teriparatide]: A Different Approach

Canalis, E., A. Giustina, and J.P. Bilezikian. "Mechanisms of Anabolic Therapies for Osteoporosis." *New England Journal of Medicine* 357 (2007): 905–16.

Gallagher, J.C., H.K. Genant, G.G. Crans, et al. "Teriparatide Reduces the Fracture Risk Associated with Increasing Number and Severity of Osteoporotic Fractures." *Journal of Clinical Endocrinology & Metabolism* 90 (2005): 1583–87.

Hodsman, A.B., D.C. Bauer, D.W. Dempster, et al. "Parathyroid Hormone and Teriparatide for the Treatment of Osteoporosis: A Review of the Evidence and Suggested Guidelines for Its Use." *Endocrine Review* 26 (2005): 688–703.

Jiang, Y., J.J. Zhao, B.H. Mitlak, et al. "Recombinant Human Parathyroid Hormone (1-34) [Teriparatide] Improves Both Cortical and Cancellous Bone Structure." *Journal of Bone and Mineral Research* 18 (2003): 1932–41.

Marcus, R., O. Wang, J. Satterwhite, and B. Mitlak. "The Skeletal Response to Teriparatide Is Largely Independent of Age, Initial Bone Mineral Density, and Prevalent Vertebral Fractures in Postmenopausal Women with Osteoporosis." *Journal of Bone and Mineral Research* 18 (2003): 18–23.

Neer, R.M., C.D. Arnaud, J.R. Zanchetta, et al. "Effect of Parathyroid Hormone (1–34) on Fractures and Bone Mineral Density in Postmenopausal Women with Osteoporosis." *New England Journal of Medicine* 344 (2001): 1434–41.

Tashjian, A.H. Jr, and R.F. Gagel. "Teriparatide [Human PTH(1-34)]: 2.5 Years of Experience on the Use and Safety of the Drug for the Treatment of Osteoporosis." *Journal of Bone and Mineral Research* 21 (2006): 354–65.

Prolia [Denosumab]: In a Class of Its Own

Cummings, S.R., J. Martin, M.R. McClung, et al. "Denosumab for Prevention of Fractures in Postmenopausal Women with Osteoporosis." *New England Journal of Medicine* 361 (2009): 756–65.

Eastell, R., C. Christiansen, and A. Grauer. "Effects of Denosumab on Bone Turnover Markers in Postmenopausal Osteoporosis." *Journal of Bone and Mineral Research* 26 (2011): 530–37.

Genant, H.K., K. Engelke, D.A. Hanley, et al. "Denosumab Improves Density and Strength Parameters as Measured by QCT of the Radius in Postmenopausal Women with Low Bone Mineral Density." *Bone* 47 (2010): 131–39.

Hiligsmann, M., and J. Reginster. "Potential Cost-Effectiveness of Denosumab for the Treatment of Postmenopausal Osteoporotic Women." *Bone* 47 (2010): 34–40.

Combination Therapy: Are Two Really Better than One?

Black, D.M., J.P. Bilezikian, K.E. Ensrud, et al. "One Year of Alendronate after One Year of Parathyroid Hormone (1–84) for Osteoporosis." *New England Journal of Medicine* 353 (2005): 555–65.

Cosman, F., J. Nieves, M. Zion, L. Woelfert, M. Luckey, and R. Lindsay. "Daily and Cyclic Parathyroid Hormone in Women Receiving Alendronate." *New England Journal of Medicine* 353 (2005): 566–75.

Deal, C., M. Omizo, E.N. Schwartz, et al. "Combination Teriparatide and Raloxifene Therapy for Postmenopausal Osteoporosis: Results From a 6-Month Double-Blind Placebo-Controlled Trial." *Journal of Bone and Mineral Research* 20 (2005): 1905–11.

Ettinger, B., J. San Martin, G. Crans, and I. Pavo. "Differential Effects of Teriparatide on Bone Mineral Density after Treatment with Raloxifene or Alendronate." *Journal of Bone and Mineral Research* 19 (2004): 745–51.

Greenspan, S.L., N.M. Nesnick, and R.A. Parker. "Combination Therapy with Hormone Replacement and Alendronate for Prevention of Bone Loss in Elderly Women." *Journal of the American Medical Association* 289 (2003): 2525–33.

Harris, S.T., E.F. Eriksen, M. Davidson, et al. "Effect of Combined Risedronate and Hormone Replacement Therapies on Bone Mineral Density in Postmenopausal Women." *Journal of Clinical Endocrinology & Metabolism* 86 (2001): 1890–97.

Johnell, O., W.H. Scheele, Y. Lu, et al. "Additive Effects of Raloxifene and Alendronate on Bone Density and Biochemical Markers of Bone Remodeling in Postmenopausal Women with Osteoporosis." *Journal of Clinical Endocrinology & Metabolism* 87 (2002): 985–92.

Making a Choice: How Do the Medicines Compare?

Ettinger, B., E. Barrett-Connor, L.A. Hoq, J.P. Vader, and R.W. Dubois. "When Is It Appropriate to Prescribe Postmenopausal Hormone Therapy?" *Menopause* 13 (2006): 404–410.

Off-Label Uses: What Else Is Being Treated?

Aspenberg, P., H.K. Genant, T. Johansson, et al. "Teriparatide for Acceleration of Fracture Repair in Humans: A Prospective, Randomized, Double-Blind Study of 102 Postmenopausal Women with Distal Radial Fractures." *Journal of Bone and Mineral Research* 2010: 401–14.

Knopp, J.A., B.M. Diner, M.Blitz, et al. "Calcitonin for Treating Acute Pain of Osteoporotic Vertebral Compression Fractures: A Systematic Review of Randomized, Controlled Trials." *Osteoporosis International* 16 (2005): 1281–90.

Langdahl, B.L., G. Rajzbaum, F. Jakob, et al. "Reduction in Fracture Rate and Back Pain and Increased Quality of Life in Postmenopausal Women Treated with Teriparatide: 18-Month Data from the European Forsteo Observational Study (EFOS)." *Calcified Tissue International* 85 (2009): 484–93.

Lyritis, G.P., and G. Trovas. "Analgesic Effects of Calcitonin." *Bone* 30 (2002): 71S–74S.

Nevitt, M.C., P. Chen, R.K. Dore, et al. "Reduced Risk of Back Pain Following Teriparatide Treatment: A Meta-Analysis." *Osteoporosis International* 17 (2006): 273–80.

Hot Topics: Cocktail Party Conversations

Allen, M.R. "Bisphosphonates and Osteonecrosis of the Jaw: Moving from the Bedside to the Bench." *Cells Tissues Organs* 189 (2009): 289–94.

Barrett-Connor, E., A. S. Swern, C. M. Hustad, et al. Forthcoming. "Alendronate and Atrial Fibrillation: A Meta-Analysis of Randomized Placebo-Controlled Clinical Trials." *Osteoporosis International*.

Black, D.M., M.P. Kelly, H.K. Genant, et al. "Bisphosphonates and Fractures of the Subtrochanteric or Diaphyseal Femur." *New England Journal of Medicine* 362 (2010): 1761–71.

Brookhart, M.A., J. Avorn, J.N. Katz, et al. "Gaps in Treatment among Users of Osteoporosis Medications: The Dynamics of Noncompliance." *American Journal of Medicine* 120 (2007): 251–56.

Cardwell, C.R., C.C. Abnet, M.M. Cantwell, et al. "Exposure to Oral Bisphosphonates and Risk of Esophageal Cancer." *Journal of the American Medical Association* 304 (2010): 657–63.

Curtis, J.R., A.O. Westfal, H. Cheng, et al. "Risk of Hip Fracture after Bisphosphonate Discontinuation: Implications for a Drug Holiday." *Osteoporosis International* 19 (2008): 1613–20.

Dell, R., D. Greene, S. Ott, et al. "A Retrospective Analysis of All Atypical Femur Fractures Seen in a Large California HMO from the Years 2007 to 2009." *Journal of Bone and Mineral Research* 25 (2010): S1201.

Goh, S.K., K.Y. Yang, J.S. Koh, et al. "Subtrochanteric Insufficiency Fractures in Patients on Alendronate Therapy: A Caution." *Journal Bone Joint Surgery, British volume.* 89 (2007): 349–53.

Green, J., G. Czanner, G. Reeves, et al. "Oral Bisphosphonates and Risk of Cancer of Oesophagus, Stomach, and Colorectum: Case-Control Analysis within a UK Primary Care Cohort." *British Medical Journal* 341 (2010): c4444.

Greenspan, S.L., R.D. Emkey, H.G. Bone, et al. "Significant Differential Effects of Alendronate, Estrogen, or Combination Therapy on the Rate of Bone Loss after Discontinuation of Treatment of Postmenopausal Osteoporosis: A Randomized, Double-Blind, Placebo-Controlled Trial." *Annals of Internal Medicine* 137 (2002): 875–83.

Iizuka, T., and M. Matsukawa. "Potential Excessive Suppression of Bone Turnover with Long-Term Oral Bisphosphonate Therapy in Postmenopausal Osteoporotic Patients." *Climacteric* 11 (2008): 287–95.

Khosla, S., D. Burr, J. Cauley, et al. "Bisphosphonate-Associated Osteonecrosis of the Jaw: Report of a Task Force of the American Society for Bone and Mineral Research." *Journal of Bone and Mineral Research* 22 (2007): 1479–91.

Kim, S.Y., S. Schneeweiss, J.N. Katz, et al. "Oral Bisphosphonates and Risk of Sub-trochanteric or Diaphyseal Femur Fractures in a Population-Based Cohort." *Journal of Bone and Mineral Research* 26 (2011): 993–1001.

Odvina, C.V., J.E. Zerwekh, D.S. Rao, et al. "Severely Suppressed Bone Turnover: A Potential Complication of Alendronate Therapy." *Journal of Clinical Endocrinology & Metabolism* 90 (2005): 1294–1301.

Shane, E., D. Burr, P.R. Ebeling, et al. "Atypical Subtrochanteric and Diaphyseal Femoral Fractures: Report of a Task Force of the American Society for Bone and Mineral Research." *Journal of Bone and Mineral Research* 25 (2010): 2267–94.

Sorenson, H.T., S. Christensen, F. Mehnert, et al. "Use of Bisphosphonates among Women and Risk of Atrial Fibrillation and Flutter: Population Based Case-Control Study." *British Medical Journal* 336 (2008): 813–16.

Stock, J.L., N.H. Bell, C.H. Chesnut III, et al. "Increments in Bone Mineral Density of the Lumbar Spine and Hip and Suppression of Bone Turnover Are Maintained after Discontinuation of Alendronate in Postmenopausal Women." *American Journal of Medicine* 103 (1997): 291–97.

Novel Medicines: What Is in the Pipeline?

Arey, B., R. Seethala, Z. Ma, et al. "A Novel Calcium-Sensing Receptor Antagonist Transiently Stimulates Parathyroid Hormone Secretion in Vivo." *Endocrinology* 146 (2005): 2015–22.

Bone, H.G., M.R. McClung, C. Roux, et al. "Odanacatib, A Cathepsin-K Inhibitor for Osteoporosis: A Two-Year Study in Postmenopausal Women with Low Bone Density." *Journal of Bone and Mineral Research* 25 (2010): 934–37.

Cosman, F., N.E. Lane, M.A. Bolognese, et al. "Effect of Transdermal Teriparatide Administration on Bone Mineral Density in Postmenopausal Women." *Journal of Clinical Endocrinology & Metabolism* 95 (2010): 151–58.

Paszty, C., C.H. Turner, and M.K. Robinson. "Sclerostin: A Gem from the Genome Leads to Bone-Building Antibodies." *Journal of Bone and Mineral Research* 25 (2010): 1897–1904.

Stoch, S.A., S. Zajic, J. Stone, et al. "Effect of the Cathepsin K Inhibitor Odanacatib on Bone Resorption Biomarkers in Healthy Postmenopausal Women: Two Double-Blind, Randomized, Placebo-Controlled Phase I Studies." *Clinical Pharmacology and Therapeutics* 86 (2009): 175–82.

Investigational SERMs: A Promise of an Ideal Estrogen

Cummings S.R., K. Ensrud, P.D. Delmas, et al. "PEARL Study Investigators: Lasofoxifene in Postmenopausal Women with Osteoporosis." *New England Journal of Medicine* 362 (2010): 686–96.

De Villiers, T., A. Chines, S. Palacios, et al. "Safety and Tolerability of Bazedoxifene in Postmenopausal Women with Osteoporosis: Results of a 5-Year, Randomized, Placebo-Controlled Phase 3 Trial." *Osteoporosis International* 22 (2011): 567–76.

Kharode Y., P.V.N. Bodine, C.P. Miller, et al. "The Pairing of a Selective Estrogen Receptor Modulator, Bazedoxifene, with Conjugated Estrogens as a New Paradigm for the Treatment of Menopausal Symptoms and Osteoporosis Prevention." *Endocrinology* 149 (2008): 6084–91.

Lindsay R., J.C. Gallagher, R. Kagan, et al. "Efficacy of Tissue-Selective Estrogen Complex of Bazedoxifene/Conjugated Estrogens for Osteoporosis Prevention in At-Risk Postmenopausal Women." *Fertility and Sterility* 92 (2009): 1045–52.

Lobo R.A., J.V. Pinkerton, M.L.S. Gass, et al. "Evaluation of Bazedoxifene/Conjugated Estrogens for the Treatment of Menopausal Symptoms and Effects on Metabolic Parameters and Overall Safety Profile." *Fertility and Sterility* 92 (2009): 1025–1038.

McClung, M.R., E. Siris, S. Cummings, et al. "Prevention of Bone Loss in Postmenopausal Women Treated with Lasofoxifene Compared with Raloxifene." *Menopause* 13 (2006): 377–86.

Miller, P.D., A.A. Chines, C. Christiansen, et al. "Effects of Bazedoxifene on BMD and Bone Turnover in Postmenopausal Women: 2-Yr Results of a Randomized, Double-Blind, Placebo- and Active-Controlled Study." *Journal of Bone and Mineral Research* 23 (2008): 525–35.

Silverman, S.L., C. Christiansen, H.K. Genant, et al. "Efficacy of Bazedoxifene in Reducing New Vertebral Fracture Risk in Postmenopausal Women with Osteoporosis: Results from a 3-Year, Randomized, Placebo- and Active-Controlled Clinical Trial." *Journal of Bone and Mineral Research* 23 (2008): 1923–34.

Other Medicines: Available Elsewhere But Not in the United States

Blake, G.M., and I. Fogelman. "Theoretical Model for the Interpretation of BMD Scans in Patients Stopping Strontium Ranelate Treatment." *Journal of Bone and Mineral Research* 21 (2006): 1417–24.

Blake, G.M., E.M. Lewiecki, D.L. Kendler, et al. "A Review of Strontium Ranelate and its Effect on DXA Scans." *Journal of Clinical Densitometry* 10 (2007): 113–19.

Cummings, S.R., B. Ettinger, P.D. Delmas, et al. "The Effects of Tibolone in Older Postmenopausal Women." *New England Journal of Medicine* 359 (2008): 697–708.

Meunier, P., C. Roux, S. Ortolani, et al. "Effects of Long-Term Strontium Ranelate Treatment on Vertebral Fracture Risk in Postmenopausal Women with Osteoporosis." *Osteoporosis International* 20 (2009): 1663–73

Meunier, P.J., C. Roux, E. Seeman, et al. "The Effects of Strontium Ranelate on the Risk of Vertebral Fracture in Women with Postmenopausal Osteoporosis." *New England Journal of Medicine* 350 (2004): 459–68.

Modelska, K., and S. Cummings. "Tibolone For Postmenopausal Women: Systematic Review of Randomized Trials." *Journal of Clinical Endocrinology & Metabolism* 87 (2002): 16–23.

Reginster, J.Y., E. Seeman, M.C. De Vernejoul, et al. "Strontium Ranelate Reduces the Risk of Nonvertebral Fractures in Postmenopausal Women with Osteoporosis:

Treatment of Peripheral Osteoporosis (TROPOS) Study." *Journal of Clinical Endocrinology & Metabolism* 90 (2005): 2816–22.

Fosteum: A Food Product by Prescription

Anna, R., M. Cannata, M. Atteritano, et al. "Effects of the Phytoestrogen Genistein on Hot Flushes, Endometrium, and Vaginal Epithelium in Postmenopausal Women: A 1-Year Randomized, Double-Blind, Placebo-Controlled Study." *Menopause* 14 (2007): 648–55.

Marini, H., L. Minutoli, F. Polito, et al. "Effects of the Phytoestrogen Genistein on Bone Metabolism in Osteopenic Postmenopausal Women." *Annals of Internal Medicine* (2007): 839–47.

Morabito, N., A. Crissafulli, C. Vergara, et al. "Effects of Genistein and Hormone-Replacement Therapy on Bone Loss in Early Postmenopausal Women: A Randomized Double-Blind Placebo-Controlled Study." *Journal of Bone and Mineral Research* 17 (2002): 1904–12.

Soy: Pass the Tofu?

Alekel, D.L., M.D. Van Loan, K.J. Koehler, et al. "The Soy Isoflavones for Reducing Bone Loss (SIRBL) Study: A 3-Y Randomized Controlled Trial in Postmenopausal Women." *American Journal of Clinical Nutrition* 91 (2010): 218–30.

Atkinson, C., J.E. Compston, N.E. Day, et al. "The Effects of Phytoestrogen Isoflavones on Bone Density in Women: A Double Blind, Randomised, Placebo-Controlled Trial." *American Journal of Clinical Nutrition* 79 (2004): 326–33.

Lagari, V.S., and S. Levis. "Phytoestrogens and Bone Health." *Current Opinion in Endocrinology, Diabetes, and Obesity* 17 (2010): 546–53.

Liu, J., S. Ho, Y. Su, et al. "Effect of Long-Term Intervention of Soy Isoflavones on Bone Mineral Density in Women: A Meta-Analysis of Randomized Controlled Trials." *Bone* 44 (2009): 948–53.

Ma, D., L. Qin, P. Wang, et al. "Soy Isoflavone Intake Increases Bone Mineral Density in the Spine of Menopausal Women: Meta-Analysis of Randomized Controlled Trials." *Clinical Nutrition* 27 (2008): 57–64.

Newton, K., A. LaCroix, L. Levy, et al. "Soy Protein and Bone Mineral Density in Older Men and Women: A Randomized Trial." *Maturitas* 55 (2006): 270–77.

Taku, K., M. Melby, M. Kurzer, et al. "Effects of Soy Isoflavone Supplements on Bone Turnover Markers in Menopausal Women: Systematic Review and Meta-Analysis of Randomized Controlled Trials." *Bone* 47 (2010): 413–23.

Wong, W. W., R. D. Lewis, F. M. Steinberg, et al. "Soy Isoflavone Supplementation and Bone Mineral Density in Menopausal Women: A 2-Y Multicenter Clinical Trial." *American Journal of Clinical Nutrition* 90 (2009): 1433–39.

Strontium Citrate (refer to section titled "Other Medicines")

Natural Products: Still More Questions to Be Answered

Barrett-Connor, E., D. Kritz-Silverstein, and S.L. Edelstein. "A Prospective Study of Dehydroepiandrosterone Sulfate (DHEAS) and Bone Mineral Density in Older Men and Women." *American Journal of Epidemiology* 137 (1993): 201–06.

Byard, R.W. "A Review of the Potential Forensic Significance of Traditional Herbal Medicines." *Journal of Forensic Science* 55 (2010): 89–92.

Hyun, T.H., E. Barrett-Connor, and D.B. Milne. "Zinc Intakes and Plasma Concentrations in Men with Osteoporosis: The Rancho Bernardo Study." *American Journal of Clinical Nutrition* 80 (2004): 715–21.

Lin, C., J. Sun, S. Sheu, et al. "The Effect of Chinese Medicine on Bone Cell Activities." *American Journal of Chinese Medicine* 30 (2002): 271–85.

Periera, J., J. Modesto-Filho, M. Agra, et al. "Plant and Plant-Derived Compounds Employed in Prevention of the Osteoporosis." *Acta Farmaceutica Bonaerense* 21 (2002): 223–34.

Putnam, S., A. Scutt, K. Bicknell, et al. "Natural Products as Alternative Treatments for Metabolic Bone Disorders and for Maintenance of Bone Health." *Phytotherapy Research* 21 (2007): 99–112.

Strause, L., P. Saltman, K.T. Smith, et al. "Spinal Bone Loss in Postmenopausal Women Supplemented with Calcium and Trace Minerals." *Journal of Nutrition* 124 (1994): 1060–64.

Tannenbaum, C., E. Barrett-Connor, G.A. Laughlin, and R.W. Platt. "A Longitudinal Study of Dehydroepiandrosterone Sulphate (DHEAS) Change in Older Men and Women: The Rancho Bernardo Study." *European Journal of Endocrinology* 151 (2004): 717–25.

Vestergaard, P., N.R. Jorgensen, P. Schwarz, and L. Mosekilde. "Effects of Treatment with Fluoride on Bone Mineral Density and Fracture Risk—A Meta-Analysis." *Osteoporosis International* 19 (2008): 257–68.

Yang, Q., S. Populo, J. Zhang, et al. "Effect of Angelica Sinensis on the Proliferation of Human Bone Cells." *Clinica Chimica Acta* 324 (2002): 89–97.

Vibration Therapy: Good, Good, Good, Good Vibrations

Hannan, M.T., D.M. Cheng, E. Green, et al. "Establishing the Compliance in Elderly Women for Use of a Low-Level Mechanical Stress Device in a Clinical Osteoporosis Study." *Osteoporosis International* 15 (2004): 918–26.

Judex, S., and C.T. Rubin. "Is Bone Formation Induced by High-Frequency Mechanical Signals Modulated by Muscle Activity?" *Journal of Musculoskeletal and Neuronal Interactions* 10 (2010): 3–11.

Kiiski, J., A. Heinonen, T. L. Järvinen, et al. "Transmission of Vertical Whole Body Vibration to the Human Body." *Journal of Bone and Mineral Research* 23 (2008): 1318–25.

Ozcivici, E., Y.K. Luu, B. Adler, et al. "Mechanical Signals as Anabolic Agents in Bone." *Nature Reviews Rheumatology* 6 (2010): 50–59.

Roelants, M., C. Delecluse, S. Swinnen, et al. "Effect of 6-Month Whole Body Vibration Training on Hip Density, Muscle Strength, and Postural Control in Postmenopausal Women: A Randomized Controlled Pilot Study." *Journal of Bone and Mineral Research* 19 (2004): 352–59.

Rubin, C.T., E. Capilla, Y.K. Luu, et al. "Adipogenesis Is Inhibited by Brief, Daily Exposure to High-Frequency, Extremely Low-Magnitude Mechanical Signals." *Proceedings of the National Academy of Sciences* 104 (2007): 17879–84.

Schoenau, E., and O. Fricke. "Mechanical Influences on Bone Development in Children." *European Journal of Endocrinology* 159 (2008): S27–S31.

Xie, L., J.M. Jacobson, E.S. Choi, et al. "Low-level Mechanical Vibrations Can Influence Bone Resorption and Bone Formation in the Growing Skeleton." *Bone* 39 (2006): 1059–66.

Physical Measures: Integrating Movement

Lee, M.S., M.H. Pittler, B.C. Shin, and E. Ernst. "Tai Chi for Osteoporosis: A Systematic Review." *Osteoporosis International* 19 (2008): 139–46.

Qin, L., W. Choy, K. Leung, et al. "Beneficial Effects of Regular Tai Chi Exercise on Musculoskeletal System." *Journal of Bone and Mineral Metabolism* 23 (2005): 186–90.

Ullmann, G., H.G. Williams, J. Hussey, et al. "Effects of Feldenkrais Exercises on Balance, Mobility, Balance Confidence, and Gait Performance in Community-Dwelling Adults Age 65 and Older." *Journal of Alternative and Complementary Medicine* 16 (2010): 97–105.

New Spine Fracture: Ways to Cement a Recovery

Gaitanis, I.N., A.G. Hadjipavlou, and P.G. Katonis. "Balloon Kyphoplasty for the Treatment of Pathological Vertebral Compressive Fractures." *European Spine Journal* 14 (2005): 250–60.

Grafe, I.A., K. Da Fonseca, J. Hillmeier, et al. "Reduction of Pain and Fracture Incidence after Kyphoplasty: 1-Year Outcomes of a Prospective Controlled Trial of Patients with Primary Osteoporosis." *Osteoporosis International* 16 (2005): 2005–2012.

Kallmes, D.F., B.A. Comstock, P.J. Heagerty, et al. "A Randomized Trial of Vertebroplasty for Osteoporotic Spinal Fractures." *New England Journal of Medicine* 361 (2009): 569–79.

Lindsay, R., S.L. Silverman, C. Cooper, et al. "Risk of New Vertebral Fracture in the Year Following a Fracture." *Journal of the American Medical Association* 285 (2001): 320–23.

Mehbod, A., S. Aunoble, J.C. Le Huec. "Vertebroplasty for Osteoporotic Spine Fracture: Prevention and Treatment." *European Spine Journal* 12 (2003): S155–S162.

Rohlmann, A., T. Zander, and G. Bergmann. "Spinal Loads after Osteoporotic Vertebral

Fractures Treated by Vertebroplasty or Kyphoplasty." *European Spine Journal* 15 (2006): 1255–64.

Theodorou, D.J., S.J. Theodorou, T.D. Duncan, et al. "Percutaneous Balloon Kyphoplasty for the Correction of Spinal Deformity in Painful Vertebral Body Compression Fractures." *Journal of Clinical Imaging* 26 (2002): 1–5.

Wardlaw, D., S. R. Cummings, J. Van Merhaeghe, et al. "Efficiency Safety of Balloon Kyphoplasty Compared with Nonsurgical Care for Vertebral Compression Fracture." *Lancet* 373 (2009): 1016–24.

Hip Fracture: What to Expect

Bruyere, O., N. Burlet, N. Harvey, et al. "Post-Fracture Management of Patients with Hip Fracture: A Perspective." *Current Medical Research and Opinion* 24 (2008): 2841–51.

Gehlbach, S.H., J.S. Avrunin, and E. Puleo. "Trends in Hospital Care for Hip Fractures." *Osteoporosis International* 18 (2007): 585–91.

Kaufman, J.D., M.E. Bolander, A.D. Bunta, et al. "Barriers and Solutions to Osteoporosis Care in Patients with a Hip Fracture." *Journal of Bone and Joint Surgery* 85 (2003): 1837–43.

How Do You Monitor Your Progress?

Clowes, J.A., N.F. Peel, and R. Eastell. "The Impact of Monitoring on Adherence and Persistence with Antiresorptive Treatment for Postmenopausal Osteoporosis: A Randomized Controlled Trial." *Journal of Clinical Endocrinology & Metabolism* 89 (2004): 1117–23.

Lewiecki, E.M., and N.B. Watts. "Assessing Response to Osteoporosis Therapy." *Osteoporosis International* 19 (2008): 1363–68.

Majumdar, S.R., J.A. Johnson, D.A. Lier, et al. "Persistence, Reproducibility, and Cost-Effectiveness of an Intervention to Improve the Quality of Osteoporosis Care after a Fracture of the Wrist: Results of a Controlled Trial." *Osteoporosis International* 18 (2007): 261–70.

Living and Coping with "Osteopenia" and Osteoporosis

Dawson-Hughes, B., A.C. Looker, A.N.A. Tosteson, et al. "The Potential Impact of New National Osteoporosis Foundation Guidance on Treatment Patterns." *Osteoporosis International* 21 (2010): 41–52.

Martin, A.R., E. Sornay-Rendu, J.M. Chandler, et al. "The Impact of Osteoporosis on Quality-of-Life: The Ofely Cohort." *Bone* 31 (2002): 32–36.

Siris, E.S., M. K. Pasquale, Y. Wang, and N.B. Watts. "Estimating Bisphosphonate Use and Fracture Reduction among US Women Aged 45 Years and Older, 2001–2008." *Journal of Bone and Mineral Research* 26 (2011): 3–11.

PART FIVE: THE BONE CONNECTION WITH COMMON PROBLEMS AND MEDICINES

Pregnancy and Breastfeeding

Hewison, M., and J.S. Adams. "Vitamin D Insufficiency and Skeletal Development in Utero." *Journal of Bone and Mineral Research* 25 (2010): 11–13.

Hollis, B.W., and C.L. Wagner. "Assessment of Dietary Vitamin D Requirements during Pregnancy and Lactation." *American Journal of Clinical Nutrition* 79 (2004): 717–26.

Johnson, D.D., C.L. Wagner, T.C. Hulsey, et al. "Vitamin D Deficiency and Insufficiency Is Common during Pregnancy." *American Journal of Perinatology* 28 (2011): 7–12.

Lenora, J., S. Lekamwasam, and M.K. Karlsson. "Effects of Multiparity and Prolonged Breast-Feeding on Maternal Bone Mineral Density: A Community-Based Cross-Sectional Study." *BioMed Central Women's Health* 9 (2009): 19.

Merewood, A., S.D. Mehta, X. Grossman, et al. "Widespread Vitamin D Deficiency in Urban Massachusetts Newborns and Their Mothers." *Pediatrics* 125 (2010): 640–47.

Naylor, K.E., P. Iqbal, C. Fledelius, et al. "The Effect of Pregnancy on Bone Density and Bone Turnover." *Journal of Bone and Mineral Research* 15 (2000): 129–37.

Pawley, N., and N.J. Bishop. "Prenatal and Infant Predictors of Bone Health: The Influence of Vitamin D." *American Journal of Clinical Nutrition* 80 (2004): 1748S–51S.

Perrine, C.G., A.J. Sharma, M.E.D. Jefferds, et al. "Adherence to Vitamin D Recommendations among US Infants." *Pediatrics* 125 (2010): 627–32.

Taylor, S.N., C.L. Wagner, and B.W. Hollis. "Vitamin D Supplementation During Lactation to Support Infant and Mother." *Journal of the American College of Nutrition* 27 (2008): 690–701.

Thomson, K., R. Morley, S.R. Grover, et al. "Postnatal Evaluation of Vitamin D and Bone Health in Women Who Were Vitamin D-Deficient in Pregnancy, and in Their Infants." *Medical Journal of Australia* 181 (2004): 486–88.

Wagner, C.L., C. Howard, T.C. Hulsey, et al. "Circulating 25-Hydroxyvitamin D Levels in Fully Breastfed Infants on Oral Vitamin D Supplementation." *International Journal of Endocrinology* (January 2010): 1–5. http://downloads.hindawi.com/journals/ije/2010/235035.pdf.

Premenopausal Women

Cohen, A., X.S. Liu, E.M. Stein, et al. "Bone Microarchitecture and Stiffness in Premenopausal Women with Idiopathic Osteoporosis." *Journal of Clinical Endocrinology & Metabolism* 94 (2009): 4351–60.

Donovan, M.A., D. Dempster, H. Zhou, et al. "Low Bone Formation in Premenopausal Women with Idiopathic Osteoporosis." *Journal of Clinical Endocrinology & Metabolism* 90 (2005): 3331–36.

Khan, A. "Premenopausal Women and Low Bone Density." *Canadian Family Physician* 52 (2006): 743–47.

Leib, E.S. "Treatment of Low Bone Mass in Premenopausal Women: When May It Be Appropriate?" *Current Osteoporosis Reports* 3 (2005): 13–18.

Rubin, M.R., D.H. Schussheim, E.S. Kurland, et al. "Idiopathic Osteoporosis in Premenopausal Women." *Osteoporosis International* 16 (2005): 526–33.

Birth Control: Pills and Shots

Beksinska, M.E., I. Kleinschmidt, J.A. Smit, et al. "Bone Mineral Density in Adolescents Using Norethisterone Enanthate, Depot-Medroxyprogesterone Acetate, or Combined Oral Contraceptives for Contraception." *Contraception* 75 (2007): 438–43.

Cromer, B.A., M. Stager, A. Bonny, et al. "Depot Medroxyprogesterone Acetate, Oral Contraceptives, and Bone Mineral Density in a Cohort of Adolescent Girls." *Journal of Adolescent Health* 35 (2004): 434–41.

Gambacciani, M., B. Cappagli, V. Lazzarini, et al. "Longitudinal Evaluation of Perimenopausal Bone Loss: Effects of Different Low Dose Oral Contraceptive Preparations on Bone Mineral Density." *Maturitas* 54 (2006): 176–80.

Hartard, M., C. Kleinmond, M. Wiseman, et al. "Detrimental Effect of Oral Contraceptives on Parameters of Bone Mass and Geometry in a Cohort of 248 Young Women." *Bone* 40 (2007): 444–50.

Kuohung, W., L. Borgatta, and P. Stubblefield. "Low-Dose Oral Contraceptives and Bone Mineral Density: An Evidence-Based Analysis." *Contraception* 61 (2000): 77–82.

Nappi, C., A. Di Spiezio Sardo, G. Acunzo, et al. "Effects of a Low-Dose and Ultra-Low-Dose Combined Oral Contraceptive Use on Bone Turnover and Bone Mineral Density in Young Fertile Women: A Prospective Controlled Randomized Study." *Contraception* 67 (2003): 355–59.

Reed, S.D., D. Scholes, A.Z. LaCroix, et al. "Longitudinal Changes in Bone Density in Relation to Oral Contraceptive Use." *Contraception* 68 (2003): 177–82.

Menstrual Problems: No Periods and Endometriosis

Chlouber, R.O., D.L. Olive, and E.A. Pritts. "Investigational Drugs for Endometriosis." *Expert Opinion on Investigational Drugs* 15 (2006): 399–407.

Devleta, B., B. Adem, and S. Senada. "Hypergonadotropic Amenorrhea and Bone Density: New Approach to an Old Problem." *Journal of Bone and Mineral Metabolism* 22 (2004): 360–64.

Lawson, E.A., D. Donoho, K.K. Miller, et al. "Hypercortisolemia Is Associated with Severity of Bone Loss and Depression in Hypothalamic Amenorrhea and Anorexia Nervosa." *Journal of Clinical Endocrinology and Metabolism.* 94 (2009): 4710–16.

Olive, D.L., S.R. Lindheim, and E.A. Pritts. "New Medical Treatments for Endometriosis." *Best Practice & Research Clinical Obstetrics and Gynaecology* 18 (2004): 319–28.

Wiksten-Almströmer, M., A.L. Hirschberg, and K. Hagenfeldt. "Reduced Bone Mineral Density in Adult Women Diagnosed with Menstrual Disorders During Adolescence." *Acta Obstetricia et Gynecologica* 88 (2009): 543–49.

Eating Disorders: Anorexia and Bulimia

Ecklund, K., S. Vajapeyam, H.A. Feldman, et al. "Bone Marrow Changes in Adolescent Girls with Anorexia Nervosa." *Journal of Bone and Mineral Research* 25: 298–304.

Fenichel, R.M., and M.P. Warren. "Anorexia, Bulimia, and the Athletic Triad: Evaluation and Management." *Current Osteoporosis Reports* 5 (2007): 160–64.

Golden, N.H., E.A. Iglesias, M.S. Jacobson, et al. "Alendronate for the Treatment of Osteopenia in Anorexia Nervosa: A Randomized, Double-Blind, Placebo-Controlled Trial." *Journal of Clinical Endocrinology & Metabolism* 90 (2005): 3179–85.

Konstantynowicz, J., H. Kadziela-Olech, M. Kaczmarski, et al. "Depression in Anorexia Nervosa: A Risk Factor for Osteoporosis." *Journal of Clinical Endocrinology & Metabolism* 90 (2005): 5382–85.

Legroux-Gérot, I., J. Vignau, M. D'Herbomez, et al. "Evaluation of Bone Loss and Its Mechanisms in Anorexia Nervosa." *Calcified Tissue International* 81 (2007): 174–82.

Lucas, A.R., L.J. Melton, C.S. Crowson, et al. "Long-Term Fracture Risk among Women with Anorexia Nervosa: A Population-Based Cohort Study." *Mayo Clinic Proceedings* 74 (1999): 972–77.

Mehler, P.S., and T.D. MacKenzie. "Treatment of Osteopenia and Osteoporosis in Anorexia Nervosa: A Systematic Review of the Literature." *International Journal of Eating Disorders* 42 (2009): 195–201.

Miller, K.K., E.E. Lee, E.A. Lawson, et al. "Determinants of Skeletal Loss and Recovery in Anorexia Nervosa." *Journal of Clinical Endocrinology & Metabolism* 91 (2006): 2931–37.

Misra, M., D.K. Katzman, J. Cord, et al. "Bone Metabolism in Adolescent Boys with Anorexia Nervosa." *Journal of Clinical Endocrinology and Metabolism* 93 (2008): 3029–36.

Misra, M., and A. Klibanski. "Anorexia Nervosa and Osteoporosis." *Reviews in Endocrine and Metabolic Disorders* 7 (2006): 91–99.

Intestinal Problems: Celiac Disease and Inflammatory Bowel Disease

Ali, T., D. Lam, M.S. Bronze, and M.B. Humphrey. "Osteoporosis in Inflammatory Bowel Disease." *American Journal of Medicine* 122 (2009): 599–604.

American Gastroenterological Association. "American Gastroenterological Association Medical Position Statement: Guidelines on Osteoporosis in Gastrointestinal Diseases." *Gastroenterology* 124 (2003): 791–94.

Bernstein, C.N. "Inflammatory Bowel Diseases as Secondary Causes of Osteoporosis." *Current Osteoporosis Reports* 4 (2006): 116–23.

Hardy, R., and M.S. Cooper. "Bone Loss in Inflammatory Disorders." *Journal of Endocrinology* 201 (2009): 309–20.

Sinnott, B.P., and A.A. Licata. "Assessment of Bone and Mineral Metabolism in Inflammatory Bowel Disease: Case Series and Review." *Endocrine Practice* 12 (2006): 622–29.

Thyroid Problems

Auer, J., P. Scheibner, T. Mische, et al. "Subclinical Hyperthyroidism as a Risk Factor for Atrial Fibrillation." *American Heart Journal* 142 (2001): 838–42.

Bauer, D.C., B. Ettinger, M.C. Nevitt, et al. "Risk for Fracture in Women with Low Serum Levels of Thyroid-Stimulating Hormone. *Annals of Internal Medicine* 134 (2001): 561–68.

Boyde, A., P.J. O'Shea, S. Sriskantharajah, et al. "Thyroid Hormone Excess Rather than Thyrotropin Deficiency Induces Osteoporosis in Hyperthyroidism." *Molecular Endocrinology* 21 (2007): 1095–1107.

Lakatos, P. "Thyroid Hormones: Beneficial or Deleterious for Bone?" *Calcified Tissue International* 73 (2003): 205–09.

Schneider D.L., E.L. Barrett-Connor, and D.J. Morton. "Thyroid Hormone Use and Bone Mineral Density in Elderly Women: Effects of Estrogen." *Journal of the American Medical Association* 271 (1994): 1245–49.

Schneider, D.L., E.L. Barrett-Connor, and D.J. Morton. "Thyroid Hormone Use and Bone Mineral Density in Elderly Men." *Archives of Internal Medicine* 155 (1995): 2005–2007.

Svare, A., T.L. Nilsen, S. Forsmo, et al. "Hyperthyroid Levels of TSH Correlate with Low Bone Mineral Density: The HUNT 2 Study." *European Journal of Endocrinology* 161 (2009): 779–86.

Turner, M.R., X. Camacho, H.D. Fischer, et al. "Levothyroxine Dose and Risk of Fractures in Older Adults: Nested Case-Control Study." *British Medical Journal* 342 (2011): d2238.

Weight Loss, Including Surgery for Weight Loss (Gastric Bypass)

Carlin, A.M., D.S. Rao, A.M. Meslemani, et. al. "Prevalence of Vitamin D Depletion among Morbidly Obese Patients Seeking Gastric Bypass Surgery." *Surgery for Obesity and Related Diseases* 2 (2006): 98–103.

Carrasco, F., M. Ruz, P. Rojas, et al. "Changes in Bone Mineral Density, Body Composition, and Adiponectin Levels in Morbidly Obese Patients after Bariatric Surgery." *Obesity Surgery* 19 (2009): 41–46.

Holbrook, T.L., and E. Barrett-Connor. "The Association of Lifetime Weight and Weight Control Patterns with Bone Mineral Density in an Adult Community." *Bone Mineral* 20 (1993): 141–49.

Salamone, L.M., J.A. Cauley, D.M. Black, et al. "Effect of a Lifestyle Intervention on

Bone Mineral Density in Premenopausal Women: A Randomized Trail." *American Journal of Clinical Nutrition* 70 (1999): 97–103.

Vilarrasa, N., J.M. Gómez, I. Elio, et al. "Evaluation of Bone Disease in Morbidly Obese Women after Gastric Bypass and Risk Factors Implicated in Bone Loss." *Obesity Surgery* 19 (2009): 860–66.

Steroid Use: Prednisone

Curtis, J.R., A.O. Westfall, J.J. Allison, et al. "Longitudinal Patterns in the Prevention of Osteoporosis in Glucocorticoid-Treated Patients." *Arthritis and Rheumatism* 52 (2005): 2485–94.

Ferguson, G.T., P.M.A. Calverley, J.A. Anderson, et al. "Prevalence and Progression of Osteoporosis in Patients with COPD: Results from the Towards a Revolution in COPD Health Study." *Chest* 136 (2009): 1456–65.

Gonnelli, S., C. Caffarelli, S. Maggi, et al. "Effect of Inhaled Glucocorticoids and 2 Agonists on Vertebral Fracture Risk in COPD Patients: The EOLO Study." *Calcified Tissue International* 87 (2010): 137–43.

Grossman, J.M., R. Gordon, V.K. Ranganath, et al. "American College of Rheumatology 2010 Recommendations for the Prevention and Treatment of Glucocorticoid-Induced Osteoporosis." *Arthritis Care & Research* 62 (2010): 1515–26.

Licata, A.A. "Systemic Effects of Fluticasone Nasal Spray: Report of 2 Cases." *Endocrine Practice* 11 (2005): 194–96.

Marystone, J.F., E.L. Barrett-Connor, and D.J. Morton. "Inhaled and Oral Corticosteroids: Their Effect on Bone Mineral Density in Older Adults." *American Journal of Public Health* 85 (1995): 1693–95.

Ramsey-Goldman, R. "Missed Opportunities in Physician Management of Glucocorticoid-Induced Osteoporosis?" *Arthritis and Rheumatism* 46 (2002): 3115–20.

Rehman, Q., and N.E. Lane. "Effect of Glucocorticoids on Bone Density." *Medical and Pediatric Oncology* 41 (2003): 212–16.

Reid, D.M., J.P. Devogelaer, K. Saag, et al. "Zoledronic Acid and Risedronate in the Prevention and Treatment of Glucocorticoid-Induced Osteoporosis (HORIZON): A Multicentre, Double-Blind, Double-Dummy, Randomized Controlled Trial." *Lancet* 373 (2009): 1253–63.

Saag, K.G., E. Shane, S. Boonen, et al. "Teriparatide or Alendronate in Glucocorticoid-Induced Osteoporosis." *New England Journal of Medicine* 357 (2007): 2028–39.

Saag, K.G., R. Emkey, T.J. Schnitzer, et al. "Alendronate for the Prevention and Treatment of Glucocorticoid-Induced Osteoporosis." *New England Journal of Medicine* 339 (1998): 292–99.

Sambrook, P.N. "Glucocorticoid-Induced Osteoporosis." *International Journal of Rheumatic Diseases* 11 (2008): 381–85.

Van Staa, T.P., H.G.M. Leufkens, L. Abenhaim, et al. "Use of Oral Corticosteroids and Risk of Fractures." *Journal of Bone and Mineral Research* 15 (2000): 993–1000.

Rheumatoid Arthritis

Cohen, S.B., R.K. Dore, N.E. Lane, et al. "Denosumab Treatment Effects on Structural Damage, Bone Mineral Density, and Bone Turnover in Rheumatoid Arthritis." *Arthritis and Rheumatism* 58 (2008): 1299–309.

Dolan, A.L., C. Moniz, H. Abraha, et al. "Does Active Treatment of Rheumatoid Arthritis Limit Disease-Associated Bone Loss?" *Rheumatology* 41 (2002): 1047–51.

Lodder, M.C., Z. de Jong, P.J. Kostense, et al. "Bone Mineral Density in Patients with Rheumatoid Arthritis: Relation between Disease Severity and Low Bone Mineral Density." *Annals of the Rheumatic Diseases* 63 (2004): 1576–80.

Phillips, K., A. Aliprantis, and J. Coblyn. "Strategies for the Prevention and Treatment of Osteoporosis in Patients with Rheumatoid Arthritis." *Drugs and Aging* 23 (2006): 773–79.

Schett, G., S. Hayer, J. Zwerina, et al. "Mechanisms of Disease: The Link Between RANKL and Arthritic Bone Disease." *Nature Clinical Practice Rheumatology* 1 (2005): 47–54.

Diabetes

Ahmed, L.A., R.M. Joakimsen, G.K. Berntsen, et al. "Diabetes Mellitus and the Risk of Non-Vertebral Fractures: The Tromsø Study." *Osteoporosis International* 17 (2006): 495–500.

Kahn, S.E., B. Zinman, J.M. Lachin, et al. "Rosiglitazone-Associated Fractures in Type 2 Diabetes: An Analysis from a Diabetes Outcome Progression Trial (ADOPT)." *Diabetes Care* 31 (2008): 845–51.

Kahn, S. E., S. M. Haffner, M. A. Heise, et al. "Glycemic Durability of Rosiglitazone, Metformin, or Glyburide Monotherapy." *New England Journal of Medicine* 355 (2006): 2427–43

Lazarenko, O.P., S.O. Rzonca, W.R. Hogue, et al. "Rosiglitazone Induces Decreases in Bone Mass and Strength That Are Reminiscent of Aged Bone." *Endocrinology* 148 (2007): 2669–80.

Loke, Y.K., S. Singh, and C.D. Furberg. "Long-Term Use of Thiazolidinediones and Fractures in Type 2 Diabetes: A Meta-Analysis." *Canadian Medical Association Journal* 180 (2009): 32–39.

Moyer-Mileur, L.J., H. Slater, K.C. Jordan, and M.A. Murray. "IGF-1 and IGF-Binding Proteins and Bone Mass, Geometry, and Strength: Relation to Metabolic Control in Adolescent Girls with Type 1 Diabetes." *Journal of Bone and Mineral Research* 23 (2008): 1884–91.

Räkel, A., O. Sheehy, E. Rahme, et al. "Osteoporosis among Patients with Type 1 and Type 2 Diabetes." *Diabetes & Metabolism* 34 (2008): 193–205.

Rosen, C.J. "Sugar and Bone: A Not-So Sweet Story." *Journal of Bone and Mineral Research* 23 (2008): 1881–83.

Rzonca S.O., L.J. Suva, D. Gaddy, et al. "Bone Is a Target for the Antidiabetic Compound Rosiglitazone." *Endocrinology* 145 (2004): 401–406.

Schwartz, A.V., D.E. Sellmeyer, E.S. Strotmeyer, et al. "Diabetes and Bone Loss at the Hip in Older Black and White Adults." *Journal of Bone and Mineral Research* 20 (2005): 596–603.

Shockley, K.R., O.P. Lazarenko, P.J. Czernik, et al. "PPAR 2 Nuclear Receptor Controls Multiple Regulatory Pathways of Osteoblast Differentiation from Marrow Mesenchymal Stem Cells." *Journal of Cellular Biochemistry* 106 (2009): 232–46.

Vestergaard, P. "Discrepancies in Bone Mineral Density and Fracture Risk in Patients with Type 1 and Type 2 Diabetes—A Meta-Analysis." *Osteoporosis International* 18 (2007): 427–44.

Yamamoto, M., T. Yamaguchi, M. Yamauchi, et al. "Diabetic Patients Have an Increased Risk of Vertebral Fractures Independent of BMD or Diabetic Complications." *Journal of Bone and Mineral Research* 24 (2009): 702–709.

Zinman, B., S. M. Haffner, W. H. Herman, et al. "Effect of Rosiglitazone, Metformin, and Glyburide on Bone Biomarkers in Patients with Type 2 Diabetes." *Journal of Clinical Endocrinology & Metabolism* 95 (2010): 134–42.

Heartburn and Reflux: "GERD"

Abrahamsen, B., P. Eiken, and R. Eastell. "Proton Pump Inhibitor Use and the Antifracture Efficacy of Alendronate." *Archives of Internal Medicine* (2011). Published online February 14, 2011. doi:10.1001/archinternmed.2011.20.

Coté, G.A., and C.W. Howden. "Potential Adverse Effects of Proton Pump Inhibitors." *Current Gastroenterology Reports* 10 (2008): 208–14.

Fournier, M.R., L.E. Targownik, and W.D. Leslie. "Proton Pump Inhibitors, Osteoporosis, and Osteoporosis-Related Fractures." *Maturitas* 64 (2009): 9–13.

Gray, S.L., A.Z. LaCroix, J. Larson, et al. "Proton Pump Inhibitor Use, Hip Fracture, and Change in Bone Mineral Density in Postmenopausal Women: Results from the Women's Health Initiative." *Archives of Internal Medicine* 170 (2010): 765–71.

Katz, M.H. "Failing the Acid Test: Benefits of Proton Pump Inhibitors May Not Justify the Risks for Many Users." *Archives of Internal Medicine* 170 (2010): 747–48.

Sipponen, P., and M. Harkonen. "Hypochlorhydric Stomach: A Risk Condition for Calcium Malabsorption and Osteoporosis?" *Scandinavian Journal of Gastroenterology* 45 (2010): 133–38.

Yu, E.W., T. Blackwell, K.E. Ensrud, et al. "Acid-Suppressive Medications and Risk of Bone Loss and Fracture in Older Adults." *Calcified Tissue International* 83 (2008): 251–59.

Depression

Diem, S.J., T.L. Blackwell, K.L. Stone, et al. "Use of Antidepressants and Rates of Hip Bone Loss in Older Women: The Study of Osteoporotic Fractures." *Archives of Internal Medicine* 167 (2007): 1240–45.

Haney, E.M., B.K. Chan, S.J. Diem, et al. "Association of Low Bone Mineral Density with Selective Serotonin Reuptake Inhibitor Use by Older Men." *Archives Internal Medicine* 167 (2007): 1246–51.

Haney, E. M., S. J. Warden, and M. M. Bliziotes. "Effects of Selective Serotonin Reuptake Inhibitors on Bone Health in Adults: Time for Recommendations about Screening, Prevention and Management?" *Bone* 46 (2010): 13–17.

Mezuk, B., W.W. Eaton, and S.H. Golden. "Depression and Osteoporosis: Epidemiology and Potential Mediating Pathways." *Osteoporosis International* 19 (2008): 1–12.

Mussolino, M.E., B.S. Jonas, and A.C. Looker. "Depression and Bone Mineral Density in Young Adults: Results from NHANES III." *Psychosomatic Medicine* 66 (2004): 533–37.

Richards, J.B., A. Papaioannou, J.D. Adachi, et al. "Effect of Selective Serotonin Reuptake Inhibitors on the Risk of Fracture." *Archives of Internal Medicine* 167 (2007): 188–94.

Robbins, J., C. Hirsch, R. Whitmer, et al. "The Association of Bone Mineral Density and Depression in an Older Population." *Journal of the American Geriatrics Society* 49 (2001): 732–36.

Rosen, C.J. "Serotonin Rising–the Bone, Brain, Bowel Connection." *New England Journal of Medicine* 360 (2009): 957–59.

Vestergaard, P., L. Rejnmark, and L. Mosekilde. "Selective Serotonin Reuptake Inhibitors and Other Antidepressants and Risk of Fracture." *Calcified Tissue International* 82 (2008): 92–101.

Westbroek, I., A. Van der Plas, K. de Rooij, et al. "Expression of Serotonin Receptors in Bone." *Journal of Biological Chemistry* 276 (2001): 28961–68.

Yadav, V.K., J.H. Ryu, N. Suda, et al. "Lrp5 Controls Bone Formation by Inhibiting Serotonin Synthesis in the Duodenum." *Cell* 135 (2008): 825–37.

Yirmiya, R., and I. Bab. "Major Depression Is a Risk Factor for Low Bone Mineral Density: A Meta-Analysis." *Biological Psychiatry* 66 (2009): 423–32.

Breast Cancer

Brufsky, A., A. Bundred, R. Coleman, et al. "Integrated Analysis of Zoledronic Acid for Prevention of Aromatase Inhibitor–Associated Bone Loss in Postmenopausal Women with Early Breast Cancer Receiving Adjuvant Letrozole." *Oncologist* 13 (2008): 503–14.

Bundred, N.J., I.D. Campbell, N. Davidson, et al. "Effective Inhibition of Aromatase Inhibitor–Associated Bone Loss by Zoledronic Acid in Postmenopausal Women with Early Breast Cancer Receiving Adjuvant Letrozole." *Cancer* 112 (2008): 1001–1010.

Chlebowski, R.T., Z. Chen, J.A. Cauley, et al. "Oral Bisphosphonate Use and Breast Cancer Incidence in Postmenopausal Women." *Journal of Clinical Oncology* 28 (2010): 3582–90.

Coleman, R.E., J. Body, J.R. Gralow, et al. "Bone Loss in Patients with Breast Cancer Receiving Aromatase Inhibitors and Associated Treatment Strategies." *Cancer Treatment Reviews* 34 (2008): S31–S42.

Diel, I.J., E.F. Solomayar, S.D. Costa, et al. "Reduction in New Metastases in Breast

Cancer with Adjuvant Clodronate Treatment." *New England Journal of Medicine* 339 (1998): 357–63.

Eidtmann, H., R. DeBoer, N. Bundred, et al. "Efficacy of Zoledronic Acid in Postmenopausal Women with Early Breast Cancer Receiving Adjuvant Letrozole: 36-Month Results of the ZO-FAST Study." *Annals of Oncology* 21 (2010): 2188–94.

Ellis, G.K., H.G. Bone, R. Chlebowski, et al. "Randomized Trial of Denosumab in Patients Receiving Adjuvant Aromatase Inhibitors for Nonmetastatic Breast Cancer." *Journal of Clinical Oncology* 26 (2008): 4875–82.

Fromigue, O., N. Kheddoumi, and J.J. Body. "Bisphosphonates Antagonize Bone Growth Factors' Effects on Human Breast Cancer Cells Survival." *British Journal of Cancer* 89 (2003): 178–84.

Gnant, M., and H. Eidtmann. "The Anti-Tumor Effect of Bisphosphonates ABCSG-12, ZO-FAST and More." *Critical Reviews in Oncology/Hematology* 74, Supplement 1 (2010): S2–S6.

Gnant, M., B. Mlineritsch, W. Schippinger, et al. "Endocrine Therapy Plus Zoledronic Acid in Premenopausal Breast Cancer." *New England Journal of Medicine* 360 (2009): 679–91.

Hadji, P., J.J. Body, M.S. Aapro, et al. "Practical Guidance for the Management of Aromatase Inhibitor–Associated Bone Loss." *Annals of Oncology* 19 (2008): 1407–16.

Hillner, B., J. Ingle, R.T. Chlebowski, et al. "American Society of Clinical Oncology 2003 Update on the Role of Bisphosphonates and Bone Health Issues in Women with Breast Cancer." *Journal of Clinical Oncology* 21 (2003): 4042–57.

Hines, S.L., B. A. Mincey, J.A. Sloan, et al. "Phase III Randomized, Placebo-Controlled, Double-Blind Trial of Risedronate for the Prevention of Bone Loss in Premenopausal Women Undergoing Chemotherapy for Primary Breast Cancer." *Journal of Clinical Oncology* 27 (2009): 1047–53.

Hortobagyi, G.N., R.L. Theriault, A. Lipton, et al. "Long-Term Prevention of Skeletal Complications of Metastatic Breast Cancer with Pamidronate: Protocol 19 Aredia Breast Cancer Study Group." *Journal of Clinical Oncology* 16 (1998): 2038–44.

Jones, D.H., T. Nakashima, O.H. Sanchez, et al. "Regulation of Cancer Cell Migration and Bone Metastasis by RANKL." *Nature* 440 (2006): 692–96.

Kritz-Silverstein, D., D.L. Schneider, and J. Sandwell. "Breast Cancer and Bone Mass in Older Women: Is Bone Density Prescreening for Mammography Useful?" *Osetoporosis International* 17 (2006): 1196–1206

Lester, J., D. Dodwell, E. McCloskey, et al. "The Causes and Treatment of Bone Loss Associated with Carcinoma of the Breast." *Cancer Treatment Reviews* 31 (2005): 115–42.

Mundy, G.R. "Metastasis to Bone: Causes, Consequences, and Therapeutic Opportunities." *Nature Reviews Cancer* 2 (2002): 584–93.

Ooi, L.L., Y. Zheng, K. Stalgis-Bilinski, and C.R. Dunstan. "The Bone Remodeling Environment Is a Factor in Breast Cancer Bone Metastasis." *Bone* 48 (2011): 66–70.

Stopeck, A.T., A. Lipton, J.J. Body, et al. "Denosumab Compared with Zoledronic Acid for the Treatment of Bone Metastases in Patients with Advanced Breast Cancer: A Randomized, Double-Blind Study." *Journal of Clinical Oncology* 28 (2010): 5132–39.

Van Poznak, C., R. A. Hannon, J. R. Mackey, et al. "Prevention of Aromatase Inhibitor–Induced Bone Loss Using Risedronate: The Sabre Trial." *Journal of Clinical Oncology* 28 (2010): 967–75.

Prostate Cancer

Aapro, M., P.A. Abrahamsson, J.J. Body, et al. "Guidance on the Use of Bisphosphonates in Solid Tumours: Recommendations of an International Expert Panel." *Annals of Oncology* 19 (2008): 420–32.

Brown, J.E., C.S. Thomson, S.P. Ellis, et al. "Bone Resorption Predicts for Skeletal Complications in Metastatic Bone Disease." *British Journal of Cancer* 89 (2003): 2031–37.

Brown, J.E., R.J. Cook, P. Major, et al. "Bone Turnover Markers as Predictors of Skeletal Complications in Prostate Cancer, Lung Cancer, and Other Solid Tumors." *Journal of the National Cancer Institute* 97 (2005): 59–69.

Brunder, J.M., J.Z. Ma, J.W. Basler, et al. "Prevalence of Osteopenia and Osteoporosis by Central and Peripheral Bone Mineral Density in Men with Prostate Cancer during Androgen-Deprivation Therapy." *Urology* 67 (2006): 152–55.

Fizazi, K., M. Carducci, M. Smith, et al. "Denosumab versus Zoledronic Acid for Treatment of Bone Metastases in Men with Castration-Resistant Prostate Cancer: A Randomized, Double-Blind Study." *Lancet* 377 (2011): 813–22.

Preston, D.M., P. Harding, R.S. Howard, et al. "Androgen Deprivation in Men with Prostate Cancer Is Associated with an Increased Rate of Bone Loss." *Prostate Cancer and Prostatic Diseases* 5 (2002): 304–10.

Saad, F., C.S. Higano, O. Sartor, et al. "The Role of Bisphosphonates in the Treatment of Prostate Cancer: Recommendations from an Expert Panel." *Clinical Genitourinary Cancer* 4 (2006): 257–62.

Shahinian, V.B., Y.F. Kuo, J.L. Freeman, and J.S. Goodwin. "Risk of Fracture after Androgen Deprivation for Prostate Cancer." *New England Journal of Medicine* 352 (2005): 154–56.

Smith, M.R., B. Egerdie, N.H. Toriz, et al. "Denosumab in Men Receiving Androgen-Deprivation Therapy for Prostate Cancer." *New England Journal of Medicine* 361 (2009): 745–55.

Smith, M.R., F.J. McGovern, A.L. Zietman, et al. "Pamidronate to Prevent Bone Loss during Androgen-Deprivation Therapy for Prostate Cancer." *New England Journal of Medicine* 345 (2001): 948–55.

Smith, M.R., J. Eastham, D.M. Gleason, et al. "Randomized Controlled Trial of Zoledronic Acid to Prevent Bone Loss in Men Receiving Androgen Deprivation Therapy for Nonmetastatic Prostate Cancer." *Journal of Urology* 169 (2003): 2008–2012.

Srinivas, S., I. Perkash, M.K. Terris, et al. "Progressive Decrease in Bone Density over 10 Years of Androgen Deprivation Therapy in Patients with Prostate Cancer." *Urology* 57 (2001): 127–32.

Long-Term Care Setting: Assisted Living and Nursing Facilities

Bischoff-Ferrari, H.A., B. Dawson-Hughes, A. Platz, et al. "Effect of High-Dosage Cholecalciferol and Extended Physiotherapy on Complications after Hip Fracture: A Randomized Controlled Trial." *Archives of Internal Medicine* 170 (2010): 813–20.

Cameron, I.D., and S. Kurrle. "Preventing Falls in Elderly People Living in Hospitals and Care Homes." *British Medical Journal* 334 (2007): 53–54.

Chandler, J.M., S.I. Zimmerman, C. J. Girman, et al. "Low Bone Mineral Density and Risk of Fracture in White Female Nursing Home Residents." *Journal of the American Medical Association* 284 (2000): 972–77.

Colón-Emeric, C., K.W. Lyles, D.A. Levine, et al. "Prevalence and Predictors of Osteoporosis Treatment in Nursing Home Residents with Known Osteoporosis or Recent Fracture." *Osteoporosis International* 18 (2007): 553–59.

Davis, G.C., T.L. White, and A. Yang. "A Bone Health Intervention for Older Adults Living in Residential Settings." *Research in Nursing & Health* 29 (2005): 566–75.

Flicker, L., R.J. MacInnis, M.S. Stein, et al. "Should Older People in Residential Care Receive Vitamin D to Prevent Falls? Results of a Randomized Trial." *Journal of the American Geriatrics Society* 53 (2005): 1881–88.

Greenspan, S.L., D.L. Schneider, M.R. McClung, et al. "Alendronate Improves Bone Mineral Density in Elderly Women with Osteoporosis Residing in Long-Term Care Facilities. A Randomized, Double-Blind, Placebo-Controlled Trial." *Annals of Internal Medicine* 136 (2002): 742–46.

Kiel, D.P., J. Magaziner, S. Zimmerman, et al. "Efficacy of a Hip Protector to Prevent Hip Fracture in Nursing Home Residents: The HIP PRO Randomized Controlled Trial." *Journal of the American Medical Association* 298 (2007): 413–22.

Lyles, K.W., C.S. Colón-Emeric, J.S. Magaziner, et al. "Zoledronic Acid in Reducing Clinical Fracture and Mortality after Hip Fracture." *New England Journal of Medicine* 357 (2007): 1799–1809.

Index

Actonel (risedronate), 175, 177, 185–93, 230–33, 236–38, 245–53, 334, 346, 368–71, 374, 397, 400, 411–12
  dosing instructions, 190
  effectiveness in clinical trials, 188–89
  side effects, 189, 247–53
  summary snapshot, 186–87
Actos (pioglitazone), 44, 379–83
African Americans, 21–23, 42, 134, 148–49, 207, 329, 417
alcohol, 22, 44–45, 78, 124, 28, 333, 404, 423, 426, 428
alendronate. *See* Fosamax
alkaline phosphatase, 90, 162
  bone-specific, 89–90, 162
almonds, 124–25, 128, 132, 138, 418
amenorrhea, 339–42, 345
American Academy of Orthopedic Surgeons, 249, 435
American Academy of Pediatrics, 154, 329
American Cancer Society, 402
American College of Obstetricians and Gynecologists, 338
American College of Rheumatology (ACR), 369–71, 435
American Gastroenterological Association, 351, 471
American Society for Bone and Mineral Research (ASBMR), 247, 462–63
American Society of Anesthesiologists, 285
Amgen, 52, 226, 257, 405
amino acids, 119
annual doctor's visit or check-up, 26, 57–61, 171, 311–14, 319–22
anorexia nervosa, 343–47
antidepressants, 347, 390–93
  tricyclic, 390
  selective serotonin receptor uptake inhibitors (SSRIs), 44, 238, 333, 347, 390–93
antiendomysial antibody, 313, 349
Aprela (bazedoxifene with Premarin), 258–62
Arimidex (anastrozole), 44, 396–98
Aromasin (exemestane), 396–97
aromatase inhibitors (AIs), 92, 316, 396–401
arthritis, 15, 43, 59, 82, 165, 300, 363, 373–75
  degenerative or osteoarthritis, 15, 165, 373–74
  rheumatoid, 43, 45, 59, 165, 363, 373–75
Asians, 21, 42, 45, 72, 207, 273–75, 332, 417
assisted living facilities, 407–413
Association of Oral and Maxillofacial Surgeons, 248
asthma, 363, 366
Atelvia (risedronate), 175, 177, 187–92, 236–37, 245–53, 411–12
atrial fibrillation, 202, 252, 304, 356
Avandia (rosiglitazone), 379–83

back pain, 34, 242, 244, 292–301
  acute spine fracture, 242–44, 294–303
  off-label medicine use, 218, 242–44
Baylink, Dr. David, 283
bazedoxifene, 258–62
beer, 78, 124, 151, 283, 423
Besser, Dr. Richard, 249
biomechanics, 38, 298

481